Artificial Intelligence in Sports, Movement, and Health

Carlo Dindorf · Eva Bartaguiz · Freya Gassmann ·
Michael Fröhlich
Editors

Artificial Intelligence in Sports, Movement, and Health

Springer

Editors
Carlo Dindorf
Department of Sports Science
University of Kaiserslautern-Landau
Kaiserslautern, Rheinland-Pfalz, Germany

Eva Bartaguiz
Department of Sports Science
University of Kaiserslautern-Landau
Kaiserslautern, Rheinland-Pfalz, Germany

Freya Gassmann
Methods of Empirical Social Research
University of Kaiserslautern-Landau
Kaiserslautern, Rheinland-Pfalz, Germany

Michael Fröhlich
Department of Sports Science
University of Kaiserslautern-Landau
Kaiserslautern, Rheinland-Pfalz, Germany

ISBN 978-3-031-67255-2 ISBN 978-3-031-67256-9 (eBook)
https://doi.org/10.1007/978-3-031-67256-9

This Springer imprint is published by the registered company Springer Nature Switzerland AG
The registered company address is: Gewerbestrasse 11, 6330 Cham, Switzerland

Editorial

Artificial Intelligence (AI) is driving revolutionary advancements and is transforming the landscape in sports, movement, and health. Rapid advancements are continuously reshaping these domains. As we embark on this journey, we recognize that while this book offers a snapshot of significant AI applications, the evolving nature of technology ensures that new breakthroughs will continually emerge beyond what we currently grasp. With this book, we aim to empower readers with knowledge and enhance the understanding of the transformative potential of AI in sports, movement, and health.

To begin our exploration, we delve into the broader realm of **Digital Transformations: AI's Role in Sports Science**. We commence with Lenhard (Chap. 1), who investigates the profound impact of AI on sports science. His work delves into its role in digitization and mathematization while also pondering the philosophical implications inherent in this transformation. Furthermore, Lenhard unravels the effects AI has on scientific practices within the field. Next, Latzel and Glauner (Chap. 2) shed light on the future of academic writing empowered by AI. Their inquiry explores how AI is reshaping research and writing across various disciplines, focusing on sports science. Our discourse concludes with Menges (Chap. 3), who examines the application of AI in endurance sports. She showcases how AI-driven technologies are revolutionizing training and how AI assists coaches and athletes in decision-making processes beyond training, encompassing elements such as race selection and strategy formulation.

AI has the power to enhance medical and health-related aspects in sports contexts, which we want to focus on in the part **AI in Medical and Health Aspects of Sports**. It is important to note that the focus of this part is not on general applications in the healthcare sector, which encompasses a myriad of other works. Instead, within the scope of this book, the focus is on movement-related health aspects, which significantly intersect with sports science. Kemmler (Chap. 4) starts the part by exploring cutting-edge fall prevention strategies and how AI-based fall technology revolutionizes fall prevention for older adults. Find out how sensor-based AI concepts enhance safety and effectiveness in training, even in unsupervised settings. This is followed by

Owen, Owen, and Evan's (Chap. 5) chapter, showcasing the future of injury prevention through the lens of AI technology. It is presented how AI not only enhances prediction accuracy but also enriches our comprehension of the multifaceted factors influencing sports-related injuries. Afterward, we want to have a look at doping in sports, a persistent issue that involves the misuse of prohibited substances to boost performance. In this context, the paper of Rahman and Maass (Chap. 6) explores the use of generative modeling to create synthetic blood sample data, aiming to enhance anti-doping analysis. A method is proposed not only for data augmentation but also to address ethical concerns regarding athletes' biological data.

After examining medical and health implications of AI, our attention turns to the realm of **Human-Computer Interaction** (HCI). Speicher and Berndt (Chap. 7) illuminate HCI's crucial role, offering insights into how AI influences athletic performance, injury management, and healthcare. They advocate for integrating human-centered design principles to elevate user engagement and outcomes in the evolving field. Subsequently, Gillmann (Chap. 8) describes the significance of comprehending and visually representing uncertainty in sporting data. She provides an overview of how uncertainty-aware visualization can contribute to enhancing the reliability and decision-making process of Machine Learning (ML) predictions in sports.

Transitioning, the discourse shifts towards **Motion Capture and Feedback Systems**. Stetter and Stein (Chap. 9) focus on the applications of ML for biomechanical analysis of human movements and the associated challenges. They show how the three major ML paradigms supervised, unsupervised, and reinforcement learning are used in biomechanics and how ML can support the understanding of human movements. Baldinger, Lippmann, and Senner (Chap. 10) give an overview of current technologies and applications focusing on markerless motion capture technologies. Furthermore, they complement this with findings from their studies on the validity of the technologies and conclude the main challenges for future research.

Through **Practical Examples of Machine Learning and Predictive Analytics**, the final part showcases how AI is reshaping the future of sports and unlocking new realms of performance optimization and strategic insights. Vives, Lázaro, Guzmán, Crespo, and Martínez-Gallego (Chap. 11) explore the recent evolution of ML techniques and their potential impact on tennis performance analysis, including a practical example showcasing predictive modeling results, leveraging new technologies like Hawk-Eye and tracking systems. The discussion then transitions to another perspective on tennis by Randrianasolo (Chap. 12), which focuses on how sports predictions can be revolutionized with convolutional neural networks. This is exemplified by forecasting outcomes without the need for extensive historical data, as demonstrated with Men Euro 2020 and Women US Open 2021.

Smyth, Feely, Berndsen, Caulfield, and Lawlor (Chap. 13) explore how ML can enhance recreational marathon running through personalized training insights and race support by mobile devices and wearable sensors. Barbon Junior, Moura, and da Silva Torres (Chap. 14) continue delving into the potential of data-driven methodologies in soccer analysis, outlining a systematic pipeline for automating data collection, transformation, and analysis, offering insights into player interactions and performance optimization through AI. Finally, McAuley, Baker, Johnston, and Kelly (Chap. 15) offer an overview of contemporary research utilizing AI to interpret large datasets in talent identification and development processes within youth sport contexts, outlining the potential of AI to enhance recruitment strategies and highlighting key strengths, weaknesses, opportunities, and threats in this evolving field.

In light of the diverse contributions presented in this book, we have amassed a rich collection of insights, practical applications, and perspectives poised to transform the realms of sports, movement, and health. However, as we stand at this juncture of exploration and innovation, it is crucial to acknowledge that our understanding is merely a snapshot of the immense potential AI holds for these domains. The evolving nature of technology ensures that new breakthroughs will continually emerge, pushing the boundaries of what we currently grasp.

As we reflect on the book's content, it becomes evident that the research approaches and practical implementations showcased within these pages mark just the beginning. The real-world impact of AI on sports, movement, and health is yet to unfold fully. The true test lies not only in the ingenuity of AI-driven solutions but also in their integration into everyday practices and established knowledge. The gap between theory, science, and practical application must be bridged to realize the full potential of these technologies.

We hope to have given our readers a first insight into the large field of AI in sports, movement, and health. Let us remain curious and attentive to how the future of AI technology will develop in the sectors and to what extent the research approaches described will be put into practice.

July 2024

Carlo Dindorf
Eva Bartaguiz
Freya Gassmann
Michael Fröhlich

Contents

Part I
Digital Transformations: Artificial Intelligences Role in Sports Science

Chapter 1
Situating Sports Science in the Movement of Digitization

Johannes Lenhard

Abstract This chapter reflects upon how Artificial Intelligence (AI) in sports science is situated in the broader movement of digitization, which in turn takes a special place in mathematization. It addresses the question: If a field is getting into AI, what impact will this potentially have from a philosophical point of view? It argues that epistemic opacity is part-and-parcel of digitization and, all the more, of AI. This makes prediction an even more important criterion for scientific success, whereas the capability for explanation is seriously diminished. Finally, the chapter explores how the use of software leads to a new social organization of science.

Keywords Sport Science · Simulation Modeling · Epistemology · Mathematization · Digitization

1.1 Introduction

Today, digitization is predominantly discussed in terms of Artificial Intelligence (AI). This chapter will take a step back and reflect upon how AI in sports science is situated in the broader movement of digitization, which in turn takes a special place in mathematization. This chapter does not aim at providing an overview of current or future applications of AI in sports science. Other contributions to this book do this in a competent manner. Nor will it act as a philosophical naysayer—asking whether AI is "new dawn or false hope" is topical in the literature (for sports science, see Bartlett, 2006). Rather, the text that follows explores the question: If a field—sports science or any other—is getting into AI, what impact will this potentially have?

The label AI is older than recent Machine Learning (ML) methods. When the label was coined in 1956 at a meeting in Dartmouth, it should mainly avoid any association with the then popular term of cybernetics, as John McCarthy, one of the meeting organizers, reminded later (1988). In the 1950s, poponents of AI believed

J. Lenhard (✉)
Rheinland-Pfälzische Technische Universität Kaiserslautern-Landau (RPTU), Kaiserslautern, Germany
e-mail: johannes.lenhard@rptu.de

C. Dindorf et al. (eds.), *Artificial Intelligence in Sports, Movement, and Health*,
https://doi.org/10.1007/978-3-031-67256-9_1

that following explicit rules is the key to intelligence. And since the digital computer is a machine that can process such rules with ease and speed, AI was expected to overtake human intelligence in foreseeable time. It was a hard-won lesson that AI did not meet these expectations. Even chess computers, although the game is completely defined by formal rules, had somewhat limited success. When Deep Blue finally won against Kasparov, the long-term world champion, this was based not on a deeper analysis of moves, but on the large database of existing games fed into the machine. Attempts to master language, like generating a translation, proved to be a nut too hard to crack, mainly because language use persistently escaped a fully formalized grammar. To make a long story short, the optimism reversed and led to the "AI winter" of the 1980s. Actually, one can discern a first (late 1970s) and a second AI winter (late 1980s to early 1990s); for highly accessible accounts see Crevier (1993) or the entry "History of artificial intelligence" in Wikipedia. The field of AI re-oriented itself. A leading strand in the 1990s took acting in the world as the leading criterion that characterized intelligent behavior—fetching a cup of coffee without spilling it, rather than playing chess. This robotic turn produced new accounts of what characterizes intelligence, in connection with new visions of what AI is—or ought to become, see Pfeifer and Scheier (2001), or Brooks (2002), among others.

However, while the robotic turn amounts to a modest niche for AI, the recent hype is more expansive and has been called the second wave of AI, rising for more than a decade now. The first wave of symbolic AI was oriented at symbolic rules—the philosopher Haugeland (1985) labeled this approach as "good old-fashioned AI" —GOFAI. Based on this term, Smith (2019) makes a thoughtful distinction between first wave (GOFAI) and second wave (connectionist, neural network) AI. Alien to the logical-symbolic standpoint, and almost contradictory to it, the current second wave is fueled by statistical approaches, with Deep Neural Networks as the paradigm example. Now, knowledge about rules does not count as essential. On the contrary, gaps in such knowledge, even gaping craters, are compensated for by statistical analyses of extensive datasets. In short, one can connect the second wave of AI to a data turn.

A series of popular and astonishing success stories supports the second wave. Very likely, every reader knows how ML jumped from chess to Go with ease (showing the power of neural networks). Image classification made a big splash and most recently, Large Language Models (LLMs) exhibit proficiency in translating texts that was not anticipated by AI nor linguistic experts. Moreover, LLMs like ChatGPT (by the US company OpenAI), or other generative networks even increase the frenzy because many people find uses for a machine that generates text and, additionally, interfaces to these machines are readily available to all internet users (which does not mean that they come free of cost).

All these examples have in common that the rules (for classification, for language) are not explicitly modeled, but implicitly defined. What makes a bird look like a blackbird is what the images labeled with blackbird have in common—in contrast to what the images labeled differently (the non-blackbirds) have "in common". The same applies to language. The rules of grammar are by and large skipped. Instead, the machine produces sentences that are similar to sentences in the database (of course, the notion of similarity is far from trivial). A human translator would proceed very differently, or more precisely, would describe what he or she does very differently: translate words, know the grammar, consider phrasing etc. The ML method just assumes that existing translations somehow entail all this knowledge.

In short, ML makes statistical evaluation of large datasets feasible and, if one has enough data, ML arrives at surprisingly good results. Recent experience with LLMs like ChatGPT makes the case. The universal key then is data from the domain of interest, not knowledge in the sense of having a good model of what happens in this domain.

But wait a moment. The universality of AI (working with Deep Neural Networks) arises from the flexibility of these networks. Mathematically speaking, learning for these networks means to adjust a function that matches input–output behavior. With expensive computing equipment, such as employed by LLMs, literally billions of parameters are adjusted. To do this in a meaningful way, extremely large amounts of data are needed, like the 14 million hand-annotated images on ImageNet, or the vast libraries of text compiled by OpenAI (in a completely non-open way). Thus, the data turn in AI is not only a revelation of how rich implicit knowledge contained in data might be, at the same time, data present a new bottleneck.

Availability and quality of data replace knowledge about rules as the bottleneck. The question is, which fields have adequate data available? There is no formal rule of how many one needs. Optimism reigns and speaking about "exciting possibilities" has become topical for many publications (see, for instance, Torgler, 2020). However, it is not straightforward to distinguish enthusiastic promises from scientific achievements. For instance, Perl noted that in actual practice sufficiently many data are almost never available (Perl 2009, 33).

To the extent that data are the key (other than complicated theories), and that tools for analysis are accessible through software packages, the AI movement is attractive for science and commerce alike. Sports science is a case in point. For instance, Dindorf et al. (2023) warn that scientific research should hurry up to not lag behind commercial application. It is a widespread belief that AI in sports science is driven by commercial application at least as much as by (scientific) modeling. Overviews like that of Chmait and Westerbeek (2021) take *Moneyball* (Lewis, 2003) as the starting point for AI in sports science because it provides a striking and impactful example of how to create data and (commercially) use them.

The following text has three parts. Section 1.2 locates AI in the context of digitization and in the broader history of mathematization. It starts with the famous book-of-nature verdict by Galileo and suggests that ML indicates a profound turn in mathematization. Section 1.3 concentrates on epistemology and argues that epistemic opacity is part-and-parcel of digitization and, all the more, of AI. This makes prediction an even more important criterion for scientific success, whereas the capability for explanation is seriously diminished. The final Sect. 1.4 explores how the use of software leads to a new social organization of science.

1.2 Mathematization—Digitization—Artificial Intelligence

First a paragraph about terminology. The terminology is complicated by the overlap of different traditions. AI is dealing with tasks that would count as based on intelligence if achieved by a human, like playing chess, finding the route back home, recognizing a face, or writing an essay. As was mentioned in the introduction, AI started with manipulating logical rules. The recent successes of AI by and large came from Deep Learning, i.e., from the use of multilayered Artificial Neural Networks (ANNs). At the same time, ML is a label that normally comprises not only these methods, but also Random Forests, among others. Thus, both AI and ML sometimes claim ownership for Deep Neural Networks. In the following, we ignore these complications and assume that AI refers to a set of methods that typically involve the use of multi-layer ANNs.

These can exhibit extremely versatile input–output behavior, depending on the setting of their parameters. Mathematically, such networks approximate an unknown function—think of image classification that is a map from the set of images into a set of labels—with the help of very many adjustable parameters. Current LLMs, for instance, work with billions of such parameters. They are true Behemoths of approximation that are said to "learn" because the parameter adjustment is a process that is guided by a set of training data. The machinery of approximation iteratively finds parameter settings that match these data better and better and in this sense the model learns from the data.

A most important observation is that AI does not simply help to solve problems, but rather influences how problems are formulated. Simply deploying computers to solve existing problems would fail, because the problems are usually not in the right form to be tackled by a computer. Thus, the intention of using AI influences how researchers perceive and formulate problems. Researchers aim at posing problems in a way that makes them amenable to AI.

This point is not particular to AI, rather applies to using computer methods in general. In fact, it generalizes beyond the computer to all sorts of instrumentation. It has been part of scientific activity all the time, or better—and even more general—part of how humans act. They use instruments and these instruments shape the way they see the world and identify solvable problems. A saying of unknown origin captures the point: "If the only tool you have is a hammer, it is tempting to treat everything as if it were a nail." (The entry "Law of the instrument" on Wikipedia presents a brief selection of possible origins of this saying.) The computer and, most recently, Deep Learning, is scientific instrumentation that exerts such influence in a particularly strong way.

If one discerns the objects that populate the world from the instruments that one uses to investigate these objects, then the case of AI comprises (at least) two layers. Computers are instruments to find out something about how mathematical or formal structures behave. But at the same time, one can see mathematical structures as instruments to find out something about how objects in the world behave. Thus, there are two layers, or two embeddings—AI as part of digitization and digitization as part of mathematization.

A most famous starting point for reasoning about mathematization is Galileo's verdict that the book of nature is written in mathematical symbols. From the seventeenth century on, there was a forceful movement in modern science towards mathematization, i.e. conceiving of nature in mathematical ways (Mahoney, 1998). Galileo's viewpoint rests on the metaphysical assumption that the world is as it is, and that one can find out some of the facts with the help of mathematical methods (and maybe in no other way). Importantly, the world is like a book, everything about nature is written there. That means, scientists are deciphering the book, not writing it. And since mathematical knowledge is the most certain knowledge, the great promise of mathematization is that certainty and truth go hand in hand.

This promise was daring from the start, because it is more grounded in philosophical belief than in actual power. Mathematical methods require a formal framework, usually involving highly idealizing modeling assumptions, whereas in practical applications many factors contribute and interact. Admittedly, there are prime examples of idealizations that work, first of all astronomy and the movement of planets. Newton's achievements maybe created the greatest success story in science, when he showed how laws of mechanics and gravitation plus a new mathematical method (calculus) could derive the elliptical orbits of the planets in full match with observational data. From then on, mathematization was deeply entrenched in the development of science. Still today, mathematical methods count as a pivotal indicator of something being scientific. Much has changed since the seventeenth century. A most obvious point is that computers redefined the arsenal of mathematical instruments.

Let us concentrate on simulation as a major area of computer instrumentation. Basically, we follow the main thesis in Lenhard (2019) that "computer and simulation modelingreally do form a new type of mathematical modeling." (2) Four features of simulation modeling together make it a novel type, namely an explorative and iterative type of modeling.

Experimenting. Simulation experiments build a particular class of experiments. Usually, experiments are described as seeking an answer from nature. Although the question an experiment poses may require extensive theoretical design, like a gigantic tunnel full of high-tech equipment under the lake Geneva (CERN), there remains an important sense in which experiments are not determined by theory, even if they are theory-laden. In the example: does the CERN particle collider register traces of the Higgs particle or not? Simulation experiments are different because they evaluate the model behavior that results from the assumptions (and the implementation) already made. In a way, they question the model-plus-computation part, not nature. Although they differ from ordinary experiments, these computer-experiments still deserve to be counted as experiments because they seek an answer to a question by observing a designed process of open ending. For instance, running a weather model ten times and counting how often it rains in Kaiserslautern, in this way determining the so-called probability of rain.

The exploratory variant of experimentation is particularly relevant for simulation modeling. Here, the focus is on the process of building a model. Often, the model is not only motivated by some theoretical consideration, but by how it behaves. Deep Learning is an excellent example. The ANN is controlled by parameter adjustments, but the values of these parameters usually do not have a meaning. Their value cannot be determined out of theoretical considerations. They are adjusted over the course of repeated experiments that explore the model behavior. "Model assumptions with effects that are hard or even impossible to survey can be tested, varied, and modified by applying iterative experimental procedures. Modeling and experimenting agree to engage in an exploratory cooperation. Such cooperation regularly employs artificial elements" (Lenhard, 2019, 133).

Artificial elements. The parameterizations in Deep Learning are a prime example, but artificial elements are significant for almost all computational methods. Let me replace a full argumentation with an example. If a model is expressed in the language of continuous mathematics, it must be discretized before a computer can evaluate it. There are various approaches to discretization, all need to be designed so that the dynamics of the discrete model closely matches the dynamics of the original continuous model. "When controlling the performance of discrete models (i.e., for instrumentalist—though unavoidable—reasons), artificial components are included. Experiments are necessary to adapt the dynamics of a simulation model, because one cannot judge whether these artificial elements are adequate without such experimental loops. This grants simulation modeling an instrumental aspect that blurs the representation relation and hence weakens the explanatory power" (ibid., 133).

Plasticity. "This denotes the high level of adaptability in a simulation model's dynamics. The structural core of such a model is often no more than a schema that requires—and allows—further specification before simulating particular patterns and phenomena" (ibid., 134). Again, Deep Learning is a prime example. The neural network usually is almost completely generic. Whether it can be used for image classification or language generation essentially depends on the data and the parameter assignments over the course of learning, i.e., iterated exploratory experimentation. Both structure and specification are necessary to determine the dynamic properties of a model.

Epistemic opacity. "This arises because models are becoming more complex in several respects. The course of dynamic events encompasses an enormous number of steps, so that the overall result cannot be derived from the structure. Instead, it emerges from model assumptions and the parameter assignments chosen during runtime. Additionally, important properties of the dynamics result from the specifications and adaptations made while developing the model. This reveals a fundamental difference compared to the traditional concept of mathematical modeling and its concern with epistemic transparency" (ibid., 134). The expectation was that formal modeling makes graspable what happens in the model and, because the model is about the world, what happens in the world. In essence, this is the promise of reading the book of nature. With simulation modeling, and more generally computer-based modeling, the essential feature of the model is its flexibility. The *new promise* is that, with suitable adaptation machinery, the model can be made to match observed data and phenomena. And exactly the adaptation machinery *creates opacity.*

These characteristics are not independent of each other, but support and reinforce each other. Therefore, they are not just a group of features, but form a distinct type. Simulation modeling is carried out in an explorative and iterative manner, in a process that partly uses and partly compensates for the above-mentioned components (opacity).

Computing instrumentation and the concept of modeling affect each other. One direction seems obvious. Mathematical models support the design and development of computers in various ways. But the other direction is at least as important: by using computers as an instrument, mathematical modelling is channeled. First and foremost, this channeling represents an epistemological shift. Traditionally, mathematical modeling has been performed by human subjects actively modeling to gain insight, control, or whatever. The channelling effect comes about because an additional technological level is added: the modelling must find a balance, namely to compensate for those (extra) transformations that are caused by the use of the computer - that is, as a rule, to neutralize them to a certain extent through further, additional constructions within the model.

The ANNs used in Deep Learning have served as examples throughout the analysis. Lenhard (2019) discusses more and different examples in the same framework. What are typical features of ANNs? They are a special type of model because they are constructed almost independently from the sort of phenomenon they are supposed to capture. They have a very generic model structure. A simple observation is that these networks are often displayed, but all pictures look essentially the same. In fact, the structure does not represent the target phenomena. Therefore, one can call ANNs structurally underdetermined. At the same time, they contain an extremely large number of parameters whose adjustment makes the overall behavior so versatile that it can approximate an almost arbitrary function. In other words, the model behavior depends completely on the specification (of parameters). This is in strong contrast to the traditional idea of model construction where the structure is supposed to capture the phenomena and parameters are for fine-tuning.

From a formal and abstract standpoint, iteration is the typical action connected with ANNs. Their construction is often meaningless, in the sense that elements in the construction do not have an interpretation in terms of the target domain—no champion of Go was necessary to build the network that—when trained over and over by playing games against itself—later beat the world champion reliably. All the more does parameter adjustment matter. And this happens iteratively, i.e. in each learning step each parameter is adjusted—and learning steps are themselves iterated. From a hardware point of view, such procedure requires to execute large masses of simple iterations.

Finally, ANNs stand for a turn in mathematization. Now, mathematization is not about the book of nature. It is not a tool for representing the world. Instead, mathematics is used as a tool to construct and control the gigantic approximation machines that ANNs are. Jost (2017) argues that mathematization now is concerned with the mathematization of tools. How can such inward-looking turn result in something that is successful in real-world tasks like image classification or language generation?

Basically, these successes are grounded in a fundamentally instrumentalist approach, namely a statistical treatment of patterns—irrespective of what these patterns mean.

1.3 Epistemology: Opacity and Understanding

Black box modeling deals solely with input–output behavior, whereas its counterpart, white box modeling, is concerned also with the inner workings of the model. Obviously, a black box model cannot explain why the modeled system behaves as it behaves. For this reason, it is a widely shared goal to replace opaque models that have a black box character by white box, transparent models. A good example is Perl (1997) who diagnoses that modeling is targeting systems of increasing complexity and that this complexity prohibits the sort of analysis possible with white box models. Perl expresses the hope that approaches like neural networks might open up a new way for understanding complex systems (Perl, 1997, 302).

About 25 years ago, the opinion was widely shared that new computational methods might bring new ways of understanding complex systems. However, the quick evolution of ANNs brought predictive successes that come together with utterly opaque models. One can still insist on the goal of making these models transparent to an extent that allows one to explain their prediction. Not very astonishingly, and in response to the successes of ANNs, there is a recent call to develop "Explainable AI" (XAI). However, opacity is part-and-parcel of simulation in general (Humphreys, 2004; Lenhard, 2019) and of Deep Learning in particular—as has been argued above. Up to now, XAI remains an open field for research whose success (or failure) can only be judged in the future.

If one is accepting that opacity is an unwanted, but unavoidable condition for using AI, how does the promise of AI (and digitization in more general) look like? From a historical and philosophical perspective, prediction challenges the search for an explanation. This tension has been a constant companion to the entire discussion about explanation since the beginning of modernity—or actually even longer: ever since mathematics played any role whatsoever in considerations of epistemology and practice. A basic viewpoint is that the ability to predict shows something important. In some way, whatever is able to give good predictions has got something right about the world, or about that fraction of the world under investigation. And this something is the fundament and the true source of the predictive capability.

Remarkably, the new methods seem to turn this upside down: Prediction happens on the basis of a method, or a generic model, whose representational properties are in question or even inaccessible. Is understanding still possible? Understanding is a central but somewhat vague and multifaceted notion in epistemology. A couple of decades ago, understanding sometimes was taken to be antonymous to explanation. There is a vast literature in philosophy of science dealing with explanation, whereas understanding is covered considerably less. Books like the one by de Regt et al. (2009) indicate a change—understanding now is on the agenda in philosophy of science.

In a way, simulation models can provide understanding at a certain standard. Scientists might conduct iterated simulation experiments and create visualizations and in this way sound out how how the input–output dynamics looks like. In doing so they can orient themselves in the model—even if parts of the dynamics are not transparent to them. Of course, this kind of familiarity with the model does not meet the high epistemic demands that are normally placed on mathematical models (cf. Russell's (1905) concept of knowledge by acquaintance). However, this lower standard is still sufficient if the aim is a controlled intervention. In other words, simulation models might remain epistemically opaque, but still provide means to control the dynamics.

A typical example is the possible breakdown of the meridional overturning circulation MOC, i.e. the Gulf Stream. Researchers investigate how the MOC behaves under varying conditions (in the simulation model), like temperature increase. Their goal is to understand how robust it is. But understanding here means the opposite of Feynman's case. Whereas he wanted to know behavior without calculation, getting a picture of the MOC is based on large amounts of calculations. Similarly, structural engineering has changed its face with computational modeling. Daring constructions can be admired that could not have been planned without calculating their structural stability via computer models. Engineers understand how such constructions behave, but in a very pragmatic sense that does not presuppose epistemic transparency.

Of course, one could question whether the pragmatic notion should be called understanding at all. We hence face two options: First, does simulation eliminate understanding in the practices of sciences and engineering, or second, do simulation practices replace a strong notion of understanding by a weaker, pragmatic notion? If one accepts that the complexity of simulation models makes epistemic opacity unavoidable, whereas at the same time, these models still are good for interventions and predictions, then the question is: Will this co-existence lead to a new conception or re-definition of scientific understanding? Devising an answer to this question still is a task for philosophy of science.

Thus, the argumentation leads to a twofold claim. First, that simulations can facilitate acquaintance with, and orientation in, model behavior even when the model dynamics itself remain (partially) opaque. And secondly, simulations change mathematical modeling in an important way: Theory-based understanding and epistemic transparency recede into the background, while a kind of pragmatic understanding comes to the fore that is oriented towards intervention and prediction rather than theoretical explanation.

1.4 Software and How Expertise is Organized

If researchers want to use simulations or other computational methods, especially ML, they have to have available appropriate infrastructure. Everybody immediately thinks of a computer terminal, rightly so. However, in this context infrastructure is far more comprehensive. As a concept, infrastructure is so interesting because it captures, or allows to capture, how modern societies, technology, and regulation are interconnected, see Edwards (2002). Having it available is demanding, in terms of costly technology, and actually using it also demanding, in terms of what sort of questions should be asked in which ways.

One of these infrastructure elements is data. The strength of ANNs unfolds when they statistically identify correlations. The prominent successes have a twofold root. Firstly, ANNs can work through amounts of data that were considered unfeasible not long ago. This data-digestive ability rests on a combined achievement of hardware, such as the use of graphical processing units, and software. Secondly, the sensitivity of ANNs to delicate traces of correlations is of use only when there are really many data available. Else all the parameters and optimization procedures remain idle, or worse, lead to spurious signals. This makes ANNs *data-hungry*. Therefore, researchers are strongly motivated to formulate questions about areas where massive data are available or can be produced. In an apt analysis, Perl (2009) had pointed out that ANN methods in sport science suffer from the fact that they need more data than are available. For a statement that computer methods will lead to data-centered 4th paradigm science, see Hey et al. (2009). It is surely not coincidental that this book comes out of Microsoft, a major company involved in data business.

A second element is the networked character of the entire research workflow. Data such as comprehensive image inventories from the internet are usually not stored locally. One can argue that Google or other companies build gigantic computing centers that duplicate and store the entire internet. But this only strengthens the case, because ordinary researchers must connect to these data storages. Moreover, parts of the actual computation are often outsourced, too. When learning and adjusting the parameters, researchers typically work with a software suite such as TensorFlow (Abadi et al., 2015) that runs on a platform maintained by Google. Thus, the exploratory—iterative mode of modeling—specifying the parameters in iterated learning steps—has been adopted by a new networked and centralized infrastructure. Although it is centralized, it is readily available (or those parts of it are that some company thinks in its interest to make available). Moreover, the exploratory part is automated; it consists in adjusting the parameters almost entirely independently from the modelers, thus contributing to opacity.

Software should be distinguished from computing as a third element of the infrastructure. Classically, creating software that adequately operationalizes research questions is a key component of scientific expertise. In the 1980s and 1990s, the motto was that computing expertise should become part of particular fields, like sports science, because a division between software developer and user would no longer work (Lames et al., 1997, p. 30) In one sense, this motto has been fulfilled. Today, everyone is working with computers. However, in an important sense, something very different happened. Software packages became available that made it easy, or at least doable, for many users to do computational science *without* being experts in actually developing the software. This division of labor amounts to a fundamental shift in how expertise is socially organized. For example, Johnson and Lenhard describe in Chap. 4 of (2024) how quantum chemical simulations are employed by researchers who are specialists in such software, but not in quantum chemical theory. Software and the way in which its uses are organized are a new research topic shared by history, sociology and philosophy of science, see for instance Haigh (2013), Hocquet and Wieber (2021), Johnson and Lenhard (2024).

In AI, a highly visible feature of social organization is that there is a host of competitions set up to achieve a given predictive task to the best degree or with the lowest failure rate (as on the platform Kaggle). Such competitions attract attention from various groups and have established an arena independent of academia (notwithstanding the fact that typical participants have had contact with universities). When data and software are provided on the internet, participants can act independently from resources provided by a university or other academic institution. These competitions function as a market from which big companies recruit scientists and programmers.

Importantly, the methodology together with the infrastructure create a new situation when it comes to policy and regulation. The quality of predictions depends on the quality of the (training) data. Because the quality of data is (still) ill defined, main actors take the quantity of data as a proxy. Today, data such as those that Tesla collects while developing its automated car count as a commercial treasure (not to mention Facebook and other actors in the field). Whereas the collected data are proprietary, government interventions such as regulating when a car has to apply its brakes depend on access to these data. And therefore, practice is heading for a conflict as far as regulatory measures—or better, their justifiability—is concerned.

Finally, a short wrap-up concerning the point raised at the beginning of this chapter: If a field is getting into AI, what effects will that potentially have? Overall, digitization brings about new research instruments. The wide distribution and uptake is depending on a comprehensive infrastructure that makes the use of software possible also for non-experts and also directs new research toward fields and questions that lend themselves to these new instruments. Concretely, since data are a potential bottleneck, creativity is required from the researchers to address questions for which they have available or can produce sufficient amounts of data. Philosophically, simulation and AI methods come with epistemic opacity. They yield predictions, but tend to be unpromising regarding explanations.

References

Abadi, M, Agarwal, A., Barham, P., Brevdo, E., Chen, Z., Citro, C., Corrado, G.S., Davis, A., Dean, J., Devin, M., Ghemawat, S., Goodfellow, I., Harp, A., Irving, G., Isard, M., Jozefowicz, R., Jia, Y., Kaiser, L., Kudlur, M., Levenberg, J, … Zheng, X. (2015). *TensorFlow: Large-scale machine learning on heterogeneous systems.* Software available from tensorflow.org

Bartlett, R. (2006). Artificial intelligence in sports biomechanics: New dawn or false hope? *Journal of Sports Science & Medicine, 5*(4), 474–479.

Brooks, R. A. (2002). *Flesh and machines: How robots will change us.* Pantheon Books.

Chmait, N., & Westerbeek, H. (2021). Artificial intelligence and machine learning in sport research: An introduction for non-data scientists. *Frontiers in Sports and Active Living, 3.* https://doi.org/10.3389/fspor.2021.682287

Crevier, D. (1993). *AI: The tumultuous history of the search for artificial intelligence*. Basic Books.
de Regt, H., Leonelli, S., & Eigner, K. (2009). *Scientific understanding*. University of Pittsburgh Press.
Dindorf, C., Bartaguiz, E., Gassmann, F., & Fröhlich, M. (2023). *Künstliche Intelligenz in Sport und Sportwissenschaft. Potenziale, Herausforderungen und Limitationen*. Springer Spektrum.
Edwards, P. N. (2002). Infrastructure and modernity: Force, time, and social organization in the history of sociotechnical systems. In T. J. Misa, P. Brey, & A. Feenberg (Eds.), *Modernity and technology* (pp. 185–226). The MIT Press. https://doi.org/10.7551/mitpress/4729.003.0011
Haigh, T. (2013). Software and souls; programs and packages. *Communications of the ACM, 56*(9), 31–34. https://doi.org/10.1145/2500131
Haugeland, J. (1985). *Artificial intelligence: The very idea*. The MIT Press.
Hey, T., Tansley, S., Tolle, K., & Gray, J. (2009). *The fourth paradigm: Data-intensive scientific discovery*. Microsoft Research. https://www.microsoft.com/en-us/research/publication/fourth-paradigm-data-intensive-scientific-discovery/
Hocquet, A., & Wieber, F. (2021). Epistemic issues in computational reproducibility: Software as the elephant in the room. *European Journal for Philosophy of Science, 11*(2). https://doi.org/10.1007/s13194-021-00362-9
Humphreys, P. (2004). *Extending ourselves. Computational science, empiricism, and scientific method*. Oxford University Press.
Johnson, A., & Lenhard, J. (2024). *Cultures of prediction*. The MIT Press.
Jost, J. (2017). Object oriented models versus data analysis—Is this the right alternative? In J. Lenhard & M. Carrier (Eds.), *Mathematics as a tool* (Vol. 327, pp. 253–286). Springer International Publishing. https://doi.org/10.1007/978-3-319-54469-4_14
Lames, M., Miethling, W.-D., & Perl, J. (1997). Interessenlagen und Perspektiven. In J. Perl, M. Lames, & W.-D. Miethling, *Informatik im Sport: Ein Handbuch* (pp. 27–30). Hofmann.
Lenhard, J. (2014). Disciplines, models, and computers: The path to computational quantum chemistry. *Studies in History and Philosophy of Science Part A, 48*, 89–96.
Lenhard, J. (2019). *Calculated surprises*. Oxford University Press.
Lewis, M. (2003). *Moneyball: The art of winning an unfair game*. W. W. Norton & Company.
Mahoney, M. S. (1998). The mathematical realm of nature. In D. Garber & M. Ayers (Eds.), *The Cambridge history of seventeenth century philosophy* (pp. 702–755). Cambridge University Press.
McCarthy, J. (1988). Review of the question of artificial intelligence. *Annals of the History of Computing, 10*(3), 224–229.
Perl, J. (1997). Ausblick. In J. Perl, M. Lames, & W.-D. Miethling, *Informatik im Sport. Ein Handbuch* (pp. 299–303). Hofmann.
Perl, J. (2009). Musteranalyse im Sportspiel mit Hilfe Neuronaler Netze. In J. Perl, M. Lames, C. Augste, O. Cordes, C. Dreckmann, C. Görsdorf & M. Siegle (Eds.), *Gegenstand und Anwendungsfelder der Sportinformatik* (Vol. 189, pp. 33–40). Czwalina Verlag.
Pfeifer, R., & Scheier, C. (2001). *Understanding intelligence*. The MIT Press.
Russell, B. (1905). On Denoting. *Mind, XIV*(4), 479–493. https://doi.org/10.1093/mind/XIV.4.479
Smith, B. C. (2019). *The promise of artificial intelligence*. The MIT Press.
Torgler, B. (2020). Big data, artificial intelligence, and quantum computing in sports. In S. L. Schmidt (Ed.), *21st century sports: How technologies will change sports in the digital age* (pp. 153–173). Springer. https://doi.org/10.1007/978-3-030-50801-2

Chapter 2
Artificial Intelligence in Sport Scientific Creation and Writing Process

Richard Latzel and Patrick Glauner

Abstract This chapter examines the transformative role of Artificial Intelligence (AI) tools in enhancing academic research and writing, with a focus on their application within sports science. It highlights the integration of technologies such as ChatGPT, Grammarly, and other generative AI tools into the academic landscape, demonstrating their impact on improving learning environments, promoting academic integrity, and streamlining administrative tasks. Through a detailed exploration of AI's contributions to literature research, data management, analysis, visualization, and writing support, the chapter delves into the efficiencies and depths these tools bring to academic work. It also addresses the limitations and challenges of AI integration, emphasizing the crucial balance between technological advancements and the indispensable value of human expertise in scholarly research. This discussion underscores AI's potential to facilitate innovation in academic writing and research, marking a significant shift towards more efficient, insightful, and comprehensive scholarly work if applied properly.

Keywords ChatGPT · AI · Scholarly Work

Declaration of the Use of Artificial Intelligence Tools in This Book Chapter

In the development of this book chapter, we selectively utilized Artificial Intelligence (AI) tools, primarily to support and enhance the writing process. This declaration outlines the extent and manner of AI tool integration within our work, emphasizing our approach to leveraging technology while ensuring the integrity and originality of our scholarly contribution.

1. **Literature Research**: We incorporated AI tools, specifically ResearchRabbit and Elicit, to assist in the initial stages of literature research. These platforms facilitated the identification of relevant studies and provided insights that informed our understanding of the topic. It is important to note that while these tools

R. Latzel (✉) · P. Glauner
Deggendorf Institute of Technology, Deggendorf, Germany
e-mail: richard.latzel@th-deg.de

C. Dindorf et al. (eds.), *Artificial Intelligence in Sports, Movement, and Health*,
https://doi.org/10.1007/978-3-031-67256-9_2

were helpful, they complemented a broader manual research effort, ensuring a comprehensive and nuanced review of existing literature.

2. **Writing Assistance**: The primary application of AI in the creation of this chapter was in the realm of writing support. Tools like ScholarAI and ChatGPT were used to enhance the clarity, grammar, and coherence of our text. These AI-driven aids offered suggestions for language improvement, helping us refine our argumentation and presentation. However, the critical evaluation of these suggestions and the final writing decisions were made by us, the authors, to maintain the academic integrity and intellectual rigor of our work.
3. **Originality and Integrity**: Despite the availability of AI-based plagiarism detection tools, we chose to ensure the originality of our content through manual verification and adherence to best practices in scholarly writing. This approach was guided by our commitment to academic ethics and the production of work that is both authentic and contributes meaningfully to the field.

By detailing the use of AI tools in the composition of this chapter, we aim to transparently acknowledge the role of technology in facilitating our academic writing process. The integration of AI was done with careful consideration, ensuring that it served to augment our capabilities as researchers and writers, rather than diminish the scholarly value of our contribution. The insights, interpretations, and conclusions presented in this chapter are the result of our professional judgment and expertise, underscored by a judicious application of AI for specific, supportive tasks in the writing process.

2.1 Introduction

The integration of Artificial Intelligence (AI) tools like ChatGPT, Grammarly, and other generative AI models into academic writing and educational platforms has been the subject of various studies, highlighting both their advantages and potential drawbacks. These tools have been shown to potentially enhance the learning environment by providing personalized tutoring, automating essay grading, facilitating translation, and creating interactive learning environments. AI tools have also been acknowledged for their role in promoting academic integrity through plagiarism detectors and assisting in administrative tasks like grading and feedback provision. This technological advancement has notably reduced the paperwork and workload for instructors, allowing them more time to dedicate to instruction and content dissemination (Duymaz & Tekin, 2023; Escalante et al., 2023).

This chapter explores the benefits and limitations of AI tools for academic research and writing, providing insights into their practical application in sports science and other academic fields. It includes a brief overview of AI tools' basic functionality before delving into their potential benefits in academic literature research, data analysis and management, and academic writing.

2.2 Overview of Artificial Intelligence

AI aims to automate human decision-making. AI has become one of the most transformative technologies of our time, reshaping industries, augmenting human capabilities, and pushing the boundaries of what machines can do. Typical tasks include learning, reasoning, problem-solving, perception, and language understanding (Russell & Norvig, 2021).

Historical sketch

The journey of AI began in the mid-twentieth century, with the term "artificial intelligence" being coined in 1955 by John McCarthy and others in a proposal for the Dartmouth Conference for the following year (McCarthy et al., 1955). This period marked the optimistic beginnings of AI, with researchers setting ambitious goals for machines to mimic human intelligence. Early AI research largely focused on symbolic approaches, attempting to encode human knowledge into machines. However, the complexity of human cognition proved to be a formidable challenge, leading to the realization that achieving true AI would require more than just programming explicit rules.

Machine Learning

The rise of Machine Learning (ML) in the latter part of the twentieth century marked a significant shift in the AI landscape. ML is a subset of AI that focuses on developing algorithms that enable computers to learn from and make predictions or decisions based on data. This approach diverged from the rule-based methods, offering a new pathway to achieving AI through data-driven learning (Bishop, 2006). The field of ML can broadly be divided into three so-called "pillars":

- Supervised learning: learn to predict a label y, i.e. a class (classification) or quantity (regression), from input data X.
- Unsupervised learning: find hidden relationships, such as clusters or lower dimensional representations, in the input data X.
- Reinforcement learning: learn which action to take in which state to achieve the best outcome.

Deep Learning

Deep Learning involves (Artificial) Neural Networks with many layers (hence "deep") that learn representations of data with multiple levels of abstraction. This approach has enabled significant advances in computer vision, natural language processing, and other areas requiring complex feature extraction in recent years (Bishop & Bishop, 2024).

Natural Language Processing

Natural Language Processing (NLP) is a domain of AI focused on the interaction between computers and humans using natural language. The goal of NLP is to enable computers to understand, interpret, and generate human languages. Techniques in NLP have evolved from rule-based systems to ML and sophisticated Deep Learning models, significantly improving the ability of machines to process and understand human language.

Large Language Models and prompt engineering

Large Language Models (LLMs), such as ChatGPT, represent the cutting edge of NLP. These models are trained on vast text datasets, learning to predict the next token in a sequence given the preceding tokens. This training enables them to generate coherent and contextually relevant text, translate languages, answer questions, and even write code. Prompt engineering has emerged as a crucial skill in leveraging LLMs, involving designing inputs (prompts) that guide these models to produce the desired output. It requires an understanding of the model's capabilities and limitations, creativity, and strategic thinking.

2.3 Role of Artificial Intelligence-Supported Tools in Literature Research

In the evolving landscape of academic research, Artificial Intelligence (AI) tools have emerged as pivotal instruments, reshaping the way research and analysis of data is conducted and findings are compiled. Some of the key advantages AI tools can offer in academic research are (Chubb et al., 2022; Pinzolits, 2023):

1. **Efficiency and Time Management**: AI tools, when used in the right way, can markedly reduce the time researchers spend on literature reviews and data analysis. They can quickly sift through extensive databases to identify relevant research papers, abstracts, and even specific sections within papers that address particular research questions. This capability allows researchers to focus more on analysis and less on the time-consuming process of finding information.
2. **Comprehensive Literature Analysis**: With access to vast databases of peer-reviewed articles, AI tools enable researchers to conduct thorough literature reviews. Some tools offer literature mapping features that help identify related research, references, and recommended readings, ensuring that researchers have a comprehensive understanding of their topic.
3. **Detailed Research Insights**: Beyond just identifying relevant papers, AI tools can analyze the full text of research documents. This deep dive into the content provides detailed insights into methodologies, results, and discussions, which are crucial for understanding the nuances of each study. Some tools can extract and summarize information from multiple research papers at once and might even aid in the development of a well-informed hypothesis and research design.

4. **Accessibility to Information**: AI tools make it easier for researchers and students to access and digest complex academic material (von Garrel & Mayer, 2023). AI tools can answer specific questions about a paper or summarize it in less elaborate language, hence simplifying the process of extracting valuable information.

However, there are some general limitations of AI tools in academic research that need to be considered:

1. **Quality and Relevance of Sources**: While these tools can retrieve a vast amount of literature, the relevance and quality of sources may vary. Researchers and students must still apply critical thinking to assess the validity and applicability of the information to their specific research questions.
2. **Contextual Understanding**: AI tools may not fully grasp the context or nuances of certain research areas, especially those involving complex human behaviors or subjective interpretations. This means that while they can provide data, the researcher must contextualize and interpret these findings within the broader scope of their study.
3. **Dependency and Skill Development**: There is a risk that heavy reliance on AI tools could impact the development of traditional research skills. Researchers, teachers and students must balance the use of AI with the cultivation of critical thinking, analytical skills, and hands-on research experiences (BaHammam, 2023).

In the following, a few AI tools available today shall be briefly presented and their potential applicability as well as limitations for literature research outlined.

At the time of compiling this chapter, none of the AI tools presented required any sort of financial transaction for use. However, it cannot be guaranteed that these tools will remain free of charge. Some already charge users for improved or updated functionalities, such as OpenAI, which offers its GPT-3.5 model free of charge but charges for the use of GPT-4.

Comprehensive user guides and tutorials for the AI tools are provided on their official websites, and are accessible to users. Additionally, video tutorials on how to utilize these tools are available on online video platforms such as YouTube.

2.3.1 ResearchRabbit

Functionalities and Benefits:

ResearchRabbit acts as a personal research assistant, helping researchers find relevant papers and stay updated with the latest research. It uses AI to learn from the user's interactions and preferences and natural language processing (NLP) which allows users to create collections of papers and receive personalized recommendations, similar to the curated playlists of music streaming services. The tool also provides personalized digests of the latest papers related to users' collections and offers interactive visualizations to explore networks of papers and co-authorships, providing new insights and opportunities for exploration. These networks can be displayed as spider webs (Fig. 2.1) or as a list in chronological order (Fig. 2.2), which could be particularly useful in situations where researchers want to limit their search to a certain point in time (e.g. conducting a Meta-Analysis on a certain topic of only the most recent literature). Typically, the more papers are included in a project, the more dense the connections between these papers and the network itself. However, the network of relevant papers typically expands with every paper added to a project, hence the researcher is advised to carefully select and deselect papers in a project.

Practical Applications:

In sports science, ResearchRabbit could be invaluable for discovering emerging trends and methodologies by creating collections focused on specific areas of interest. It is particularly useful for researchers looking to establish a comprehensive background for their study or seeking to identify gaps in the current literature.

Limitations:

While ResearchRabbit simplifies finding relevant literature, it may have a learning curve regarding its interface and maximizing its features. Additionally, it is more focused on discovery and recommendation rather than in-depth analysis of papers, which means researchers still need to critically evaluate the suggested literature for quality and relevance. Lastly, while the graphical representation of the findings does provide a concise visualization of the literature currently used and potentially of interest, one can quickly get lost in playing around with the networks. Rather than streamlining the search for relevant academic papers, this could lead to actually spending even more time searching.

2.3.2 Elicit

Functionalities and Benefits:

Elicit is known for its robust literature review capabilities, facilitating the exploration of research questions by automatically summarizing research papers and extracting relevant data points. It aids in hypothesis generation and testing by analyzing vast amounts of literature to identify trends, gaps, and consensus within specific research fields. Elicit leverages language models to efficiently locate relevant academic papers, eliminating the need for precise keyword matching. This user-friendly interface allows users to engage with the tool through simple queries, making it particularly beneficial for early-stage researchers and students who are just beginning to navigate the complexities of scientific writing. This intuitive approach not only simplifies the research process but also enhances learning opportunities for those new to academic environments.

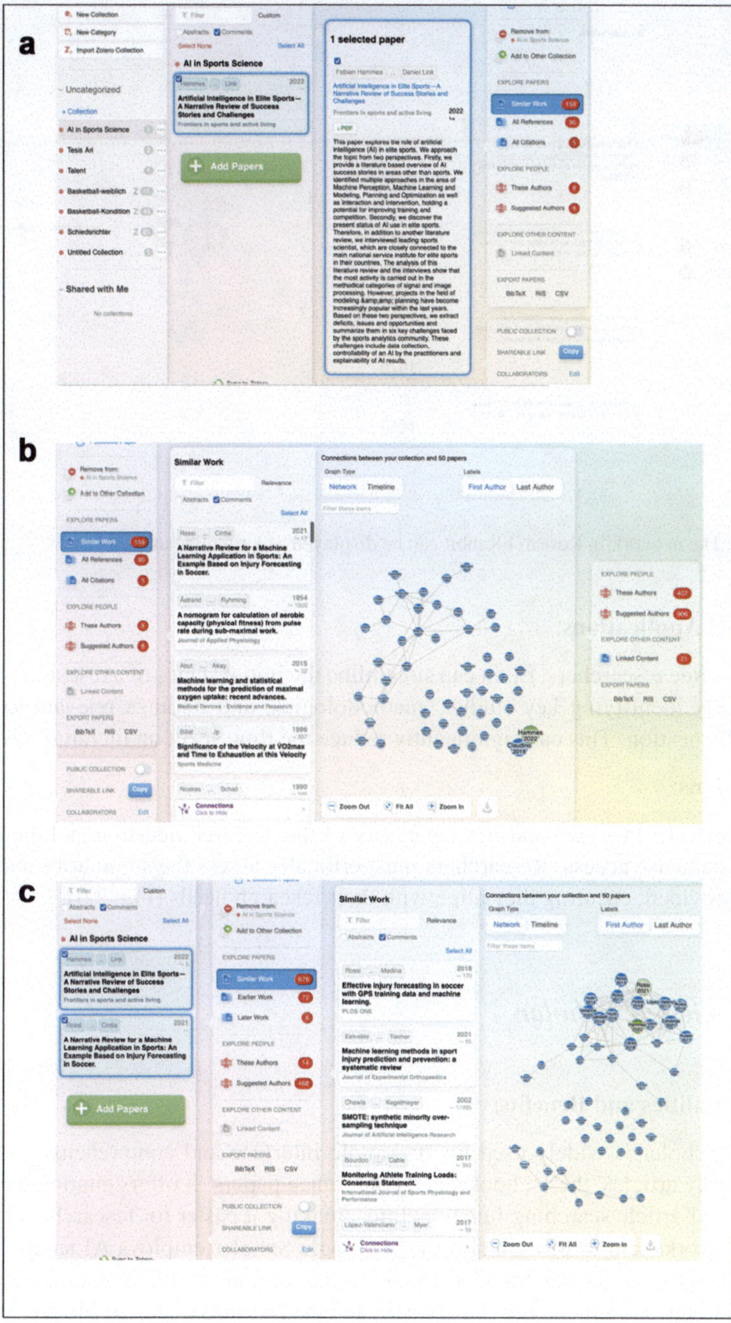

Fig. 2.1 Once a paper is added to a project in ResearchRabbit (**a**), a network of similar studies is created (**b**), with more papers being added to the project, the network changes and evolves (**c**)

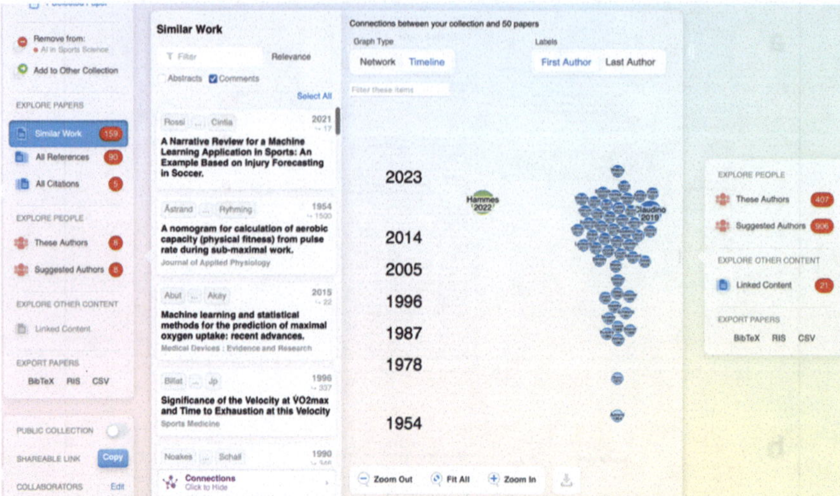

Fig. 2.2 The network in ResearchRabbit can be displayed as a timeline as well

Practical Applications:

For academic researchers, Elicit can streamline the initial stages of a research project by quickly identifying key studies, methodologies, and findings relevant to their research question. This can significantly reduce the time spent on literature reviews.

Limitations:

Elicit's effectiveness depends on the clarity of the research question and the tool's current database access. Researchers must critically assess the summaries and data points provided, ensuring they align with their research needs (Fig. 2.3).

2.3.3 *Google Scholar*

Functionalities and Benefits:

Google Scholar is widely used for its simple interface and comprehensive access to scholarly articles, thesis, books, and conference papers. It offers citation tracking and related-article searching functionalities, making it easier for researchers to find seminal works and follow citation trails. Google Scholar employs AI technologies similar to those used in the broader Google Search Engine. It utilizes neural mapping, Natural Language Processing (NLP), ML, and the Multitask Unified Model (MUM) to enhance its search capabilities. These technologies collectively work to refine search results, contextualize information, and offer concise summaries.

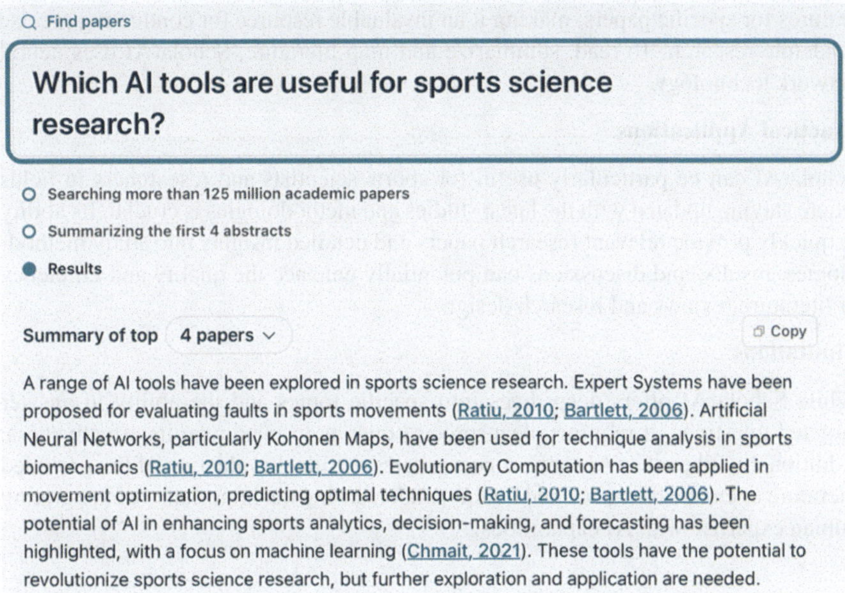
Find papers
Which AI tools are useful for sports science research?
Searching more than 125 million academic papers
Summarizing the first 4 abstracts
Results
Summary of top 4 papers
Copy
A range of AI tools have been explored in sports science research. Expert Systems have been proposed for evaluating faults in sports movements (Ratiu, 2010; Bartlett, 2006). Artificial Neural Networks, particularly Kohonen Maps, have been used for technique analysis in sports biomechanics (Ratiu, 2010; Bartlett, 2006). Evolutionary Computation has been applied in movement optimization, predicting optimal techniques (Ratiu, 2010; Bartlett, 2006). The potential of AI in enhancing sports analytics, decision-making, and forecasting has been highlighted, with a focus on machine learning (Chmait, 2021). These tools have the potential to revolutionize sports science research, but further exploration and application are needed.

Fig. 2.3 Elicit answers a research question by summarizing relevant papers

Practical Applications:

Its broad access makes it a fundamental tool for conducting preliminary literature searches and citation analysis in nearly any academic field, including sports science. Google Scholar is particularly useful for identifying highly cited works that define a research area.

Limitations:

Google Scholar may include non-peer-reviewed sources in its search results, requiring researchers to verify the credibility of their sources. Furthermore, its algorithm prioritizes highly cited papers, which could overshadow newer, less-cited research that might be equally relevant.

2.3.4 ScholarAI

Functionalities and Benefits:

ScholarAI specializes in providing comprehensive access to a wide array of academic papers, leveraging advanced search algorithms to find relevant literature based on specific inquiry keywords. It offers detailed analysis capabilities, including abstract searches, full-text analysis for in-depth research insights, and question-answering features for specific papers, making it an invaluable resource for conducting precise academic research. To read, summarize and map literature, ScholarAI uses neural network technology.

Practical Applications:

ScholarAI can be particularly useful for sports scientists and researchers in fields where staying updated with the latest studies and methodologies is crucial. Its ability to quickly provide relevant research papers and detailed insights into study methodologies, results, and discussions can potentially enhance the quality and efficiency of literature reviews and research design.

Limitations:

While ScholarAI offers deep dives into specific topics and the ability to answer targeted questions, it requires clear, precise queries to maximize its effectiveness. Additionally, like other AI tools, it necessitates a critical evaluation of the provided literature to ensure relevance and quality, underscoring the importance of integrating human expertise with AI capabilities.

2.3.5 *Summary of Artificial Intelligence Tools in Literature Research*

The landscape of AI tools for academic research is diverse, with each tool offering distinct advantages to researchers. From ResearchRabbit's personalized recommendations and interactive visualizations, Elicit's robust literature review and hypothesis testing capabilities, Google Scholar's broad access to scholarly materials and citation tracking, to ScholarAI's detailed research insights and targeted question-answering features, these tools collectively represent a powerful suite of resources that can potentially enhance academic research efficiency and depth. One suggested strategy for using AI tools in the scientific writing process begins with engaging Elicit to either discover a research question or refine an existing idea. After identifying pertinent papers (skipping the initial use of Elicit if relevant papers are already known), tools such as Google Scholar, Scholar AI, and ResearchRabbit can be utilized for a comprehensive search. Subsequently, it's advisable to verify the scientific validity of these findings by consulting specialized databases like PubMed. Throughout this process, ResearchRabbit's graphical representation of the literature and its integration with citation management programs like Zotero can be instrumental in organizing the literature and ensuring accurate citation in the thesis or paper draft. This approach streamlines the research process, leveraging the strengths of each AI tool to enhance the efficiency and depth of literature exploration and review.

However, the practical application of these tools underscores the need for a balanced approach, combining their advanced technological capabilities with the researcher's critical thinking and expertise. While AI tools offer unparalleled ease in sourcing relevant papers, automating literature reviews, and ensuring up-to-date citations, they are not without limitations. The potential for recommending non-relevant literature, the need for manual verification, and the importance of critical assessment remain paramount.

In essence, the integration of AI tools into academic research workflows opens new horizons for efficiency, knowledge discovery, and innovation. However, their limitations highlight the indispensable value of human judgment, ensuring that research outcomes not only benefit from the breadth and speed of AI but also reflect the depth and discernment that come with scholarly expertise.

2.4 Data Management, Analysis, and Visualization

Data management, analysis, and visualization form the backbone of AI and ML projects, enabling data scientists and researchers to derive insights, make informed decisions, and effectively communicate findings. The enormous growth in data volume and complexity has underscored the importance of efficient data handling and interpretation methods, making these disciplines critical in the context of AI and ML. Those data sets are substantially larger than those used in other empirical research projects.

Data management

In AI and ML projects, data management is crucial for the actual training of models, as the quality and quantity of data directly impact model performance. Data management in AI and ML encompasses the practices, architectural techniques, and tools for achieving consistent access to data in a way that is both efficient and secure. It involves data collection, storage, organization, and governance. The goal is to ensure data quality and accessibility for analysis and processing. Effective data management supports the iterative process of model development, enabling the refinement of datasets and the integration of new data sources to improve model accuracy and relevance.

Data analysis

Data analysis in AI and ML involves processing and examining datasets to discover patterns, test hypotheses, or make inferences. It is a critical step that directly influences model development and outcomes. Techniques range from statistical analysis to complex ML algorithms. In the context of AI, data analysis helps in feature selection, where relevant variables are identified for model training. It also plays a role in evaluating model performance through metrics. Through data analysis, researchers can identify trends, outliers, and correlations that inform the development and refinement of AI models.

Data visualization

Data visualization is the graphical representation of information and data. By using visual elements like charts, graphs, and maps, data visualization tools provide an accessible way to see and understand trends, outliers, and patterns in data. In AI and ML, visualization is not just a tool for presenting results but also a critical component of exploratory data analysis (EDA). Visualizations can reveal insights into the data that might not be apparent from raw data alone, making it easier for stakeholders to understand complex models or predictions. It also aids in diagnosing issues in model performance by highlighting data imbalances, errors in classification, or areas where the model is underfitting or overfitting.

Exploratory data analysis

In the context of AI and ML, exploratory data analysis (EDA) is a preliminary step before model building, where data scientists explore the data through visualizations and statistics to understand and interpret its characteristics, quality, and structure. EDA is crucial for identifying the most relevant features, understanding the distribution of data, and making informed decisions about data preprocessing and model selection.

EDA uses a variety of techniques (mostly graphical) to (Tukey, 1977):

- Maximize insight into a data set;
- Uncover underlying structure;
- Extract important variables;
- Detect outliers and anomalies;
- Test underlying assumptions;
- Develop parsimonious models; and
- Determine optimal factor settings.

Together, data management, analysis, visualization, and exploratory data analysis constitute essential processes in AI and ML projects. They enable the efficient handling of data, uncover insights that guide model development, and ensure that findings are communicated effectively. As AI and ML continue to evolve, the role of these disciplines will only grow in importance, driving advancements and innovation in the field. Furthermore, AI tools can be used to support those steps, e.g. DALL·E for visualization of data, but there are also other approaches to partially automate EDA (Patel et al., 2023).

2.5 Writing Support Through Artificial Intelligence

In the realm of academic writing, AI-powered tools such as Grammarly, ProWritingAid, DeepL, and ChatGPT play pivotal roles in enhancing writing quality, refining grammar, spelling, and style. These tools are designed not just to correct errors but also to improve the overall coherence and eloquence of academic texts, making them beneficial for researchers, students, and academics alike. Like the other AI tools previously discussed, the following tools also offer free versions with basic functionalities. However, for access to more powerful features or higher usage limits, users are usually required to opt for paid versions. All of the tools presented primarily use NLP for grammar checking, style editing and writing suggestions.

User-friendly interfaces are provided by these tools, and their intuitive usage often makes specific tutorials unnecessary for basic writing support. Effective outcomes can be significantly enhanced by crafting appropriate prompts for ChatGPT. Additionally, the "Grammarly Handbook," which outlines grammatical rules and provides examples of correct and incorrect usage, is made available on Grammarly's own website, aiding users in refining their writing skills.

Grammarly

Grammarly stands out for its comprehensive feedback on grammar, spelling, punctuation, sentence structure, style, and vocabulary enhancement. Its technology assists both learners and teachers by providing immediate modifications and reducing the workload of checking and evaluating writing. Studies have shown that Grammarly can significantly improve students' writing skills by offering precise corrections and suggestions across various error categories. However, it is crucial to note that while Grammarly excels in correcting language use, it may provide misleading feedback, struggle with checking bibliographies, and fail to evaluate context and content accurately. Thus, integrating Grammarly's feedback with careful review and critical feedback from educators is essential for achieving the best results in academic writing (Zinkevich & Ledeneva, 2021).

ProWritingAid

ProWritingAid, similar to Grammarly, offers detailed analysis of writing style, grammar, and errors. It provides suggestions for improvement, focusing on readability, sentence length variation, and overused words, which are crucial for academic writing. The tool is particularly helpful in making academic writing more concise and impactful. However, like all AI tools, it requires the user to critically assess the suggestions to ensure they align with the intended message and academic standards.

DeepL

DeepL is renowned for its translation accuracy, which could be beneficial for academic writers working with sources in multiple languages or needing to translate their work. Beyond translation, DeepL offers suggestions for enhancing sentence construction, making it a valuable tool for non-native English speakers aiming to polish their academic writing. To achieve high-quality translations, DeepL employs Machine Translation (MT) based on Deep Learning and neural networks. This advanced approach allows DeepL to consider the entire context of a sentence, rather than translating word by word. This method ensures that translations are not only accurate but also contextually appropriate, capturing the nuances of the source text more effectively. However, the limitation lies in its primary function as a translator; while it ensures grammatical accuracy and fluency, the depth of stylistic or content-specific advice may not be as comprehensive as other dedicated writing aids.

ChatGPT

ChatGPT, powered by advanced language models, assists in generating coherent and contextually relevant text, making it a helpful tool for drafting and revising academic writing. It can provide outlines, summaries, and even detailed sections of academic papers. Nonetheless, users must remain vigilant about the accuracy of the information provided and ensure it meets the rigorous standards of academic integrity and originality (Homolak, 2023).

Practical Applications and Limitations

These AI writing tools are invaluable for enhancing the clarity, coherence, and correctness of academic texts. They serve as initial screening layers for grammatical and stylistic errors, allowing writers to focus on the content's depth and originality. However, the integration of AI tools in academic writing represents a balance between leveraging technology for enhanced language precision and maintaining the critical, analytical approach characteristic of scholarly work. As these tools continue to evolve, their potential to support the academic community will undoubtedly expand. However, these tools should complement rather than replace the meticulous review processes typical of scholarly work.

2.6 Conclusion

The integration of AI tools into the academic research and writing process heralds a new era of efficiency and innovation in sports science and beyond. These tools offer unparalleled support in literature research, data analysis, writing assistance, and more, enhancing the overall quality and depth of academic work. However, the essence of successful AI integration lies in the symbiotic relationship between technology and human expertise. While AI tools can provide a foundation of efficiency and accessibility, the nuanced understanding and critical analysis inherent to human researchers remain irreplaceable. Furthermore, efficiency and quality of academic writing are not always enhanced with the use of AI tools, especially in less experienced scholars and researchers (Bašić et al., 2023).

As we continue to explore and expand the boundaries of knowledge, the judicious application of AI in academic research will undoubtedly serve as a catalyst for discovery and innovation. The future of sports science, enriched by AI, promises advancements that are not only technologically driven but also deeply rooted in the critical, analytical approach characteristic of scholarly work. However, the rise of (generative) AI tools in scientific writing calls for transparent declaration upon usage (Tang et al., 2023).

References

BaHammam, A. (2023). Balancing innovation and integrity: The role of AI in research and scientific writing. *Nature and Science of Sleep, 15*, 1153–1156. https://doi.org/10.2147/NSS.S455765

Bašić, Ž., Banovac, A., Kružić, I., & Jerković, I. (2023). ChatGPT-3.5 as writing assistance in students' essays. *Humanities and Social Sciences Communications, 10*(1), 750. https://doi.org/10.1057/s41599-023-02269-7

Bishop, C. M. (2006). *Pattern recognition and machine learning*. Springer.

Bishop, C. M., & Bishop, H. (2024). *Deep Learning: Foundations and concepts* (1st ed.). Springer. https://doi.org/10.1007/978-3-031-45468-4

Chubb, J., Cowling, P., & Reed, D. (2022). Speeding up to keep up: Exploring the use of AI in the research process. *AI & Society, 37*(4), 1439–1457. https://doi.org/10.1007/s00146-021-01259-0

Duymaz, Y. K., & Tekin, A. M. (2023). Harnessing artificial intelligence in academic writing: Potential, ethics, and responsible use. *European Journal of Therapeutics*. https://doi.org/10.58600/eurjther1755

Escalante, J., Pack, A., & Barrett, A. (2023). AI-generated feedback on writing: Insights into efficacy and ENL student preference. *International Journal of Educational Technology in Higher Education, 20*(1), 57. https://doi.org/10.1186/s41239-023-00425-2

F. J. Pinzolits, R. (2023). AI in academia: An overview of selected tools and their areas of application. *MAP Education and Humanities, 4*(1), 37–50. https://doi.org/10.53880/2744-2373.2023.4.37

Homolak, J. (2023). Exploring the adoption of ChatGPT in academic publishing: Insights and lessons for scientific writing. *Croatian Medical Journal, 64*(3), 205–207. https://doi.org/10.3325/cmj.2023.64.205

McCarthy, J., Minsky, M. L., Rochester, N., & Shannon, C. E. (1955). A proposal for the Dartmouth summer research project on artificial intelligence. *AI Magazine, 27*(4), 12.

Russell, S. J., & Norvig, P. (2021). *Artificial intelligence: A modern approach* (4th ed.). Pearson.

Patel, H., Guttula, S., Gupta, N., & Hans, S. (2023) A data-centric AI framework for automating exploratory data analysis and data quality tasks. *ACM Journal of Data and Information Quality, 15*(4), 1–26.

Tang, A., Li, K., Kwok, K. O., Cao, L., Luong, S., & Tam, W. (2023). The importance of transparency: Declaring the use of generative artificial intelligence (AI) in academic writing. *Journal of Nursing Scholarship*. https://doi.org/10.1111/jnu.12938

Tukey, J. W. (1977). *Exploratory data analysis*. Pearson. ISBN 978-0201076165.

von Garrel, J., & Mayer, J. (2023). Artificial Intelligence in studies—Use of ChatGPT and AI-based tools among students in Germany. *Humanities and Social Sciences Communications, 10*(1), 799. https://doi.org/10.1057/s41599-023-02304-7

Zinkevich, N. A., & Ledeneva, T. V. (2021). Using Grammarly to enhance students' academic writing skills. *Professional Discourse & Communication, 3*(4), 51–63. https://doi.org/10.24833/2687-0126-2021-3-4-51-63

Chapter 3
Advancing Endurance Sports with Artificial Intelligence: Application-Focused Perspectives

Tessa Menges

Abstract As one of the key technologies in today's society, Artificial Intelligence (AI) is increasingly influencing every facet of people's daily routines, including sports training. This chapter explores the use of AI in endurance sports and how it enhances various aspects of the sporting world. AI can provide targeted assistance in athletes' training through methods such as data analysis and simulation of training scenarios. In the context of cycling, an AI system can analyze a cyclist's performance data, including factors like cadence, power output and heart rate, to identify specific areas for improvement. The AI can show the coach or the athlete training types that explicitly help the cyclist to improve his recognized weaknesses. This focused approach empowers cyclists to fine-tune their training regimens based on individual needs, ultimately contributing to heightened performance and skill refinement. In a professional context, where personalized training has long been the norm, the value lies in AI's capacity to identify weaknesses, providing insights that may surpass traditional coaching methods. This new type of intelligent data analysis can support the coach and the athlete in the decision-making process. This applies not only to training but also to the selection of races or the definition of a strategy. Specific practical examples will also be highlighted to illustrate how AI is being used in sports today. The aim is to concretize the approaches of AI in sports and explain how these tools work. In conclusion, this chapter not only serves as a compass guiding readers through the exciting intersection of AI and sports but also invites reflection on the vast potential and transformative power of technology in shaping the future of athletic pursuits.

Keywords Artificial Intelligence in Sports · Machine Learning in Sports · Artificial Intelligence Assistant · Performance Analytics · Injury Prevention · Wearable Technology · Data-Driven Decision-Making

---

T. Menges (✉)
enduco GmbH, Saarbrücken, Germany
e-mail: tessa.menges@enduco.app

C. Dindorf et al. (eds.), *Artificial Intelligence in Sports, Movement, and Health*,
https://doi.org/10.1007/978-3-031-67256-9_3

3.1 Introduction

In recent years, the surge of AI has permeated various facets of human life, bringing about a substantial shift in our perspectives and utilization of this advanced technology (Littman et al., 2021. p. 12). The rapid growth of AI has significantly altered the way we approach and integrate it into our daily activities. There's a major shift happening, with a greater focus on practical and useful applications of AI. This means AI is not just getting better; it's becoming more about real-world use cases in different areas, moving away from just theoretical or experimental ideas. Figure 3.1 captures the total number of AI patent filings from 2010 to 2021.

The changing landscape has not only affected our understanding of sports but has also transformed the methods we use to improve athletic performance and refine our practice routines. This shift includes advancements in sports science, technology, and innovative training approaches, which are reshaping how we engage with and compete in sports (Chmait & Westerbeek, 2021).

For example, in the past, talent scouts were faced with a labor-intensive and time-consuming process of manually analyzing countless videos to identify the right player for a team. This required a deep understanding of player nuances and team dynamics. However, with the advent of AI, the scouting landscape has changed. AI algorithms can now quickly scan large amounts of video footage to quickly analyze the performance of basketball players. For example, SportVU 2.0 (Stats Perform, Germany, Düsseldorf), which uses advanced optical tracking and computer vision, extracts player and ball coordinates to generate rich performance statistics. This data, harnessed by the latest AI analysis software, offers valuable insights into player strengths, weaknesses, and overall suitability for a team. Talent scouts can now use AI as a powerful tool to streamline the scouting process, focusing on nuanced aspects

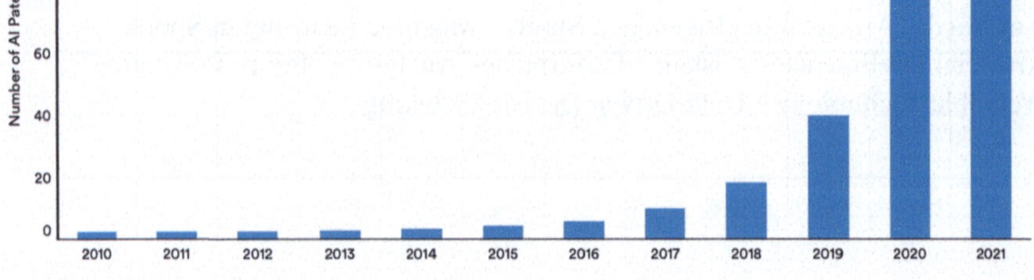

Fig. 3.1 Number of AI patent filings in the world, 2010–2021 (Clark & Perrault, 2022, Artificial Intelligence index report 2022, p. 36)

that AI might not capture, ultimately enhancing the precision and efficiency of player evaluation for college and professional organizations.

Moreover, this transformative use of AI in sports scouting draws parallels with the revolutionary concept of Moneyball. This concept introduced a groundbreaking approach to baseball team management by relying on statistical analysis to identify undervalued players around the year 2000. The common thread lies in leveraging data-driven insights to make strategic decisions, challenging conventional methods. At this time, Billy Beane, General Manager of the Oakland Athletics, brought about a groundbreaking change by incorporating statistical analysis into athlete selection. By leveraging data analytics, Beane and his team identified undervalued players based on their statistical performance rather than traditional scouting methods. This strategic shift not only enabled the "Oakland-Athletics" to compete effectively against wealthier teams but also exposed inefficiencies in the way players were traditionally valued in the sports industry (Lewis, 2004). They developed themself a guiding compass to facilitate optimal team decision-making and benefit from it.

In the pursuit of gaining a competitive edge, teams in soccer and basketball, inspired by the data-driven revolution exemplified by Moneyball, have implemented sophisticated analytics to inform decision-making. This extends beyond player recruitment to various aspects of team strategy, performance optimization and tactical planning. For instance, teams may use data analytics to analyze player movements, assess playing patterns, and identify effective strategies in specific game situations. In soccer, Rossi et al. (2018) and in basketball, Horvat et al. (2019) highlight how teams leverage data-driven insights for better player management, injury prevention, and strategic planning during matches. While player recruitment is part of the equation, the broader application of data-driven decision-making encompasses a holistic approach to enhancing team performance and gaining a strategic advantage in dynamic, fast-paced team sports. The emergence of Deep Learning (DL), a subgroup of Machine Learning (ML), in sports builds upon this foundation by introducing more advanced and nuanced methods for data analysis (Bartlett, 2006). It can process complex patterns and relationships in large data sets to continuously improve the performance of teams and individual athletes.

DL algorithms gained popularity among computer scientists between 2006 and 2010. This trend can be attributed not only to advances in computer hardware capabilities but also to a paradigm shift within the AI community towards open collaboration and data sharing. The publication of extensive datasets like ImageNet by Stanford University and the creation of open-source ML competitions stimulated innovation and exploration in the area, resulting in swift progressions in AI technologies that are fundamental to the current sports analytics environment (Chmait & Westerbeek, 2021). ImageNet is an image database organized according to the WordNet hierarchy, in which each node of the hierarchy is represented by hundreds and thousands of images. The project has been instrumental in advancing research in computer vision and DL.

The continuous evolution of sensors and wearables is crucial for providing a robust data foundation that enables comprehensive tracking of athletes. This data serves as the basis for conducting AI analysis and provides valuable insights into various aspects of an athlete's performance. The significance lies in the ability to gather real-time, precise, and extensive information about an athlete's physiological responses, movements, and overall health. By leveraging advanced sensors and wearables, coaches, sports scientists, and medical professionals can access a wealth of data, allowing for nuanced monitoring of factors such as heart rate, sleep patterns, and recovery metrics. The Sensor support has increased every year, equipped with various sensors, algorithms, and accompanying mobile apps. In the period from 2011 to 2017, the photoplethysmograph was the second most commonly used sensor, after the accelerometer, for estimating heart rate (Henriksen et al., 2018). Recent advances in mobile sensor technologies have made it possible to use privately collected data on physical activity to complement existing health data collection methods in research. Devices such as Garmin, Whoop, Oura, and Polar can now provide data on sleep and other health metrics, including heart rate variability. The Australian Institute of Sport (Dean et al., 2022) has tested the best providers against the gold standard of sleep measurement (Polysomnography, PSG) and heart rate (Electrocardiogram, ECG), as well as heart rate variability. The data obtained was highly accurate, enabling precise statements to be made about the athlete's recovery status at an affordable cost.

Furthermore, the landscape of AI accessibility and efficiency has experienced notable changes. Since 2018, the cost of training an image classification system has decreased by 63.6%, and training times have improved by 94.4% (Zhang et al., 2021). The research by Cao et al. (2017) introduces a key point detector for the body and foot, reducing inference time while maintaining accuracy. This advancement in human pose estimation, offering real-time capabilities, holds implications for diverse domains, including sports analytics and virtual environment design. As these developments unfold, collaborative efforts, sophisticated sensors, and increased AI accessibility converge to redefine the landscape of sports analytics in a dynamic and data-driven era.

This chapter demonstrates specific use cases, including AI-driven performance analytics, injury prevention strategies, and personalized training regimens. Much like a compass that adapts to changing magnetic fields, AI adapts to the evolving dynamics of each athlete, offering tailor-made solutions for optimal performance and health.

3.2 Artificial Intelligence-Based Approaches in Sport

In the contemporary landscape of sports science and performance optimization, the integration of AI stands as a seminal paradigm shift. Rajšp and Fister (2020) provide a holistic overview about the use of data analysis in different kinds of sports. The literature includes studies between 2006 and 2020 to figure out 97 studies that fulfills the requirements. Between 2006 and 2012, there was a gradual increase in research studies, with one to four being published each year. However, in 2013, there was a significant increase, with no fewer than four studies being published annually. It is

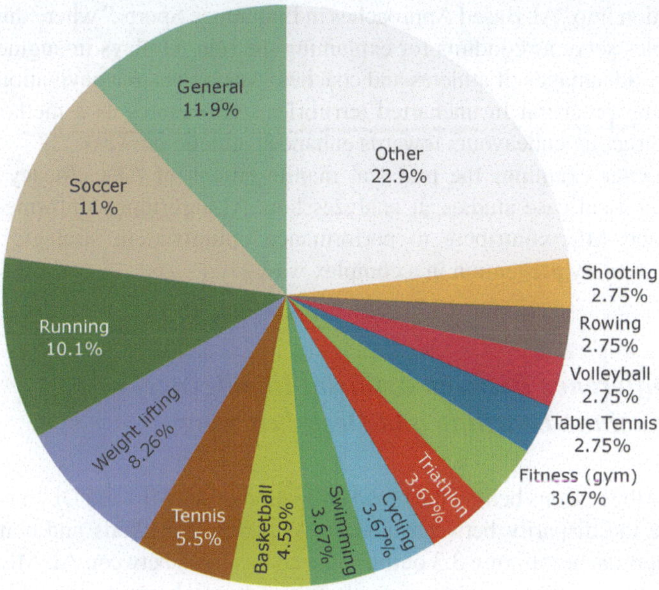

Fig. 3.2 Identified sports where intelligent data analysis methods have been used by Rajšp and Fister (2020)

worth noting that in 2018 and 2019, there was a substantial increase in the number of research studies published, with 23 and 22, studies, respectively. This trend highlights the increasing importance and focus on intelligent sports training in academic and research circles (Rajšp and Fister, 2020). Figure 3.2 displays the sports that have been most frequently researched in studies on the use of AI.

The distribution may be due to the popularity of these sports and their ability to invest in new technology. The review indicates that the majority of the studies analyzed were conducted in individual sports (54%), followed by team sports (28%) and mixed sports (17%).

- Individual Sports: These are activities where participants compete against other individuals rather than as part of a team. The listed examples include for example climbing, fitness, triathlon, running, and swimming.
- Mixed Sports: These are sports where individuals may compete both individually against others and, in certain competitions, as part of a duo or a team. Examples provided are badminton, cycling, and rowing.
- Team Sports: This category encompasses sports where individuals are consistently part of a larger team, competing against other teams. The identified team sports include basketball, cricket, football, handball, hockey, soccer, and volleyball.

It is also notable that the individual endurance sports "running", "cycling", "swimming" and also "triathlon" represent 21% of the research fields. This is why this review uses examples of cycling and running in particular. This review embarks on an exploration into "AI-Based Approaches in Endurance Sports," where three empirical examples serve as conduits for explaining the role AI plays in augmenting the competitive advantages of athletes and coaches. Analogous to a navigational instrument guiding precision in uncharted territories, AI operates as a methodological compass, directing endeavours towards enhanced athletic prowess.

This chapter examines the practical manifestations of AI's efficacy in sports through empirical case studies. It analyzes how AI algorithms, informed by data analytics and ML, contribute to performance optimization, strategic decision-making, and injury prevention in a complex way.

3.2.1 Difference Between Artificial Intelligence, Machine Learning and Deep Learning

To perceive the reasons behind the broad utilization of AI, ML, and DL, it is essential to examine the disparity between modern AI learning methods and conventional analytics approaches. Figure 3.3 outlines the connections between AI, ML, and DL.

AI is defined as the capacity of a system to accurately interpret and learn from external data and apply the acquired knowledge to achieve specific goals and solve problems through flexible adaptation. In this context, AI is primarily used as a decision-making tool for large amounts of data (Kaplan & Haenlein, 2019).

ML is a subfield of AI that employs statistical techniques to improve machine performance via experience. The method comprises multiple data iterations to unveil correlations and extract meaning from unstructured data.

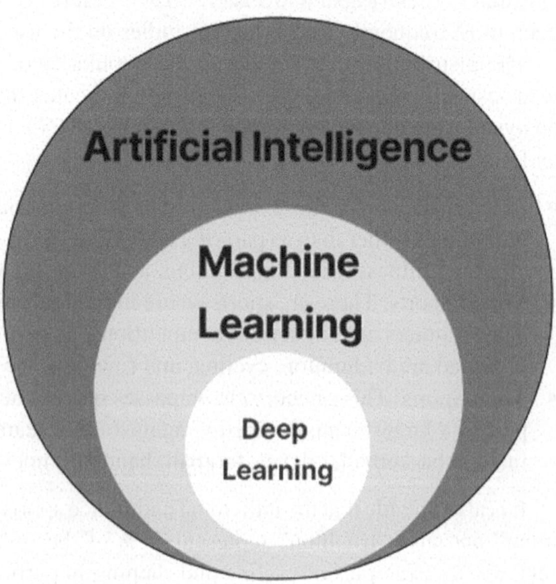

Fig. 3.3 Relationships between Artificial Intelligence, Machine Learning and Deep Learning (based on Dindorf et al. 2022, p. 9)

In ML, the types of algorithms used can be broadly classified into Supervised Learning, Unsupervised Learning, and Reinforcement Learning (Bonaccorso, 2017).

1. **Supervised Learning:** This type of ML algorithm involves learning a function that maps an input to an output based on example input–output pairs. It infers a function from labeled training data consisting of a set of training examples. In sports, Supervised Learning could be used for predicting the outcome of games based on historical data where the results of past matches are known.
2. **Unsupervised Learning:** Unlike Supervised Learning, Unsupervised Learning deals with input data without labeled responses. The system tries to learn patterns and structure from the data without reference to known or labeled outcomes. In sports, Unsupervised Learning could be utilized for player segmentation or team profiling based on playing styles or statistics without any predefined categories.
3. **Reinforcement Learning:** This type of learning is about taking suitable action to maximize reward in a particular situation. It is employed by various software and machines to find the best possible behavior or path it should take in a specific situation. Through experimentation and interaction with its surroundings, an agent formulates a strategy that recommends the optimal course of action to achieve the highest long-term rewards from any given situation. This approach effectively becomes a decision-making strategy that adjusts and advances as the agent gains knowledge from new encounters.

DL represents an advanced form of ML, delving into more intricate levels of data processing. The primary objective of DL is to employ algorithms in constructing Neural Networks are capable of solving complex problems. Neural Networks are models inspired by the structure and functioning of the human brain. They consist of layers of artificial neurons connected to each other. These connections have weights that are adjusted during training to improve the network. This approach is especially valuable for addressing issues that would otherwise demand intricate rules when approached through traditional methods. Notably, DL finds application in tasks such as speech, image, and text recognition and processing. Its ability to discern intricate patterns and features within vast datasets makes it a powerful tool for tackling challenges that extend beyond the scope of conventional approaches.

The following section provides examples of AI applications and explains how AI, ML, or DL are used in the field of cycling and running.

3.2.2 Data-Driven Team Strategy in Road Cycling

For the past 150 years, road cycle racing has stood as an organized and competitive team sport (Mignot, 2016). In this athletic endeavour, teams of cyclists engage in a series of races throughout the year. During these races, teammates collaborate, with the overall team performance determined by the first member to cross the finish line. The team is collectively dedicated to propelling one of its cyclists to victory as swiftly as possible.

Typically consisting of around thirty cyclists, each team is limited to a smaller group of participants in individual races, usually ranging from 8 to 10 cyclists. The composition of the top ten cyclists can vary drastically depending on the course profile. Whether the competition course is flat or hilly can make a significant impact. Each competition is characterized by a distinct blend of factors, including length, gradients, and surfaces (e.g., asphalt with or without pebbles, and cobblestones). Another distinctive feature in cycling is the interplay between teams and individual competitors. While teamwork is crucial, only one individual can emerge victorious (except in events like team time trials), creating a dynamic among team members. The team's coach, relying on recent workout performances and considering race-specific conditions, selects the participants for each race (U.C. Internationale, 2022). The coach generally devises a scheduling plan for the upcoming season's races, followed by creating a tailored workout schedule for each cyclist. Nonetheless, this plan frequently undergoes alterations prior to each race, and the coach might opt to field a different cyclist than initially planned, contingent upon the recent workout performances of the athletes. For instance, relevant information may include the athlete's recent distance covered, history of illness or injury, and average caloric expenditure.

Contemporary cyclists utilize an array of gadgets and wearable devices to track extensive data, including comprehensive details such as overall elevation gain, distance covered, heart rate measurements, cadence, power, estimated energy expenditure, total workout duration, and additional metrics. The raw data is transmitted to health and fitness software applications, which often employ ML or AI to analyze the data.

The coach can monitor and assess the overall health and performance data of each of the 30 athletes through access to the data. AI is used to navigate through the mass of data and support the coach in making decisions about the allocation of cyclists to races.

Sagi et al. (2022) introduces a method called RaceFit, a recommendation system for assigning cyclists to race stages. The goal is to determine, based on historical coaching decisions, which cyclists from a team are best suited for a particular race stage. The methodology utilizes a form of Supervised Learning approach known as Binary Classifier. The algorithm is trained with a dataset containing examples of the two classes it is meant to distinguish, such as 'positive' and 'negative'. The aim is to teach the algorithm to recognise patterns in the training data so that it can then predict which of the two classes it belongs to for new, untrained data. In RaceFit, the Binary Classifier is used to predict a cyclist's participation in a race stage. The classifier is trained using examples that match a cyclist with a stage, and the label indicates whether or not the cyclist participated (Fig. 3.4).

For the classification properties of the race stage (distance, elevation gain, etc.), cyclists characteristics (weight, height, age, and statistics from the Pro Cycling Stats website), and summarized workout data from the cyclist in five weeks leading up to the race stage were included. This is because they assumed that coaches make their final decisions before that week, allowing cyclists time to prepare and travel to the race location.

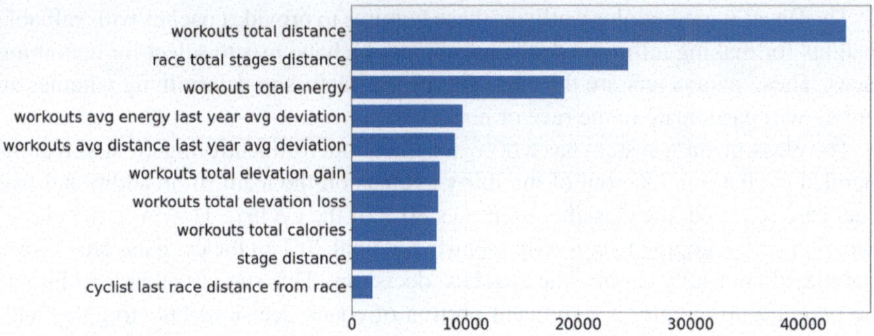

Fig. 3.4 Most correlated features used by the algorithm RaceFIT (Sagi et al., 2022, p. 9)

The most important features used by the algorithm to predict the athletes in the next race are the following listed in the order of their importance:

- Total Distance in last five weeks: This is the most crucial factor, indicating how much distance cyclists covered in their recent workouts. It reflects their training intensity and helps identify those who train hard. It can also highlight cyclists dealing with injuries not directly reported.
- Race's Total Distance: The distance of the upcoming race plays a significant role. Longer distances might require higher endurance, affecting the decision on which cyclists to choose.
- Workouts Total Energy: Reflects the overall energy expended in recent workouts, offering insights into the rider's fitness levels. It indicates how hard the last workouts were for the cyclists.
- Cyclist Workouts Energy: Integrates the power produced by the cyclist in watts with the average duration of recent workouts. High values indicate a cyclist's suitability for the upcoming race, considering both energy production and long distances.
- Difference in Cyclists Distance Relative to Annual Mean: Measures changes in a cyclist's recent distance compared to their average annual distance. It helps identify both improvements and potential performance reductions, possibly due to recent injuries.
- Elevation Gain and Elevation Loss: Describe changes in elevation during workouts. As some races are in mountainous areas while others are on plains. These features influence the decision-making, considering the race's terrain.
- Calories Burned During Workouts: Implies workout intensity, similar to, energy produced. It helps gauge the effort cyclists put into recent training sessions.
- Stage Distance: Identifies races with very long distances, requiring higher endurance and more energy expenditure than others.
- Geographic Constraint (Distance to Current Race Location from Last Race Location): Reflects the distance from the cyclist's last race location to the current race location. Coaches tend to assign cyclists to nearby races to minimize travel.

The RaceFit methodology utilizes these features to provide coaches with valuable insights for making informed decisions about which cyclists to select for upcoming races. These parameters are the most significant factors in determining whether an athlete will participate in the race or not.

The classification system has a 60% accuracy rate for identifying the first recommended cyclist in a race out of the thirty cyclists on the team. If an additional five riders are required, the classifier identifies 80% of the cyclists. However, the classifiers find it challenging to correctly identify the final 20% of the cyclists. This shows that they do not fully capture the coaches' decisions. This suggests that RaceFit has the potential to identify a significant portion of coach decisions but struggles with the last 20%.

For these reasons, it is important to rely on the coach's decision in addition to the RaceFiT tool, especially when selecting the last 20% of the team. The tool can assist the coach in selecting athletes from a group of five people. It is an objective and precise method that can aid in the decision-making process. It is important to keep the selection of features as small as possible. Using too many parameters requires more data to achieve valid results.

3.2.3 *Prediction of Real-Time Track Cycling Performance*

Having gained insight into the classic discipline of road cycling, characterized by long distances and varied terrains, let's now shift the focus to a specialized branch of the sport—track cycling. While road cycling often revolves around endurance and tactical skills, Track Cycling stands out with its short, intense races on specially designed velodromes. Track cycling consists of several disciplines, such as Sprint, Keirin, Omnium, Pursuit, and Team Sprint. Each discipline has its own unique rules and challenges. In Sprint, two riders compete directly against each other, while Keirin involves riders following a pacing vehicle before sprinting. Omnium is a multi-event discipline that includes races like Scratch Race and Elimination Race. The pursuit sees two riders starting on opposite sides of the velodrome, attempting to catch each other. Team Sprint is a team event with three riders per team. Analyzing and predicting Track Cycling events involve distinct individual physiological factors and strategies that differ from those in road cycling.

For the coach, it becomes even more crucial to understand the current state of an individual athlete, especially when the athlete can't rely on other team members. This personalized insight, coupled with real-time performance estimations during a Track Cycling event, empowers the coach to make informed decisions, strategically adjust race tactics, and optimize training plans based on the unique requirements of each athlete. The ability to monitor and analyze real-time data enhances the coach's capacity to provide timely feedback, prevent potential overexertion, and motivate athletes effectively. Overall, having access to estimated real-time performance data amplifies the coach's capabilities, enabling a more tailored and effective approach to individualized athlete development in the dynamic context of Track Cycling events.

Sudin et al. (2018) utilizes the Fuzzy Inference System (FIS) and Adaptive Neuro-Fuzzy Inference System (ANFIS) for performance classification, and a prediction is proposed.

An FIS is based on fuzzy logic and rules derived from human experts or empirical values (Blej & Azizi, 2016). The fuzzy features are represented by linguistic variables, such as "fast", "slow", "high", and "low". These fuzzy features are used in sets of rules to draw conclusions. An FIS possesses a static structure (IF–THEN rules), and the parameters need to be configured manually. The FIS provides the advantage of decreased computational workload and time. Therefore, this model is well-suited for integration into optimization processes and other adaptive techniques like Genetic Algorithm (GA) and Adaptive Neural Network (ANN) (Sudin et al., 2018). Section 2.4 provides a detailed explanation of genetic algorithms (Fig. 3.5).

The ANFIS is, in contrast an extension that offers an adaptive learning capability through the integration of ANN. ANFIS can automatically adapt the structure and parameters of the fuzzy model to better fit the data (Dewan et al., 2016). It combines the fuzzy logic of a FIS with the learning ability of a Neural Network. The adaptation takes place through training with existing data, whereby the system learns the optimum parameters itself (Zounemat-Kermani & Teshnehlab, 2008).

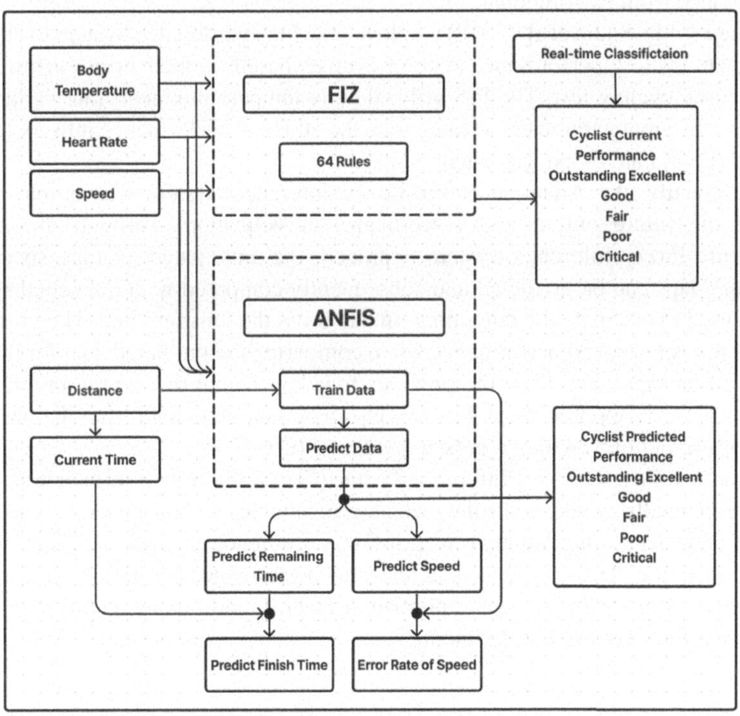

Fig. 3.5 Overall diagram for FIS and ANFIS-based systems (based on Sudin et al., 2018, p. 10)

For example, suppose we use an ANFIS (Adaptive Neuro-Fuzzy Inference System) and a FIS (Fuzzy Inference System) to predict a cyclist performance in a race. Here are two fuzzy features that could be considered in both systems:

1. Fitness level of the athlete (fuzzy feature):

FIS: Linguistic variables could represent fitness level, e.g. "very fit", "fit", "average". The fuzzy rules would define how these linguistic variables influence performance.

ANFIS: Here, the ANFIS adaptively learns how different fitness levels influence performance by learning the relationships between the linguistic variables and performance from existing training data.

2. Fatigue of the athlete (fuzzy characteristic):

FIS: Linguistic variables could represent different degrees of fatigue, such as "rested", "slightly fatigued", and "fatigued". The fuzzy rules would define how these levels of fatigue affect performance.

ANFIS: Here, ANFIS adaptively learns how different degrees of fatigue affect performance by learning the link between the linguistic variables for fatigue and performance from existing data.

In their study, Sudin et al. (2018) employed the Fuzzy Inference System to classify the current cycling performance state of cyclists based on their prior performance in an indoor cycling test. The FIS utilized body temperature, heart rate variability, and speed as input parameters to categorize the athletes' performance into six levels: Critical, Poor, Fair, Good, Excellent, Outstanding.

Additionally, the Adaptive Neuro-Fuzzy Inference System was employed to predict the future output and performance classification. Through the Adaptive Neuro-Fuzzy Inference System approach, the anticipated average speed for upcoming laps can be predicted and subsequently compared with the actual speed. This is used to calculate the remaining time to cross the finishing line. The predictor demonstrates improved performance when comparing the predicted data for the last lap based on input data from the previous four laps (1 out of 5) with a regression value of 0.87, as opposed to the last two laps based on input data from the previous three laps (2 out of 5) with a regression value of 0.76.

In track cycling, the Fuzzy Inference System (FIS) simplifies performance analysis through manually configured rules, which are suitable for optimization processes. On the other hand, the Adaptive Neuro-Fuzzy Inference System (ANFIS), which leverages Neural Networks, excels in real-time performance prediction. This allows coaches to estimate future laps, optimize strategies, and enhance athlete training plans for more effective development.

3.2.4 Wearables and Adaptable Training Plans

Athlete tracking and monitoring is an area in which AI excels. Wearable devices fitted with AI algorithms are capable of monitoring biometric data, including heart rate, sleep patterns, and muscle fatigue, to offer valuable insights for coaches and athletes to optimize performance and recovery.

Injury prevention is one of the vital applications of AI in sports. In the context of predicting sports injuries using supervised Machine Learning, wearable devices can be used to collect data on athletes' movements during training and competition. Furthermore, by analyzing movement patterns and biomechanical data, AI models can identify areas that could lead to overtraining and injuries. The trackers collect various data like distance covered, pace, maximal speed, number of sprints, sprint distances, intensity, time in red zone, accelerations, and total stress load. This data alongside the historical medical data that is collected by physiotherapists and club doctors, is then tagged with instances where injuries have occurred. A Supervised Learning algorithm, such as a Decision Tree or Neural Network, can be trained on this dataset to identify patterns that often precede injuries. Zadeh et al. (2021), examine the applications of wearable technology in sports. Once trained, the model can predict the likelihood of injury given the athlete's current data. For example, if a particular movement pattern or load is known to correlate with a high risk of a knee injury, the model can alert coaches and medical staff to a high-risk situation, allowing preventative measures to be taken, such as modifying training intensity or providing targeted interventions.

The study by Bowen et al. (2016) investigates the correlation between physical workload and injury risk in elite youth football players. The study reveals that higher workloads are associated with an increased risk of injury. This suggests that workloads can serve as a metric in an AI model for injury prediction. Hullin et al. (2016) conducted another study that assesses the Acute Chronic Workload Ratio (ACWR) in Rugby League players. The ACWR is a metric used in sports science and athletic training to assess the balance between short-term (acute) and long-term (chronic) workloads. It compares the recent training load (acute workload) with the average training load over a longer period (chronic workload). The study found that a higher ACWR raises the risk of injury. This, along with other related variables, has potential importance in using ML for injury prediction.

With the rise of accessibility and accurate wearable measurements, fitness apps are now using AI to generate personalized training recommendations and adaptive plans in individual sports. These plans are based on data such as heart rate, training metrics, sleep patterns, and exertion levels. Through data analytics, AI can recognize patterns and identify trends to create a customized training plan according to the athletes' goal (Fister & Fister, 2019). For example, an athlete trains too intensively in one session, the AI will automatically adjust the next day's training.

For instance, enduco is a company that utilizes an athletes' training data like acute stress and recovery data to recommend through an AI-based algorithm the best course of action for improving their performance or achieving a specific goal.

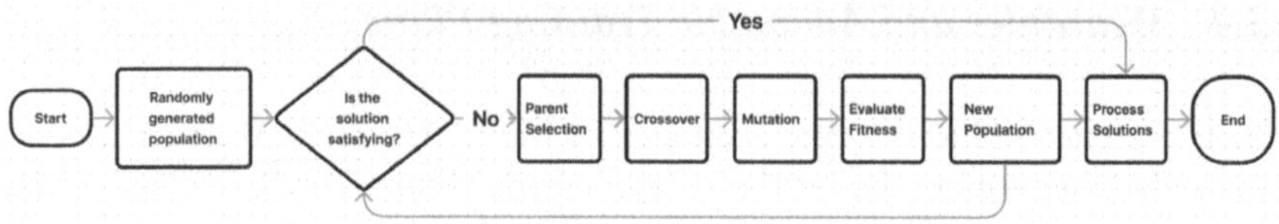

Fig. 3.6 Workflow of a genetic algorithm (based on Ariyaratne & Silva, 2022)

Enduco analyzed user data to make assumptions about an athlete's training needs and performance development. Using optimized heuristics, the basic principles of an effective training plan are defined based on expert knowledge and current research. Heuristics address the challenges posed by time constraints, information availability, and processing capacity. The essence of heuristics, as described by Kahneman (2011), lies in their role as adaptive mechanisms that enable rapid and resource-efficient decision making. For example, the heuristic in enduco analyses the most appropriate plan for an individual athlete based on many features like intensity distribution, workload, and current fatigue.

An effective training plan for a marathon should consider different intensities and allow for sufficient recovery periods between training sessions. For instance, it may be important to avoid intensive training for more than two consecutive days to prevent overtraining and injury. The heuristic may suggest including various intensities to improve maximal oxygen uptake or achieve an economical metabolic rate before the aerobic-anaerobic threshold. It can be supplemented by numerous rules in addition to these examples.

The application of a heuristic can lead to quick, acceptable solutions but is not necessarily aimed at guaranteeing the best possible result. Heuristics are often suboptimal, quick approaches based on experience. At enduco, an optimization algorithm, such as a Genetic Algorithm (GA), is then used. A GA is a method inspired by biological evolution. This approach goes through several iterations or generations, selecting the best training plans to influence the next generation (Ariyaratne & Silva, 2022) (Fig. 3.6).

Based on Ariyaratne and Silva (2022), the GA starts in with a randomly generated population of possible solutions to a given problem. Each solution is treated as an individual and is represented by a set of parameters. To evaluate the quality of the solutions, a fitness function is used that indicates how well each individual solves the problem. If the initial results are not satisfactory, selection is based on fitness, where those with higher fitness have a greater chance of being selected. These selected individuals are then crossed to produce a new generation. Through this process, the new generations inherit traits from their parents. Occasionally, random changes (mutations) may also occur to maintain some genetic diversity in the population.

The new generation of offspring forms the next population and replaces some of the previous parents.

This cycle of selection, crossover, and mutation is repeated over many generations. Over time, the population improves as evolutionary mechanisms tend to favor better solutions (Langdon & Harman, 2014).

Enduco the training plan is evaluated using a fitness function that considers compliance with the heuristic and, for example the approximation of target times for the marathon. The algorithm converges to a training plan that effectively fulfills the heuristic and maximizes the target times for the marathon. The ability to optimize is an important feature of AI.

The continuous improvement of wearables and other devices is democratizing access to the use of AI in sports. Advanced data collection is making AI applications in endurance sports accessible to amateur athletes. This is leading to an increased willingness to use AI, as the precise data collected by improved wearables enables individual performance optimization and a better understanding of physical activity. Overall, AI in sports is becoming an integrative tool that is widely used and enhances athletic performance and well-being (Li & Xu, 2021).

3.3 Advantages and Disadvantages of Artificial Intelligence Applications in Sports for Key Stakeholders

The incorporation of AI in sports offers substantial advantages and poses notable challenges for athletes and coaches alike (Avici & Bayrakdar, 2023). Athletes experience benefits, with technological advancements contributing to significant performance improvements, reduced injury instances, and accelerated recovery times through innovations in sports medicine and technology. Moreover, coaches can provide more objective and targeted feedback, fostering skill development among athletes.

However, the increasing reliance on technology introduces potential drawbacks. The utilization of AI may compromise the confidentiality of sensitive information, raising concerns about data security and privacy. In addition, there is a risk that the line between personal and professional life will become blurred for athletes as they navigate the technological landscape. For instance, the coach can monitor the athlete's rest days and advise them against engaging in any further leisure activities. It is important to clarify the extent to which the coach is permitted to intervene in the athlete's life beyond training.

The use of AI in sports also supports coaching strategies, as mentioned in the first two examples above. They have access to advanced analytics tools that enable them to accurately analyze athletes' performance, identify patterns, and formulate more effective strategies. Informed decision-making based on comprehensive data analysis and real-time monitoring of athletes during training and competitions further enhances coaches' capabilities.

Despite these benefits, coaches also face challenges. To avoid misinterpretation of data, it is important for individuals to become familiar with the technology (Düking et al., 2020). Technical malfunctions and failures of AI systems can disrupt training sessions or competitions, which can negatively impact performance. Financial constraints can also be a hurdle, as access to cutting-edge technology can be a major burden for some teams or coaches, resulting in differences in technological support at different levels of competition. In addition, the collection and analysis of player data requires ethical guidelines to address privacy concerns and protect athlete confidentiality.

3.4 Conclusion

The use of AI in endurance sports has become more prevalent, especially in high-performance sports. The topic of AI in sports needs to be considered in a differentiated way. AI is used differently depending on whether the sport is competitive or amateur.

In high-performance sports, the proficiency of AI lies in its precise analysis of data, provision of personalized recommendations, and the simulation of realistic training scenarios. This unique skill set enables athletes and coaches to optimize their training routines, thereby enhancing overall performance.

While AI offers invaluable insights, it is essential to emphasize that it should not entirely replace human judgment. Athletes and coaches must uphold their critical thinking abilities and retain responsibility for decision-making, utilizing AI as a supportive tool. For example, the RaceFit tool (Sect. 2.2) can only provide a good estimate if the team size is more than five people. There is 80% agreement with the trainer's strategy.

The effective integration of AI into sports science may necessitate expertise, substantial financial investment, specialized infrastructure, and individuals capable of accurately interpreting results, as pointed out by Hammes et al. (2022). This could potentially create a significant advantage for athletes and teams with greater resources. In the realm of amateur sports, there is an anticipation that AI will operate autonomously, assuming the role of the coach itself.

In addition, the incorporation of AI into sports training methods introduces new and innovative approaches, as highlighted by Wei et al. (2021). For example, AI fitness applications use wearable data to evaluate an athlete's current physical state. By combining this information with the athlete's objectives, AI carefully analyses individual performance data to create tailored training programs. This personalized approach is valuable in helping athletes improve specific aspects of their performance. As Zago et al. (2021, p. 3) aptly put it: "To date, artificial intelligence does not simply provide new tools to study human motion. Rather the way we study human motion is evolving thanks to artificial intelligence." AI in sports enables coaches to make better strategic decisions based on data from many different athletes. Athletes are also provided with solutions through the continuous improvement of data collection, enabling individuals to improve their performance in relation to a goal.

References

Ariyaratne, M. K. A., & Silva, R. M. (2022). Meta-heuristics meet sports: A systematic review from the viewpoint of nature inspired algorithms. *International Journal of Computer Science in Sport, 21*(1), 49–92.

Avici, P., & Bayrakdar, A. (2023). *Revolutionizing sport—How technology is changing the sports industry? The use of developing technology in sports*, 1.

Bartlett, R. (2006). Artificial intelligence in sports biomechanics: New dawn or false hope? *Journal of Sports Science & Medicine, 5*(4), 474.

Blej, M., & Azizi, M. (2016). Comparison of Mamdani-type and Sugenotype fuzzy inference systems for fuzzy real-time scheduling. *International Journal of Applied Engineering Research, 11*(22), 11071–11075.

Bonaccorso, G. (2017). *Machine learning algorithms*. Packt Publishing Ltd.

Cao, Z., Simon, T., Wei, S. E., & Sheikh, Y. (2017). *Real-time multi-person 2D pose estimation using part affinity fields*. Proceedings of the IEEE Conference on Computer Vision and Pattern Recognition, pp. 7291–7299

Chmait, N., & Westerbeek, H. (2021). Artificial intelligence and machine learning in sport research: An introduction for non-data scientists. *Frontiers in Sports and Active Living, 3*, 63.

Clark, J., & Perrault, R. (2022). *Artificial intelligence index report 2022*. Stanford Institute for Human-Centered AI.

Dewan, M. W., Huggett, D. J., Liao, T. W., Wahab, M. A., & Okeil, A. M. (2016). Prediction of tensile strength of friction stir weld joints with adaptive neuro-fuzzy inference system (ANFIS) and neural network. *Materials & Design, 92*, 288–299.

Dindorf, C., Bartaguiz, E., Gassmann, F., & Fröhlich, M. (2022). Conceptual structure and current trends in artificial intelligence, machine learning, and deep learning research in sports: A bibliometric review. *International Journal of Environmental Research and Public Health, 20*(1), 173.

Düking, P., Fröhlich, M., & Sperlich, B. (2023). Technologische Innovation in der Trainingswissenschaft: Digitalgestützte Trainingssteuerung mittels tragbarer Sensorik. In *Bewegung, Training, Leistung und Gesundheit: Handbuch Sport und Sportwissenschaft* (pp. 991–998). Springer Berlin Heidelberg.

Fister, I., & Fister Jr, I. (2019). Generating training plans based on existing sports activities. *Computational Intelligence in Sports*, 139–180.

Hammes, F., Hagg, A., Asteroth, A., & Link, D. (2022). Artificial intelligence in elite sports—A narrative review of success stories and challenges. *Frontiers in Sports and Active Living, 4*, 861466.

Henriksen, A., Haugen Mikalsen, M., Woldaregay, A. Z., Muzny, M., Hartvigsen, G., Hopstock, L. A., & Grimsgaard, S. (2018). Using fitness trackers and smartwatches to measure physical activity in research: Analysis of consumer wrist-worn wearables. *Journal of Medical Internet Research, 20*(3), e110.

Horvat, T., Havas, L., Srpak, D., & Medved, V. (2019, September). Data-driven basketball web application for support in making decisions. In *icSPORTS* (pp. 239–244).

Kahneman, D. (2011). *Thinking, fast and slow*. Macmillan

Kaplan, A., & Haenlein, M. (2019). Siri, Siri, in my hand: Who's the fairest in the land? On the interpretations, illustrations, and implications of artificial intelligence. *Business Horizons, 62*(1), 15–25.

Langdon, W. B., & Harman, M. (2014). Optimizing existing software with genetic programming. *IEEE Transactions on Evolutionary Computation, 19*(1), 118–135.

Lewis, M. (2004). *Moneyball: The art of winning an unfair game*. W.W. Norton & Company.

Li, B., & Xu, X. (2021). Application of artificial intelligence in basketball sport. *Journal of Education, Health and Sport, 11*(7), 54–67.

Littman, M. L., Ajunwa, I., Berger, G., Boutilier, C., Currie, M., Doshi-Velez, F., Hadfield, G., Horowitz, M. C., Isbell, C., Kitano, H., Levy, K., Lyons, T., Mitchell, M., Shah, J., Sloman, S.,

Vallor, S., & Walsh, T. (2021). *Gathering strength, gathering storms: The one hundred year study on artificial intelligence (AI100) 2021 study panel report*. Stanford, CA: Stanford University. https://arxiv.org/pdf/2210.15767
Mignot, J. F. (2016). The history of professional road cycling. In *The economics of professional road cycling* (pp. 7–31). Springer.
Rajšp, A., & Fister, I. (2020). A systematic literature review of intelligent data analysis methods for smart sport training. *Applied Sciences, 10*(9).
Rossi, A., Pappalardo, L., Cintia, P., Iaia, F. M., Fernández, J., & Medina, D. (2018). Effective injury forecasting in soccer with GPS training data and machine learning. *PLoS ONE, 13*(7), e0201264.
Sagi, M., Saldanha, P., Shani, G., & Moskovitch, R. (2022). Modelling coach decisions in professional cycling teams. *Abgerufen von.* https://dtai.cs.kuleuven.be/events/MLSA22/papers/MLSA22_paper_9312.pdf
Sudin, S., Md Shakaff, A. Y., Zakaria, A., Salleh, A. F., Kamarudin, L. M., Azmi, N., & Ahmad Saad, F. S. (2018). Real-time track cycling performance prediction using ANFIS system. *International Journal of Performance Analysis in Sport, 18*(5), 806–822.
U.C. Internationale. (2022). UCI cycling regulations part I—General organisation of cycling as a sport. *Abgerufen von.* https://assets.ctfassets.net/761l7gh5x5an/wQympSG6EWlKq6o6HKw9E/d4f7039ce3bf3963b457ae35cf5449bd/1-GEN-20220301-E.pdf
Wei, S., Huang, P., Li, R., Liu, Z., & Zou, Y. (2021). Exploring the application of artificial intelligence in sports training: A case study approach. *Complexity, 2021*, 1–8.
Zadeh, A., Taylor, D., Bertsos, M., Tillman, T., Nosoudi, N., & Bruce, S. (2021). Predicting sports injuries with wearable technology and data analysis. *Information Systems Frontiers, 23*, 1023–1037.
Zago, M., Kleiner, A. F. R., & Federolf, P. A. (2021). Machine learning approaches to human movement analysis. *Frontiers in Bioengineering and Biotechnology, 8*, 638793.
Zhang, D., Mishra, S., Brynjolfsson, E., Etchemendy, J., Ganguli, D., Grosz, B., & Perrault, R. (2021). *The AI index 2021 annual report*. arXiv preprint arXiv:2103.06312
Zounemat-Kermani, M., & Teshnehlab, M. (2008). Using adaptive neuro-fuzzy inference system for hydrological time series prediction. *Applied Soft Computing, 8*(2), 928–936.

Part II
Artificial Intelligence in Medical and Health Aspects of Sports

Chapter 4
Sensors, Internet of Things and Artificial Intelligence for the Diagnosis and Prevention of Falls and Fall-Related Injuries in Older People—An Exercise-Related Perspective

Wolfgang Kemmler

Abstract Falls are the leading cause of injury, hospitalization, and accidental death in older people. Many studies provide considerable evidence that the majority of health-related aspects of fall risk can be positively affected by physical activity or, even better, dedicated exercise interventions. Artificial Intelligence (AI)-based fall technology is the most advanced fall prevention technology currently available. Sensor-based AI concepts with direct feedback options significantly increase the safety and effectiveness of conventional training concepts or e-exercise programs even in non- or only partially supervised training settings. Smart technologies also provide closer monitoring of performance development, an aspect important for the subsequent alignment of the exercise intervention. However, while the predictive ability of present technology to determine the individual risk of fall is satisfactory, current AI-based approaches do not address the identification of dedicated fall risk factors in a way that would allow a precise response through specific exercise intervention. Future research should focus on interpretable AI-based concepts that provide a deeper insight into the individual risk factor profile in order to generate comprehensive training interventions that address several risk factors in a parallel but prioritized manner.

Keywords Fall Prevention · Exercise · Older People · Sensors · Artificial Intelligence

---

W. Kemmler (✉)
Institution of Radiology, University Hospital Erlangen, Erlangen, Germany
e-mail: wolfgang.kemmler@fau.de

C. Dindorf et al. (eds.), *Artificial Intelligence in Sports, Movement, and Health*,
https://doi.org/10.1007/978-3-031-67256-9_4

4.1 Relevance of Falls and Fall-Related Injuries in Older People

The most important risk factor for fractures in the elderly is falls (Jarvinen et al., 2008). More than 95% of hip fractures are caused by falls (Parkkari et al., 1999). Falls are a common event in older people and have a significant public health impact. Numerous international cohort studies with prospective data collection showed that about one in three independently living people aged 65 years and older fall at least once a year (Lord et al., 2021). With increasing age and in other settings (emergency rooms, hospitals, care facilities) and/or with specific diseases/syndromes (e.g. dementia, Parkinson's, stroke), significantly higher fall rates are reported (Rubenstein, 2006). In Germany, around five to six million fall accidents occur every year in people over the age of 65 years (Rapp et al., 2014).

In parallel, falls are the leading cause of injury in older people and are associated with increased mortality (Gribbin et al., 2009; Sylliaas et al., 2009). Approximately 22–60% of those affected suffer physical injuries from falls, ranging from bruises, cuts, sprains, and abrasions to severe fractures or cranial injuries (Lord et al., 2021). Falls in people aged 65 years and older are, therefore, the most common cause of injury-related hospitalizations (Lord et al., 2021) and traumatic brain injuries (Harvey & Close, 2012).

The number of falls resulting in fractures is approx. 2–6% (Rubenstein & Josephson, 1992; Stubbs et al., 2014; Tinetti et al., 1988), about 1–2% of falls result in a fracture of the proximal femur (Stubbs et al., 2020) with its known severe consequences for morbidity and mortality. Of importance, with increasing age the number of fractures increases disproportionately to the frequency of falls (Evans, 1992; Kannus, 1999). According to Evans (1992), the incidence of fall-related hip fractures increases from 200:1 to 10:1 in people between the ages of 65 and 85 years. This tremendous increase in the incidence rate can only be partially attributed to decreases in bone strength. Much more biomechanically unfavorable falls with a high impact on bone must be taken into account (Komisar & Robinovitch, 2021; Sturnieks, 2021).

Falls with and without injury are determinants of loss of function in basic and instrumental activities of daily living (Kiel et al., 1991; Tinetti & Williams, 1997). Falls and repeated falls are important predictors of moving to residential care facilities (Donald & Bulpitt, 1999; Kiel et al., 1991; Tinetti & Williams, 1997).

In addition to physical injuries, the psychological consequences of falls or the anticipation of them are limiting for the individual. Up to 92% of people who have fallen (and more than 50% of older people who have not fallen!) develop a Fear of Falling (FoF) (Aoyagi, 1998; Scheffer et al., 2008). Of note, FoF is associated with poorer physical, mobility, and cognitive performance (Donoghue et al., 2013; Vellas et al., 1997). As a major consequence, activities are restricted, resulting in a downward spiral of inactivity, deconditioning, loss of confidence: all leading to a further increased risk of falls (Wijlhuizen et al., 2007). Physical, psychological, and social consequences of falls can significantly reduce the quality of life of older people (Schoene et al., 2019). Apart from the far-reaching individual consequences, the 4.3 million fragility fractures incur costs for the European health care systems of Euro 56 billion a year (Kanis et al., 2021).

4.2 Exercise Effects on Falls and Fall Related Fractures

Recent reviews of exercise interventions and falls in older adults (e.g. Sherrington et al., 2019; Wang et al., 2020; Zhao et al., 2019) have reported significant reductions of falls and fall-related injuries. The Cochrane Review by Sherrington et al. (2019) listed a relative fall risk reduction of 23% (95%-CI: 17–29%). Fall-related fractures were reduced by 27% (95%-CI: 5–44%) and fall-related medical treatment by 39% (95%-CI: 21–53%). Perhaps due to the limited statistical power, exercise effects on falls and fall-related injuries were less prominent in people with specific limitations and/or diseases. While structured exercise significantly reduces the rate of falls by 30 and 53% in people with cognitive impairments and Morbus Parkinson, respectively, no reduction of fall rate (RR: 1.01; 95%-CI: 0.90–1.14) was reported for stroke patients or after recent hospitalization however (RaR 1.16; 95%-CI: 0.88–1.52, 3 studies) (Li et al., 2021; Sherrington et al., 2017). Even more important for a more individualized exercise approach, the effectiveness of exercise on fall reduction differs with respect to the setting in which it is applied (i.e. specialized fall clinic vs. non-supervised home application). Without a doubt, adherence to the exercise program plays a crucial role in its effectiveness. Thus, the successful implementation of exercise programs for different settings should carefully consider how to achieve and maintain adequate adherence rates.

4.3 Determinants of Exercise Training in the Area of Falls and Fall-Related injuries—risk Factors for Falls

The occurrence of falls is multifactorial and the combined result of different factors. About 400 different factors have been identified as contributing to a fall in the elderly (Skelton & Dinan, 1999). These can be categorized into factors related to (a) behavior, (b) health, and (c) environment. There is considerable evidence that a large number of health-related aspects of fall risk could be positively affected by physical activity or exercise. Table 4.1 displays potentially modifiable risk factors categorized into risk factor domains (DVO, 2024).

As can be seen from Table 4.1, the large number and the complexity of fall risk factors indicate the need for comprehensive assessments, scarcely manageable with the present conventional tools comprising observations, simple tests, questionnaires, interviews and their manual acquisition and interpretation. Connected smart devices, apps, monitoring technologies, and wireless communication ideally supported by

Table 4.1 Risk factors for falls and fall-related injuries potentially modifiable by exercise programs (DVO, 2024; Lord et al., 2021)

Risk-factor domain	Risk-Factors
Postural stability and gait characteristics	• Reduced simple and choice reaction time • Inadequate reactive stepping performance • Impaired stability while standing • Impaired stability while leaning or reaching • Impaired sit-to-stand transfer • Reduced gait velocity • Changes in gait pattern (e.g. reduced step length, cadence) • Increased gait variability (cadence/step length) • Impaired voluntary/choice stepping performance • Arrhythmic head, trunk and pelvis acceleration during gait • Reduced hip extension, increased knee/hip flexion during gait
Center of mass shifts (ventral)	• Hyperkyphosis • Vertebral fractures • Assistive device
Sensoric function	• Impaired vision and eye disease (e.g. glaucoma, macular degeneration) • Impaired vestibular function (e.g. vestibulospinal reflexes) • Impaired peripheral sensation • Impaired proprioception
Neuromotor function	• Reduced maximum strength • Reduced maximum power • Reduced strength endurance • Reduced aerobic endurance • Reduced simple reaction time • Reduced choice reaction time
Cognitive function	• Enhanced executive dysfunction • Reduced information processing speed (IPS)
Psychologic aspects	• Increased concern about falls (e.g. fear of falling) • Depressive symptoms
Cardiovascular/cardiometabolic function	• Syncope, dizziness, heart rate, blood pressure fluctuations • Reduced fatigue resistance, rapid fatigability • Fall-relevant medication/polypharmacy (e.g. antihypertensiva)

Artificial Intelligence (AI) methods might be a reliable solution not only for the detection of falls but also for the identification of individual risk factors that can be addressed by individualized smart technology and AI-assisted exercise programs in different settings. However, before looking at these issues of individual risk factor assessment, the area of fall detection by new technologies will be briefly addressed as a blueprint for the growing relevance and increased evidence for the use of smart technology, Internet of Things (IoT), and AI in the area of falls in older people.

4.4 Detecting Falls by Smart Technology and Artificial Intelligence

Fall Detection Systems (FDS) might be the currently most addressed and advanced technologies in the area of fall research related to wireless technology, smart technology, and AI techniques (Gharghan & Hashim, 2024). The high relevance of FDS is based on the finding that 50–80% of fallers are unable to get up independently after a fall (Fleming & Brayne, 2008; Tinetti et al., 1993). Where no external help is to hand, longer prone times are associated with serious consequences, e.g. dehydration, injuries, admission to hospital, subsequent moves into long term care, or even death (Fleming & Brayne, 2008; Tinetti et al., 1993). Of importance, about 80% of fallers cannot or do not activate personal response alarms to summon help (Fleming & Brayne, 2008). FDS components include sensor modules, methods of data acquisition, data procession and feature extraction (i.e., reduction of information to a few core information/outcomes), falls detection per se, and alarm systems to get help from family members, caregivers, or emergency services. Nevertheless, there is no standard solution for fall detection yet (Vasoya et al., 2023), but a large variety of wearable single or multiple sensors (e.g., accelerometer, gyroscope, pressure, contact, heart rate, GPS/location, camera) or ambient sensors (e.g., kinetic/depth camera, pressure, microphones, ultrasonic, infrared, radar) (Gharghan & Hashim, 2024). The implementation of AI-based Machine (ML) or Deep Learning (DL) techniques is particularly important in the step of data procession and feature extraction. In the past few years, several studies have confirmed the high performance of different ML and particularly DL techniques (review in (Gharghan & Hashim, 2024)) for detecting falls in older people. In detail, AI-powered FDS have demonstrated sensitivity of up to 98% and a specificity of up to 99%, indicating their accuracy in identifying falls (Alharbi et al., 2023). While the high accuracy, specificity, sensitivity, and precision of AI technology metrics for the detection of a fall is undisputed, few systems have been tested under real-world conditions. Nevertheless, and although FDS focuses on a dichotomous outcome (i.e., “fall or not”), many features of sensor technology, IoT, and AI might be transferable to the more challenging identification of individual risk factors that can be addressed by exercise programs.

4.5 Identification and Consideration of Risk Factors for Falls and Fall-Related Injuries Potentially Modifiable by Exercise Programs

4.5.1 Sensor Technology

A large variety of simple and low-tech tools and tests are available for assessing fall risk factors related to health and physical fitness (Scott et al., 2007). Unfortunately, these tests are frequently not applied in clinical practice or during ongoing exercise interventions due to a lack of time, limited personnel resources, or lack of accuracy under (field-) test conditions. A good example of the latter aspect might be the habitual gait speed test in older people with a high variation of voluntary gait velocity. Using smart technologies not only offers the advantage of saving time and human resources and thus providing much denser monitoring of fall risk factors but also allows much more discrete data sampling, in some cases largely independent of participant voluntary compliance. Wearables enable the capturing of data during the user's daily activities, such as gait characteristics, without being exposed to sampling problems.

Reviewing the literature, several novel sensing technologies have been used to assess fall risk in older adults (Sun & Sosnoff, 2018). The sensor techniques used for fall detection can be classified into wearable and ambient or environmental sensors. Environmental sensor technologies are based predominately on video/depth cameras, pressure sensors, and motion sensors. More flexible and less elaborate wearable sensor-based technologies for fall risk assessment in older adults, which include inertial sensors, smartphone, video/sensitive depth camera, pressure sensors, can efficiently capture and analyze movement data and provide an easy-to-implement objective fall risk assessment (Sun & Sosnoff, 2018). Briefly introducing the tools, inertial sensors as the predominately used sensor type in fall risk assessment so far (Sun & Sosnoff, 2018), rely on accelerometers and gyroscopes and focus predominately on gait characteristics. Pressure-sensing platforms (e.g. Wii board) enable the sampling of postural stability and step/gait characteristics. Video/depth cameras provide fast and marker-less 3D motion tracking. Motion-ambient sensing, using infrared/passive infrared, ultrasound, laser, or radar, for example, usually tracks movement characteristics of different body segments to quantify the movement pattern. Mobile/smart phones with inertial sensors and sensitive depth cameras predominately focus on gait and postural stability characteristics at the moment, although other biometrical parameters (Table 4.1) can also be addressed to determine power, endurance, fatigue resistance using technologies already integrated into conventional smart phones. Wearable and ambient/environmental sensors connected in IoT systems are applied in the smart home approach that focuses on comprehensive behavior-based analysis of daily living activities and human activity recognition in frail older people.

4.5.2 *Sensors Used in Functional Tests of Falls Risk*

Sensors are increasingly being used to improve the validity and reliability of established functional tests and to derive new parameters for the discrimination of fall risk factors. As an example, a recent study (Abdollahi et al., 2024) of fall risk assessment in stroke survivors determined the prediction accuracy of four common functional tests with and without dual tasking supported by a machine learning model that used motion data from inertial sensors. In detail, the 30s balance test with eyes open/closed, Timed Up and Go (TUG), 10 m habitual gait speed, and the Sit-To-Stand test (STS) were applied with and without cognitive load (count-down from 200), while eight motion sensors with integrated 3D accelerometers, 3D gyroscopes and 3D magnetometers extracted a total of 92 spatiotemporal parameters. Data was transmitted wirelessly to customized MATLAB software for data processing and feature extraction. Applying three machine learning techniques (i.e. Support Vector Machine, Logistic Regression, Random Forest (RF)) known to demonstrate high performance during motion testing (Halilaj et al., 2018), the study revealed the highest prediction accuracy (91%) for fall discrimination when applying the RF model for data sampled during dual task balance and TUG. Further, a single motion sensor placed on the thorax shows similar high precision during the TUG and STS compared with the multiple sensor approach. Lin et al. (Lin & Wai, 2021) used the TUG test and handgrip strength i.e. current sarcopenia criteria according to the Asian Working Group of Sarcopenia (AWGS) (Chen et al., 2014), to determine fall risk in community-dwelling older adults. Gesture detection of gait and balance was conducted via AI using wearable sensors, doppler technology, 2D/3D cameras, and floor sensors. Adaptive modification of the interventional program over 3 months resulted in significant increases in gait speed (31%).

4.6 Artificial Intelligence-Based Approaches to Determining Fall Risk

Several AI-based approaches to fall prevention and prediction of fall risk in older people have been conducted during the last few years (Mohan et al., 2024). Although AI and ML techniques were also applied to determine the risk of falling, e.g. based on emotional risk factors, i.e. depression, coping strategies, anxiety, and FoF (Mohan et al., 2024), most fall prevention/prediction approaches focus on posture or gait characteristics. Indeed, due to their complexity, human posture and gait research, in particular, is subjected to AI or, more precisely, machine or deep learning techniques (Mohan et al., 2024). Liang et al. (2024), who aimed to classify fall risk in older people using an ML and Explainable AI (XAI) approach, relied on tracker-based posturographic/body sway parameters under different stance conditions. However, while the model shows high agreement with the TUG test, the discriminating ability to separate people with vs. without a previous fall history was unsatisfying. Based on this result that implies that the stance condition reflects mobility balance better than the much more complex falls with their numerous intrinsic and extrinsic risk factors, the authors (Liang et al., 2024) concluded that more comprehensive information on individual fall risk should be added to increase the accuracy of the AI-based fall risk assessment. In this context, the LINDERA mobility analysis applied an AI-based algorithm (Stamm & Heimann-Steinert, 2020) based on video analysis of individuals' gait but also a standardized questionnaire to determine fall risk on a score from 0 to 100 points. Using data from 242 senior citizens, on average 85 years old, Rabe et al. (2020) reported a high discriminative ability to distinguish fallers from non-fallers, irrespective of the learning model (e.g., Gaussian Naive Bayes Mode, Support Vector Classification or RF Model) used. Another study (Strutz et al., 2022), which compared the LINDERA concept with reference standard tests (i.e. TUG, Berg Balanced Scale, Tinetti Test) in older people, reported moderate-high correlations r = 0.46–0.59 with narrow limits of agreement. In contrast to other fall risk apps (e.g. FallSA (Singh et al., 2021), Apple iOS 15), LINDERA is deemed a medical device, thus facilitating its application in healthcare settings.

In summary, AI-based fall technology is the most advanced fall prevention technology currently available. But although the predictive ability of present technology to determine the individual risk of fall is satisfactory, it currently fails to identify dedicated risk factors related to postural stability listed in Table 4.1. This is important, however, for defining specific training aims realized by dedicated exercise programs. Nonetheless, the application of time-effective, inexpensive, and resource saving AI-based technology enables a dense monitoring of changes in fall risk and thus allows verification of the effects of exercise programs on individual fall risk by healthcare or exercise professionals or users themselves.

4.7 Effectiveness of e-interventions on Falls and Fall-Risk Factors

Many e-interventions for fall prevention include IoT technology with ambient sensors, mobile phones, tablets, or computers. These e-interventions can be roughly classified into six categories: telehealth, exergames (i.e., gamified exercise), cognitive training, (non-conventional) balance training, smart home systems, and socialized exercise. Highly relevant for the present topic, exergames typically use motion sensing technology and simultaneously address physical and cognitive aspects of balance. Due to the complex interaction of executive, attentional, and motor aspects of balance along with increased adherence thanks to its entertainment and engaging character, exergaming is regarded as offering a high fall-reducing potential (van het Reve & de Bruin, 2014). Exergames combined with telehealth are a frequent constellation in fall prevention settings. A recent systematic review and meta-analysis (Leal et al., 2023) reported significant effects on fall risk in older people (community dwelling or nursing home residents) compared with controls without intervention or even with conventional exercise training. Cognitive training, predominately applied under physically inactive conditions, focuses on executive function (Smith-Ray et al., 2014) and is frequently combined with conventional exercise. There is some evidence for a fall-reducing effect of cognitive training (Blackwood et al., 2016). Moreover it can be provided safely and with minimal supervision at home. However, while cognitive training alone did not affect falls or fall-related functional parameters (Smith-Ray et al., 2015), combined exercise and cognitive training does improve specific factors associated with falls, such as gait speed, cognitive function, and balance—at least in people with mild cognitive impairments (Lipardo et al., 2017). Socialized training includes exercise programs applied in virtual gyms specifically tailored to the needs and abilities of the participants, such as tablet-based balance, strength, or power training with motivational aspects and feedback systems. Participants exercised online in groups or were able to link to other people presently exercising. Amongst others, Harrison et al. (2024) provided evidence for the favorable effect of virtual classes (ballet or wellness) on fall-related risk factors (e.g. gait, balance, quality of life) in older women. Zhao et al. (2023), who addressed the effects of a 12-month Virtual Reality (VR) training 3×50 min/week on fall prevention and Bone Mineral Density (BMD) in hospitalized older people, reported significant effects on balance, TUG performance, functional gait assessment and, of note, BMD at the lumbar spine and femoral neck compared with a control group which conducted a 3×50 min/week low-intensity resistance type exercise. A recent scoping review on VR in effect concluded that VR, be it immersive and non-immersive, "is a valuable tool for promoting physical exercise in older adults, helping to prevent recurrent accidental falls" (Ortiz-Mallasén et al., 2024). Finally, non-conventional balance training using inertial sensors focuses on balance control by providing feedback to correct posture. However, the effects of non-conventional balance training were rarely addressed by randomized controlled trials (Chan et al., 2021). Hagedorn and Holm (2010), who compared the effects of a 12-week multi-purpose exercise-training with traditional balance training versus computer feedback balance training, failed to determine significantly superior effects of the computer feedback setting on fall-related outcomes in frail elderly people. Although the effects ranged at a similarly positive level, computer feedback balance training does offer new perspectives for a non-supervised home training program that can be carried out widely independently.

In summary, there is considerable evidence for the favorable effects of e-interventions on falls and fall-related abilities roughly in the range of conventional supervised exercise. But, unlike the latter intervention, e-interventions can be easily performed as home-training. Considering the aspect that many older people are unable or unwilling to (permanently) participate in supervised facility-based programs (Cohen-Mansfield et al., 2003; Franco et al., 2015), home-based e-interventions, supervised or not, might be a feasible training option for these people. Additionally, the zero charges or at least lower expenses for instructors, personnel, and locations, as well as potential lockdowns and/or isolation of particularly older people under epidemic conditions, underscore the increasing relevance of home-based exercise programs not only but particularly in a fall prevention concept for older people.

4.8 Advanced Application of Artificial Intelligence in Exercise Training for Fall Prevention

4.8.1 Prediction of Fall Risk and Categorization of Training Aims

An accurate assessment of an individual's fall risk is crucial for risk categorization and subsequent allocation to dedicated training courses. As an example, the present S3 guideline on "exercise and fracture prevention" suggests a risk factor categorization that includes bone strength and fall risk as the starting point for the individualized assignment of primary and secondary training objectives (Mohebbi et al., 2023). The focus of training intervention is now shifting from a "bone (strength)-oriented exercise strategy to fall prevention in people with a higher tendency to fall. Nevertheless, the present guideline remains unclear as to when a dedicated fall prevention program should be implemented in the intervention (Mohebbi et al., 2023). Considering the predictive ability of current technology to determine the individual risk of falls, more individualized exercise training—at least with respect to the prioritized training aim—should be possible. The aforementioned LINDERA "app", for example, which ranks the fall risk on a score from 0 to 100 points, might be helpful in the allocation of people to dedicated core training aims. Since the LINDERA app is a medical device increasingly used by health professionals, including general and specialized practitioners, the allocation of patients with increased fall risk to dedicated exercise programs will be supported by the German healthcare system (i.e. "Rehabilitionssport" or "Funktionstraining" according to §64 SGB IX) (Beck & Sahar, 2020).

4.8.2 Identification of Fall Risk Factors and Specific Accentuation of the Training Contents

Adding non-exercise specific modifiable risk factors (e.g. home environment, footwear) to the number of modifiable fall risk factors that can be addressed by physical exercise training (Table 4.1) will result in an almost unmanageable number of fall risk factors. In this context, sensors, IoT, and AI applied in a closely monitored, e.g. smart home, setting can be helpful for identifying and reducing general fall-risk factors (Mohan et al., 2024). However, the currently available sensor-based AI solutions for fall prevention do not provide the information that allows the dedicated risk factors listed in Table 4.1 to be specifically addressed by suitable exercise interventions. In fact, most AI-based approaches focus on a single or a few categories or risk factor domains, predominately posture or gait characteristics, to determine or categorize the fall risk as such. However, no information on the relevance of the inherent specific risk factor (e.g. reduced choice reaction time, reduced gait velocity) has been provided yet. Given that the training-specific targeting of these risk factors varies widely, a more detailed, interpretable result would be helpful for designing a more tailored exercise training package. In parallel, as already mentioned, most AI-based approaches focus on posture and gait characteristics and include information on general risk factors at best. In this context, a more comprehensive inclusion of other risk factor domains significantly modifiable by exercise programs will be helpful for the stratification of the training contents. Apart from the highly modifiable and validly quantifiable neuromotor risk factor domain, other domains involving sensoric, cognitive, psychologic, and cardiovascular/cardiometabolic risk factors should be included in the analysis in order to generate a comprehensive training schedule covering several risk factors in parallel, albeit in a prioritized manner. Particularly, the cardiovascular/cardiometabolic risk factor categorization is easily accessible by wearable sensors and/or smartphone solutions and is frequently addressed by AI solutions (Maurya et al., 2021). On the other hand, data showing the relative relevance of anxiety or FoF, for example, will be helpful for specifying the setting and type of the exercise program (Schoene et al., 2023). Thus, an AI-based risk factor stratification that provides an interpretable hierarchy of the most relevant individual fall-risk factors will be beneficial for determining training contents and methods more stringently and time efficiently.

4.8.3 Implementation in the Training Process

A key decision in training programs is the setting of the exercise program, i.e., in general, "facility-based" or "home-based". In the past, several studies have underscored the superiority of the usually supervised facility-based programs versus non-supervised home exercise programs (Fisher et al., 2021; Hoffmann et al., 2022). Applying the Otago Exercise Program, Kyrdalen et al. (2014) reported significantly higher effects on fall-related outcomes after supervised group training compared to the usual home training setting of Otago. Several aspects might contribute to this result however, the most striking limitation of non-supervised exercise in an at-home program might be the frequent lack of progression, particularly with respect to exercise intensity (Fisher et al., 2021). But now, the large and increasing variety of e-(exercise) programs with feedback systems or simple remote and online settings ensure adequate supervision of home exercise training. Moreover, feedback systems that enable accurate monitoring of the user's performance development and hence guide implementation intensity progression will also increase the effectiveness and safety of home exercise programs. This enhanced safety of home training programs, at least with respect to fall risk, proper movement, and cardiovascular/cardiometabolic side effects offered by connected wearable sensors, might serve to boost acceptance of the resource-saving and popular home training setting in the community. In terms of exercise intensity, wearable sensors provide guidance on adequate intensity in the area of cardiovascular fitness. In parallel, the "repetition in reserve" concept (Zourdos et al., 2016) combined with advanced movement sensors can be applied to prescribe and monitor exercise intensity in the area of strength and power-training, e.g. via velocity based resistance exercise (Lopez et al., 2023). Another issue closely related to the effectiveness of the training protocol is low adherence to the pre-specified exercise frequency. Alarm systems included in sensors that record physical activity and exercise are feasible responses to this problem.

Looking ahead and considering the rapid progress in this field, future sensor based AI-technology on fall prevention might soon be able to (1) identify and stratify the most relevant risk factors for falls, (2) generate optimized training strategies and detailed exercise programs for individual users, (3) apply dedicated e-programs with monitoring of individual training sessions for effectiveness and safety, (4) provide a progression of intensity once predefined thresholds are reached so as to ensure consistent overload, (5) properly apply advanced training principles (e.g. reversibility, variation, periodization) during the intervention (Donath & Faude, 2020), (6) deliver detailed information on exercise-induced changes of fall risk and lastly (7) adapt training programs to respond to lacking efficiency on relevant risk factors. Nevertheless, progress in the effectiveness and safety of home training programs will not necessarily replace supervised facility-based programs. Thanks to the training equipment they offer, facility-based training programs can address many training aims much more reliably, safely, and effectively compared with the tools available at home. This goes not only for resistance devices with their safe positioning, quantifiable intensity or load selection, and easy to handle intensity progression but in particular also for the scarcely available and highly effective (Devasahayam et al., 2023) perturbation-based balance devices (e.g. perturbating treadmills) "which apply repeated, externally applied mechanical perturbations to trigger rapid reactions to regain postural stability in a safe and controlled environment" (McCrum et al., 2022). On the other hand, sensor-based direct feedback systems, along with the AI-based algorithms installed in new generation training devices, will enable the addressing of prespecified training aims with enhanced safety and effectiveness and, at the same time, reduce the personnel demands of the intervention.

4.9 Conclusion

By way of conclusion, AI-based technology for fall prevention might play an increasingly crucial role in healthcare concepts for the elderly, which, due to the increasingly scarce personal resources, could specifically include exercise interventions.

References

Abdollahi, M., Kuber, P. M., & Rashedi, E. (2024). Dual tasking affects the outcomes of instrumented timed up and go, sit-to-stand, balance, and 10-meter walk tests in stroke survivors. *Sensors, 24*(10). https://doi.org/10.3390/s24102996

Alharbi, H. A., Alharbi, K. K., & Hassan, C. A. U. (2023). Enhancing elderly fall detection through IoT-enabled smart flooring and AI for independent living sustainability. *Sustainability, 15*(22), 15695.

Aoyagi, K. (1998). Falls among community dwelling elderly in Japan. *Journal of Bone and Mineral Research, 14*, 1468–1474.

Beck, L., & Sahar, J. (2020). Rehabilitationssport und Funktionstraining als Vehikel für ein körperliches Training für Osteoporose-Betroffene – Grundlagen. *Perspektiven und Limitationen. Osteologie, 29*(3), 227–230.

Blackwood, J., Shubert, T., Fogarty, K., & Chase, C. (2016). The impact of a home-based computerized cognitive training intervention on fall risk measure performance in community dwelling older adults, a pilot study. *The Journal of Nutrition, Health & Aging, 20*(2), 138–145. https://doi.org/10.1007/s12603-015-0598-5

Chan, J. K. Y., Klainin-Yobas, P., Chi, Y., Gan, J. K. E., Chow, G., & Wu, X. V. (2021). The effectiveness of e-interventions on fall, neuromuscular functions and quality of life in community-dwelling older adults: A systematic review and meta-analysis. *International Journal of Nursing Studies, 113*, 103784. https://doi.org/10.1016/j.ijnurstu.2020.103784

Chen, L. K., Liu, L. K., Woo, J., Assantachai, P., Auyeung, T. W., Bahyah, K. S., Chou, M. Y., Chen, L. Y., Hsu, P. S., Krairit, O., Lee, J. S., Lee, W. J., Lee, Y., Liang, C. K., Limpawattana, P., Lin, C. S., Peng, L. N., Satake, S., Suzuki, T., & . . . Arai, H. (2014). Sarcopenia in Asia: Consensus report of the Asian Working Group for Sarcopenia. *Journal of the American Medical Directors Association, 15*(2), 95–101. https://doi.org/10.1016/j.jamda.2013.11.025

Cohen-Mansfield, J., Marx, M. S., & Guralnik, J. M. (2003). Motivators and barriers to exercise in an older community-dwelling population. *Journal of Aging and Physical Activity, 11*(2), 242–253.

Devasahayam, A. J., Farwell, K., Lim, B., Morton, A., Fleming, N., Jagroop, D., Aryan, R., Saumur, T. M., & Mansfield, A. (2023). The effect of reactive balance training on falls in daily life: an updated systematic review and meta-analysis. *medRxiv*, 2022.2001. 2027.22269969.

Donald, I. P., & Bulpitt, C. J. (1999). The prognosis of falls in elderly people living at home. *Age and Ageing, 28*(2), 121–125. https://doi.org/10.1093/ageing/28.2.121

Donath, L., & Faude, O. (2020). (Evidenzbasierte) Trainingsprinzipien. In A. Güllich & M. Krüger (Eds.), *Handbuch Sport und Sportwissenschaft*. Springer.

Donoghue, O. A., Cronin, H., Savva, G. M., O'Regan, C., & Kenny, R. A. (2013). Effects of fear of falling and activity restriction on normal and dual task walking in community dwelling older adults. *Gait & Posture, 38*(1), 120–124. https://doi.org/10.1016/j.gaitpost.2012.10.023

DVO. (2024). *Körperliches Training zur Frakturprophylaxe* [*Physical exercise for fracture prevention*].

Evans, W. J. (1992). After a fall: consequences and implications of falls by old people. In B. Vellas, M. Toupet, L. Z. Rubenstein, J. L. Albarede, & J. Christen (Eds.), *Falls, balance, and gait disorders in the elderly*. Elsevier.

Fisher, J., Steele, J., Wolf, M., Androulakis-Korakakis, P., Smith, D., Giessing, J., & Wescott, W. L. (2021). The role of supervision in resistance training; An exploratory systematic review and meta-analysis. *Sportrxiv*. https://doi.org/10.51224/SRXIV.18

Fleming, J., & Brayne, C. (2008). Inability to get up after falling, subsequent time on floor, and summoning help: Prospective cohort study in people over 90. *BMJ, 337*, a2227. https://doi.org/10.1136/bmj.a2227

Franco, M., Howard, K., Sherrington, C., Ferreira, P., Rose, J., Gomes, J., & Ferreira, M. (2015). Eliciting older people's preferences for exercise programs: A best-worst scaling choice. *Journal of Physiotherapy, 61*, 34–41.

Gharghan, S. K., & Hashim, H. A. (2024). A comprehensive review of elderly fall detection using wireless communication and artificial intelligence techniques. *Measurement, 226*, 114186. https://doi.org/10.1016/j.measurement.2024.114186

Gribbin, J., Hubbard, R., Smith, C., Gladman, J., & Lewis, S. (2009). Incidence and mortality of falls amongst older people in primary care in the United Kingdom. *QJM, 102*(7), 477–483. https://doi.org/10.1093/qjmed/hcp064

Hagedorn, D. K., & Holm, E. (2010). Effects of traditional physical training and visual computer feedback training in frail elderly patients. A randomized intervention study. *Eur J Phys Rehabil Med, 46*(2), 159–168. https://www.ncbi.nlm.nih.gov/pubmed/20485221

Halilaj, E., Rajagopal, A., Fiterau, M., Hicks, J. L., Hastie, T. J., & Delp, S. L. (2018). Machine learning in human movement biomechanics: Best practices, common pitfalls, and new opportunities. *Journal of Biomechanics, 81*, 1–11. https://doi.org/10.1016/j.jbiomech.2018.09.009

Harrison, E. C., Haussler, A. M., Tueth, L. E., Baudendistel, S. T., & Earhart, G. M. (2024). Graceful gait: Virtual ballet classes improve mobility and reduce falls more than wellness classes for older women. *Frontiers in Aging Neuroscience, 16*, 1289368. https://doi.org/10.3389/fnagi.2024.1289368

Harvey, L. A., & Close, J. C. (2012). Traumatic brain injury in older adults: Characteristics, causes and consequences. *Injury, 43*(11), 1821–1826. https://doi.org/10.1016/j.injury.2012.07.188

Hoffmann, I., Shojaa, M., Kohl, M., von Stengel, S., Becker, C., Gosch, M., Jakob, F., Kerschan-Schindl, K., Kladny, B., Clausen, J., Lange, U., Middeldorf, S., Peters, S., Schoene, D., Sieber, C. C., Tholen, R., Thomasius, F. E., Bischoff-Ferrari, H., Uder, M., & Kemmler, W. (2022). Exercise reduces the number of overall and major osteoporotic fractures in adults. Does supervision make a difference? Systematic review and meta-analysis. *JBMR, 37*(11), 2132–2148. https://doi.org/10.1002/jbmr.4683

Jarvinen, T. L., Sievanen, H., Khan, K. M., Heinonen, A., & Kannus, P. (2008). Shifting the focus in fracture prevention from osteoporosis to falls. *BMJ, 336*(7636), 124–126. 336/7636/124 [pii]. https://doi.org/10.1136/bmj.39428.470752.AD

Kanis, J. A., Norton, N., Harvey, N. C., Jacobson, T., Johansson, H., Lorentzon, M., McCloskey, E. V., Willers, C., & Borgstrom, F. (2021). SCOPE 2021: A new scorecard for osteoporosis in Europe. *Archives of Osteoporosis, 16*(1), 82. https://doi.org/10.1007/s11657-020-00871-9

Kannus, P. (1999). Fall-induced injuries and death among older adults. *JAMA, 271*, 1895–1899.

Kiel, D. P., O'Sullivan, P., Teno, J. M., & Mor, V. (1991). Health care utilization and functional status in the aged following a fall. *Medical Care, 29*(3), 221–228. https://doi.org/10.1097/00005650-199103000-00004

Komisar, V., & Robinovitch, S. N. (2021). The role of fall biomechanics in the cause and prevention of bone fractures in older adults. *Current Osteoporosis Reports, 19*(4), 381–390. https://doi.org/10.1007/s11914-021-00685-9

Kyrdalen, I. L., Moen, K., Roysland, A. S., & Helbostad, J. L. (2014). The Otago exercise program performed as group training versus home training in fall-prone older people: A randomized controlled Trial. *Physiotherapy Research International, 19*(2), 108–116. https://doi.org/10.1002/pri.1571

Leal, J. C., Belo, V. S., Santos, I. M., Ferreira, R. V., de Melo, S. N., & da Silva, E. S. (2023). Exergames in older adult community centers and nursing homes to improve balance and minimize the risk of falls in older adults: a systematic review and meta-analysis. *Healthcare (Basel), 11*(13). https://doi.org/10.3390/healthcare11131872

Li, F., Harmer, P., Eckstrom, E., Ainsworth, B. E., Fitzgerald, K., Voit, J., Chou, L. S., Welker, F. L., & Needham, S. (2021). Efficacy of exercise-based interventions in preventing falls among community-dwelling older persons with cognitive impairment: Is there enough evidence? An updated systematic review and meta-analysis. *Age and Ageing, 50*(5), 1557–1568. https://doi.org/10.1093/ageing/afab110

Liang, H. W., Ameri, R., Band, S., Chen, H. S., Ho, S. Y., Zaidan, B., Chang, K. C., & Chang, A. (2024). Fall risk classification with posturographic parameters in community-dwelling older adults: A machine learning and explainable artificial intelligence approach. *Journal of Neuroengineering and Rehabilitation, 21*(1), 15. https://doi.org/10.1186/s12984-024-01310-3

Lin, K.-C., & Wai, R.-J. (2021). A feasible fall evaluation system via artificial intelligence gesture detection of gait and balance for sub-healthy community-dwelling older adults in Taiwan. *IEEE Access, 9*, 146404–146413.

Lipardo, D. S., Aseron, A. M. C., Kwan, M. M., & Tsang, W. W. (2017). Effect of exercise and cognitive training on falls and fall-related factors in older adults with mild cognitive impairment: a systematic review. *Archives of Physical Medicine and Rehabilitation, 98*(10), 2079–2096. https://doi.org/10.1016/j.apmr.2017.04.021

Lopez, P., Rech, A., Petropoulou, M., Newton, R. U., Taaffe, D. R., Galvao, D. A., Turella, D. J. P., Freitas, S. R., & Radaelli, R. (2023). Does high-velocity resistance exercise elicit greater physical function benefits than traditional resistance exercise in older adults? A systematic review and network meta-analysis of 79 trials. *Journals of Gerontology. Series A, Biological Sciences and Medical Sciences, 78*(8), 1471–1482. https://doi.org/10.1093/gerona/glac230

Lord, S. R., Sherrington, C., & Hicks, C. (2021). Epidemiology of falls and fall-related injuries. *Falls in Older People: Risk Factors, Strategies for Prevention and Implications for Practice, 3*, 3–22.

Maurya, M. R., Riyaz, N., Reddy, M. S. B., Yalcin, H. C., Ouakad, H. M., Bahadur, I., Al-Maadeed, S., & Sadasivuni, K. K. (2021). A review of smart sensors coupled with Internet of Things and Artificial Intelligence approach for heart failure monitoring. *Medical & Biological Engineering & Computing, 59*(11–12), 2185–2203. https://doi.org/10.1007/s11517-021-02447-2

McCrum, C., Bhatt, T. S., Gerards, M. H. G., Karamanidis, K., Rogers, M. W., Lord, S. R., & Okubo, Y. (2022). Perturbation-based balance training: Principles, mechanisms and implementation in clinical practice. *Front Sports Act Living, 4*, 1015394. https://doi.org/10.3389/fspor.2022.1015394

Mohan, D., Al-Hamid, D. Z., Chong, P. H. J., Sudheera, K. L. K., Gutierrez, J., Chan, H. C., & Li, H. (2024). Artificial intelligence and IoT in elderly fall prevention: A review. *IEEE Sensors Journal, 24*(4), 4181–4198.

Mohebbi, R., von Stengel, S., Kohl, M., Jakob, F., Kerschan-Schindl, K., Lange, U., Peters, S., Schöne, D., Thomasius, F., & Becker, C. (2023). Trainingsziele und Risikokategorisierung im Spannungsfeld körperliches Training und Frakturprophylaxe: Ansatzpunkte für individualisierte Trainingsprogramme. *Osteologie, 32*(3), 166–170. https://doi.org/10.1055/a-2075-7106

Ortiz-Mallasén, V., Claramonte-Gual, E., González-Chordá, V. M., Llagostera-Reverter, I., Valero-Chillerón, M. J., & Cervera-Gasch, Á. (2024). Can virtual reality help improve motor and cognitive function in active aging in older adults? A scoping review. *Healthcare, 12*(3), 356. https://doi.org/10.3390/healthcare12030356

Parkkari, J., Kannus, P., Palvanen, M., Natri, A., Vainio, J., Aho, H., Vuori, I., & Jarvinen, M. (1999). Majority of hip fractures occur as a result of a fall and impact on the greater trochanter of the femur: a prospective controlled hip fracture study with 206 consecutive patients. *Calcified Tissue International, 65*(3), 183–187. http://www.ncbi.nlm.nih.gov/entrez/query.fcgi?cmd=Retrieve&db=PubMed&dopt=Citation&list_uids=10441647

Rabe, S., Azhand, A., Pommer, W., Muller, S., & Steinert, A. (2020). Descriptive evaluation and accuracy of a mobile app to assess fall risk in seniors: Retrospective case-control study. *JMIR Aging, 3*(1), e16131. https://doi.org/10.2196/16131

Rapp, K., Freiberger, E., Todd, C., Klenk, J., Becker, C., Denkinger, M., Scheidt-Nave, C., & Fuchs, J. (2014). Fall incidence in Germany: Results of two population-based studies, and comparison of retrospective and prospective falls data collection methods. *BMC Geriatrics, 14*, 105. https://doi.org/10.1186/1471-2318-14-105

Rubenstein, L. Z. (2006). Falls in older people: Epidemiology, risk factors and strategies for prevention. *Age Ageing, 35*(Suppl. 2), ii37–ii41. https://doi.org/10.1093/ageing/afl084

Rubenstein, L. Z., & Josephson, K. R. (1992). Causes and prevention of falls in elderly people. In B. Vellas, M. Toupet, L. Z. Rubenstein, J. L. Albarede, & J. Christen (Eds.), *Falls, ballance and gait disorders in the elderly* (pp. 21–38). Elsevier.

Scheffer, A. C., Schuurmans, M. J., van Dijk, N., van der Hooft, T., & de Rooij, S. E. (2008). Fear of falling: Measurement strategy, prevalence, risk factors and consequences among older persons. *Age and Ageing, 37*(1), 19–24. https://doi.org/10.1093/ageing/afm169

Schoene, D., Gross, M., von Stengel, S., Kohl, M., Kladny, B., Gosch, M., Sieber, C. C., Peters, S., Kiesswetter, E., & Becker, C. (2023). Empfehlungen für ein körperliches Training zur Sturzprävention bei älteren, selbständig lebenden Menschen. *Osteologie, 32*(03), 183–195.

Schoene, D., Heller, C., Aung, Y. N., Sieber, C. C., Kemmler, W., & Freiberger, E. (2019). A systematic review on the influence of fear of falling on quality of life in older people: Is there a role for falls? *Clinical Interventions in Aging, 14*, 701–719. https://doi.org/10.2147/CIA.S197857

Scott, V., Votova, K., Scanlan, A., & Close, J. (2007). Multifactorial and functional mobility assessment tools for fall risk among older adults in community, home-support, long-term and acute care settings. *Age and Ageing, 36*(2), 130–139. https://doi.org/10.1093/ageing/afl165

Sherrington, C., Fairhall, N. J., Wallbank, G. K., Tiedemann, A., Michaleff, Z. A., Howard, K., Clemson, L., Hopewell, S., & Lamb, S. E. (2019). Exercise for preventing falls in older people living in the community. *Cochrane Database Systematic Review, 1*, CD012424. https://doi.org/10.1002/14651858.CD012424.pub2

Sherrington, C., Michaleff, Z. A., Fairhall, N., Paul, S. S., Tiedemann, A., Whitney, J., Cumming, R. G., Herbert, R. D., Close, J. C. T., & Lord, S. R. (2017). Exercise to prevent falls in older adults: An updated systematic review and meta-analysis. *British Journal of Sports Medicine, 51*(24), 1750–1758. https://doi.org/10.1136/bjsports-2016-096547

Singh, D. K. A., Goh, J. W., Shaharudin, M. I., & Shahar, S. (2021). A mobile app (FallSA) to identify fall risk among Malaysian community-dwelling older persons: Development and validation study. *JMIR mHealth and uHealth, 9*(10), e23663. https://doi.org/10.2196/23663

Skelton, D. A., & Dinan, S. M. (1999). Exercise for falls management: Rationale for an exercise programme aimed at reducing postural instability. *Physiotherapy Theory and Practice, 15*(2), 105–120.

Smith-Ray, R. L., Hughes, S. L., Prohaska, T. R., Little, D. M., Jurivich, D. A., & Hedeker, D. (2015). Impact of cognitive training on balance and gait in older adults. *Journals of Gerontology. Series b, Psychological Sciences and Social Sciences, 70*(3), 357–366. https://doi.org/10.1093/geronb/gbt097

Smith-Ray, R. L., Makowski-Woidan, B., & Hughes, S. L. (2014). A randomized trial to measure the impact of a community-based cognitive training intervention on balance and gait in cognitively intact Black older adults. *Health Education & Behavior, 41*(1 Suppl), 62S-69S. https://doi.org/10.1177/1090198114537068

Stamm, O., & Heimann-Steinert, A. (2020). Accuracy of monocular two-dimensional pose estimation compared with a reference standard for kinematic multiview analysis: Validation study. *JMIR mHealth and uHealth, 8*(12), e19608. https://doi.org/10.2196/19608

Strutz, N., Brodowski, H., Kiselev, J., Heimann-Steinert, A., & Muller-Werdan, U. (2022). App-based evaluation of older people's fall risk using the mHealth App Lindera mobility analysis: Exploratory study. *JMIR Aging, 5*(3), e36872. https://doi.org/10.2196/36872

Stubbs, B., Binnekade, T., Eggermont, L., Sepehry, A. A., Patchay, S., & Schofield, P. (2014). Pain and the risk for falls in community-dwelling older adults: systematic review and meta-analysis. *Archives of Physical Medicine and Rehabilitation, 95*(1), 175–187, e179. https://doi.org/10.1016/j.apmr.2013.08.241

Stubbs, B., Perara, G., Koyanagi, A., Veronese, N., Vancampfort, D., Firth, J., Sheehan, K., De Hert, M., Stewart, R., & Mueller, C. (2020). Risk of hospitalized falls and hip fractures in 22,103 older adults receiving mental health care vs 161,603 controls: A large cohort study. *Journal of the American Medical Directors Association, 21*(12), 1893–1899. https://doi.org/10.1016/j.jamda.2020.03.005

Sturnieks, D. L. (2021). Biomechanics of balance and falling. In *Falls in older people: Risk factors, strategies for prevention and implications for practice*, 105.

Sun, R., & Sosnoff, J. J. (2018). Novel sensing technology in fall risk assessment in older adults: A systematic review. *BMC Geriatrics, 18*(1), 14. https://doi.org/10.1186/s12877-018-0706-6

Sylliaas, H., Idland, G., Sandvik, L., Forsen, L., & Bergland, A. (2009). Does mortality of the aged increase with the number of falls? Results from a nine-year follow-up study. *European Journal of Epidemiology, 24*(7), 351–355. https://doi.org/10.1007/s10654-009-9348-5

Tinetti, M. E., Liu, W. L., & Claus, E. B. (1993). Predictors and prognosis of inability to get up after falls among elderly persons. *JAMA, 269*(1), 65–70. https://www.ncbi.nlm.nih.gov/pubmed/8416408

Tinetti, M. E., Speechley, M., & Gintner, S. F. (1988). Risk factors for falls among elderly persons living in the community. *New England Journal of Medicine, 319*, 1701–1707.

Tinetti, M. E., & Williams, C. S. (1997). Falls, injuries due to falls, and the risk of admission to a nursing home. *New England Journal of Medicine, 337*(18), 1279–1284. https://doi.org/10.1056/NEJM199710303371806

van het Reve, E., & de Bruin, E. D. (2014). Strength-balance supplemented with computerized cognitive training to improve dual task gait and divided attention in older adults: A multicenter randomized-controlled trial. *BMC Geriatrics, 14*, 134. https://doi.org/10.1186/1471-2318-14-134

Vasoya, H., Bhattasana, H., & Mishra, R. G. (2023). *A review of elderly fall detection systems using artificial intelligence.* 7th International Conference on Intelligent Computing and Control Systems (ICICCS).

Vellas, B. J., Wayne, S. J., Romero, L. J., Baumgartner, R. N., & Garry, P. J. (1997). Fear of falling and restriction of mobility in elderly fallers. *Age and Ageing, 26*(3), 189–193. https://doi.org/10.1093/ageing/26.3.189

Wang, Q., Jiang, X., Shen, Y., Yao, P., Chen, J., Zhou, Y., Gu, Y., Qian, Z., & Cao, X. (2020). Effectiveness of exercise intervention on fall-related fractures in older adults: A systematic review and meta-analysis of randomized controlled trials. *BMC Geriatrics, 20*(1), 322. https://doi.org/10.1186/s12877-020-01721-6

Wijlhuizen, G. J., de Jong, R., & Hopman-Rock, M. (2007). Older persons afraid of falling reduce physical activity to prevent outdoor falls. *Preventive Medicine, 44*(3), 260–264. https://doi.org/10.1016/j.ypmed.2006.11.003

Zhao, R., Bu, W., & Chen, X. (2019). The efficacy and safety of exercise for prevention of fall-related injuries in older people with different health conditions, and differing intervention protocols: A meta-analysis of randomized controlled trials. *BMC Geriatrics, 19*(1), 341. https://doi.org/10.1186/s12877-019-1359-9

Zhao, R., Zhao, X., Guan, J., Zhang, C., & Zhu, K. (2023). The effect of virtual reality technology on anti-fall ability and bone mineral density of the elderly with osteoporosis in an elderly care institution. *European Journal of Medical Research, 28*(1), 204. https://doi.org/10.1186/s40001-023-01165-9

Zourdos, M. C., Klemp, A., Dolan, C., Quiles, J. M., Schau, K. A., Jo, E., Helms, E., Esgro, B., Duncan, S., Garcia Merino, S., & Blanco, R. (2016). Novel resistance training-specific rating of perceived exertion scale measuring repetitions in reserve. *Journal of Strength and Conditioning Research, 30*(1), 267–275. https://doi.org/10.1519/JSC.0000000000001049

Chapter 5
Artificial Intelligence for Sport Injury Prediction

Robin Owen, Julian A. Owen, and Seren L. Evans

Abstract Preventing injury is a core facilitator of success in sport. Thus, vast sums of money are invested into achieving this. However, sport injury is still seen as equal parts "art" and science. Despite the best efforts of individuals, teams, and national bodies to apply scientifically-derived injury prevention strategies, millions of athletes still get injured in sport every year. Evidently, sport injury prediction is a field, which has scope for improvement. One potential way of advancing the field is the use of Artificial Intelligence (AI). It offers an opportunity to: (1) treat sporting injury as the complex phenomenon it appears to be; (2) consider the non-linear context surrounding athlete injuries; and (3) provide a supplement to practitioner reasoning, to facilitate quicker decisions. The present book chapter evaluates previous research studies' use of AI for injury prediction, assesses the unique advantages offered by AI-based analyses, and discusses challenges when attempting to utilise AI for injury prediction. Overall, the use of AI for sport injury prediction offers a fascinating opportunity. It may one day create a revolution in the field, improving not only prediction itself but also our understanding of the complex interactive factors, which govern injury in sport.

Keywords Machine Learning · Pattern Recognition · Sport Injury · Injury Prevention

5.1 Sport Injury—The Context

It is well established that participation in sports offers numerous physical and mental health benefits alongside providing opportunities for social interaction and the development of positive psychosocial health (Eime et al., 2013). However, the benefits

R. Owen
School of Health and Sport Sciences, Liverpool Hope University, Liverpool, UK

J. A. Owen (✉) · S. L. Evans
School of Psychology and Sport Science, Bangor University, Bangor, UK
e-mail: j.owen@bangor.ac.uk

C. Dindorf et al. (eds.), *Artificial Intelligence in Sports, Movement, and Health*,
https://doi.org/10.1007/978-3-031-67256-9_5

of sport participation are accompanied by a significant sport-related injury burden in both elite and recreational athletes (Emery et al., 2007; Jacobsson et al., 2012). Despite this, there is a relative paucity of research evaluating the efficacy of injury prevention strategies (Conn et al., 2003).

The exact number of sports injuries worldwide each year is challenging to determine precisely due to variations in reporting systems, definitions of sports injuries, and the vast range of sports and activities involved. Estimates suggest that sport-related injuries are common, with millions of people suffering from injuries each year, ranging from minor sprains and strains to more severe fractures, concussions, and other traumatic injuries. In context, an estimated seven million Americans and almost six million Europeans receive medical attention annually for sport-related injuries (Conn et al., 2003; Kisser & Bauer, 2012). Roughly one in five school children miss at least one day of school, while one in three working adults loses at least one workday yearly due to sport-related injuries (Conn et al., 2003; Emery et al., 2006).

Advancements in comprehending the financial strain and allocating resources toward preventing sports injuries have been constrained, partly due to difficulties in clearly defining the extent, breadth, and financial implications of the sports injury issue. An Australian research study approximated the burden of sports-related injuries over a span of seven years to amount to $265 million Australian dollars (Finch et al., 2015). In Europe, the economic assessment of health expenditures, considering both the savings generated through sports participation and the losses incurred due to injuries, suggests that 40–50% of the economic advantage is eroded by sports-related injuries (BASBO, 2001; Weiß, 2000). Many of these estimates of the direct costs represent medical related treatment costs and ignore the indirect costs, which include the immediate and future loss of income costs due to injury. Therefore, the financial cost of sport-injury is likely underestimated as indirect costs can account for approximately 46–71% of the total costs associated with injuries (Lacny et al., 2014).

The repercussions of sports injuries extend beyond mere physical and financial implications. It is widely acknowledged that there exists a significant emotional and psychological toll on athletes' mental health and well-being. This toll often manifests in the form of depression, stress, anger, and diminished self-esteem, especially among competitive athletes or those severely injured (Smith, 1996). Therefore, as sport and physical activity continues to be promoted as part of a healthy lifestyle, sport-related injuries are becoming an important public health concern.

In competitive sports, the adverse effects of injuries are typically more pronounced. It is recognised that the burden of injuries escalates with the level of competition, primarily due to greater exposure to rigorous training and competitions, leading to increased physical and psychological strain. Professional and national sports organisations are obligated to ensure the well-being of their athletes; hence, prioritising athlete welfare is crucial. Lowering the burden of injuries also becomes a notable advantage for team success, which influences commercial revenues.

Injury prediction should be a key component for injury prevention, since the successful identification of injury predictors forms the basis for effective preventive measures. Traditionally, research focusing on the prevention of sports injury is based on the "sequence of prevention", which includes injury audit (surveillance) to establish the extent and nature of the problem, identification of risk factors, and implementation of relevant prevention strategies based on these findings (van Mechelen et al., 1992). This epidemiological approach is useful as it allows researchers to identify the risk of injury (injury incidence or rate and injury burden), prevalence, and risk factors associated with injury within different sports and populations and helps to identify patterns and trends, contributing to injury occurrence. This approach has often attested that single risk factors account for the occurrence of an injury. Although this approach has uncovered numerous potential predictors of injuries using conventional statistical methods like logistic regression. Unsurprisingly, these methods have not consistently identified risk factors (Bekker & Clark, 2016). These inconsistencies underscore the complexity inherent in most human health conditions.

Fundamentally, sports injury is a multifaceted phenomenon influenced by various modifiable and non-modifiable risk factors, including biomechanical, physiological, psychological, environmental, and sociocultural aspects. To understand injury risk, we must analyse the forces, loads, and motions involved in sports activities to understand how they contribute to tissue stress, strain, and injury. We must consider the psychological factors that can modulate the physiological responses to stress and influence injury vulnerability. We must also include context and consider the influence of societal values, gender roles, coach-athlete relationships, peer interactions, and institutional practices on athlete behaviour, risk-taking, and injury reporting.

Since the "sequence of prevention" was first suggested, several models have been developed to conceptualise the complexities surrounding sports injury occurrence and that the injury has a non-linear behaviour (Bekker & Clark, 2016; Bittencourt et al., 2016; Meeuwisse, 1994; Meeuwisse et al., 2007). These models suggest that the multifaceted and intricate nature of sports injuries does not stem solely from the linear combination of isolated predictive factors but rather from the interplay often referred to as "the web of determinants" (Philippe & Mansi, 1998). These determinants may be interconnected in a nonlinear fashion, meaning that slight changes in a few determinants can result in significant and occasionally unforeseen outcomes. To comprehensively understand the complex origins of sports injuries, a complex systems approach is essential.

5.2 The Current State of Artificial Intelligence for Injury Prediction

As outlined, it is well established that sports injuries are multifactorial in nature, and very rarely are attributed to a singular variable in the line of causation; rather, sports injuries arise from multiple interactions between both modifiable (i.e. training load, strength) and non-modifiable determinants (i.e. age, previous injury history) and their non-linear fluctuations over time (Bittencourt et al., 2016; Hulme & Finch, 2015). Therefore, to accurately determine the complexity of their origin, sports injury prediction requires a complex systems approach to better understand how these intricate interactions lead to injury.

Recent advancements of Artificial Intelligence (AI) based analysis (including machine learning and pattern recognition) have lead to its introduction into the realm of sports medicine research (Ruddy et al., 2018; Van Eetvelde et al., 2021), allowing for a more robust analysis of large quantities of data to formulate prediction models of injury (Sigurdson & Chan, 2021). AI can be designed to process imbalanced datasets, which is commonplace in sports injury research as, typically there will be more athletes not sustaining an injury when compared to those sustaining an injury (Lopez-Valenciano et al., 2018; Van Eetvelde et al., 2021). Furthermore, utilising AI for sports injury research allows for the inclusion of both modifiable and non-modifiable risk factors as input features and can be used to evaluate their effectiveness in predicting injury as a binary classification outcome (injury versus no injury).

Caution is needed that we are not reverting back to over-simplistic, reductionist views of injuries, such as injuries occuring due to singular inciting events. Models which have previously been generated for targeted injury diagnoses (e.g., lower extremity injuries, lateral ankle sprains) may be of greater sensitivity within multivariate modelling when compared to grouping all injuries together, producing more interpretable and unambiguous findings for injury incidence (Henriquez et al., 2020).

Various predictive variables of sports injury have, therefore, emerged across a range of sports as a result of AI-based analyses. Within Australian Football, risk factors such as age, stature, body mass, playing position, and previous lower limb injury history were identified as predictors of hamstring strain injury, with an associated accuracy of 85% across algorithms (Ruddy et al., 2018); namely, Naive Bayes, Logistic Regression, Random Forest, Support Vector Machine, and Neural Network, which have qualities of probabilistic classification and the ability to model complex, non-linear interactions within multiple predictor variables (John & Langley, 1995; Keerthi et al., 2006; Quinlan, 1993). Utilising a similar approach with random forest algorithms in identifying lower limb musculoskeletal injuries amongst National Collegiate Athletic Association (NCAA) athletes, Rommers et al. (2020) identified hip-based strength metrics, demographic and balance variables as indicators for future injury. Furthermore, adopting a subgroup discovery approach which allows for the analysis of subsets of individuals who share common attributes for injury risk from input features (Herrera et al., 2011), de Leeuw et al. (2022) discovered that predictors of injury within elite male volleyball were fatigue, overuse, sleep, muscle soreness, and training exertion. Physical attributes such as height and weight, alongside strength, flexibility, speed, agility, and endurance features, achieved 85% precision using XGBoost in assessing injury predictors within elite youth football (Rommers et al., 2020). Pattern recognition analyses, therefore, show initial potential to provide a feasible statistical method of forecasting injuries in sport whilst being able to account for (1) modifiable and non-modifiable risk factors, (2) the time-series nature of athlete training data, (3) whilst also considering their nonlinear interactions.

5.3 Advantages of Using Artificial Intelligence for Injury Prediction

Natural sciences, such as injury prediction in sport, traditionally adhere to explanatory positivist views where understanding and generalisation of phenomena require the testing of clearly defined hypotheses (i.e., predictions) using tightly controlled methods (Kuhn, 2012). This approach inherently encourages a "reductionist" approach to research, wherein testing theoretically-based and limited-in-number predictors of phenomena is considered superior. Indeed, injury prediction research has predominantly adhered to these principles (Bekker & Clark, 2016; Bittencourt et al., 2016). However, such approaches induce a case of "survivor bias"; factors are prioritised for consideration if their relationship with injury is either known or can be clearly predicted (Lockwood, 2021). Consequently, this may prohibit the identification of new, as-of-yet unknown, factors which may affect injury in sport (Tee et al., 2020). Similarly, once a certain number of predictors is reached, it can make it difficult for researchers to fully grasp their interaction.

Concerted efforts to broaden understanding of sports injury are of particular importance given recent calls to consider sports injury as a complex phenomenon, affected by many variables and interactions (Fonseca et al., 2020; Tee et al., 2020). Explanatory positivist approaches to-date have laid the foundations for identifying modifiable and non-modifiable risk factors of injury in sport (Bahr, 2016; Rossi et al., 2021), but limitations arise from the typical utilisation of mono-dimensional approaches. Variables are often treated as static, absolute at one point in time, and subsequently ignore the complex underlying pattern of sports injuries and time-series nature of athlete status (Rossi et al., 2021). This "static" attitude to predictors, combined with assumptions of linear relationships between singular variables and injury, means that current approaches with high explanatory power do not always translate to high predictive power in relation to injury risk (Jauhianen et al., 2021; Shmueli, 2010).

Therefore, a possible means to deepening understanding of injury predictors are AI-assisted analyses. AI is particularly suited to complex problems, given its ability to: process large volumes of data; comprise partial automation to reduce time cost; provide non-linear assessment of multiple interactions; and discover useful hidden patterns in data (Pham et al., 2020; Zhuang et al., 2017). Accordingly, sports injury researchers are beginning to utilise artificial neural networks, support vector machines, gradient boosting machines, and decision tree methods (Bullock et al., 2022). Although pursuing complex analytical procedures such as these goes against fundamental scientific principles (e.g., Occam's Razor, wherein the simplest explanations are regarded as the most plausible, and should thus be pursued; Blumer et al., 1987), injury risk appears to be highly complex by nature (Fonseca et al., 2020; Tee et al., 2020) and may thus benefit from AI-assisted analyses. Specifically, AI-based approaches could demonstrate a better capacity for interpreting the highly complex and non-linear contexts surrounding each case despite their seeming contradiction with established explanatory conventions (Tee et al., 2020).

5.4 Training and Testing an Artificial Intelligence for Injury Prediction

Just like the athletes themselves, AI models require rigorous training and testing (Kanal & Chandrasekaran, 1971). "Training" entails calibrating the underlying parameters which AI models use to produce outputs from inputs. "Testing" entails evaluating the effectiveness of these models, often using a different dataset to that used in training. There are many testing/training methods, such as supervised learning, unsupervised learning, and reinforcement learning; however, a commonality among them all is a requirement for large volumes of representative data to create models which provide accurate outputs (L'heureux et al., 2017). Although the quantity and quality of training/testing data is only one of many factors which can cause undesirable bias in models, it is one of the key determinants (see Prediction model Risk of Bias Assessment Tool; Wolff et al., 2019). If an AI model is subject to insufficient volumes of relevant data during training, it is likely that these models will contain bias, which can lead to inaccurate outputs.

A recent systematic review found that 98% of AI-based analyses used to predict sporting injuries were at high or unclear risk of bias (Bullock et al., 2022). In part, this is a product of the additional challenges the field has when it comes to testing and training models; contexts surrounding injury are dynamic and not interchangeable (Tee et al., 2020). Injury can be affected by more than just match play and training load. It is highly dependent on the context surrounding an athlete. Historical, political, social, economic, scientific, cultural, and organisational factors can all affect injury likelihood and the effectiveness of preventative methods. For example, playing on hard ground out of geographical/economic necessity can increase injury likelihood (Chalmers et al., 2012). Relatedly, the contexts surrounding injury are dynamic rather than static. For example, Between 1998 and 2010, rugby union forwards have become 22% heavier, 8% taller, and 18% stronger (Lombard et al., 2015). Likewise, changes in coaching and backroom staff can produce profound changes to an athlete's recovery protocols from one year to the next (Galdino et al., 2023). A result of the complex and dynamic factors surrounding sports injury is that it makes it challenging for a single research team to collect sufficient predictors as well as sufficient volumes of data to optimally train and test AI models.

Given the challenges faced when attempting to apply AI methods to sports injury, it is not surprising that previous studies have been criticised for their generalisability and application to applied contexts (see Bullock et al., 2022). Specifically, it has been suggested that even in AI-based studies featuring low risk of bias, modest predictive performance of models means that there may be no injury prediction models which can be confidently recommended for applied practice. Going forward, it may be necessary for researchers to embrace the open science to collaborate and compile sufficiently detailed datasets. Such Open Science approaches entail intentional sharing of data (and failing that, making data freely accessible) to better build on previous studies (Vicente-Saez & Martinez-Fuentes, 2018). Precedent for the rapid advancement of AI given sufficient access to detailed datasets for testing/training can be seen in text-to-text applications such as ChatGPT, where access to a large corpus of written work throughout history has allowed impressively accurate predictions of desired text, based on user inputs (Wu et al., 2023). Researchers investigating sports injury should aim to work together to further elucidate underlying complex interactions of predictors.

5.5 Practical Implications: Pitfalls and Solutions

Although AI has the potential to become a powerful tool in injury prediction (Bullock et al., 2022), its underlying mechanisms may be too complex for applied practitioners to find useful/comprehensible themselves. Therefore, AI-based approaches may further increase the researcher-practitioner gap. This researcher-practitioner gap occurs when scientifically derived knowledge is not applied by practitioners in the field (Lenfant, 2003). The present wealth of different AI-based approaches, complex statistical metrics, and frequent requirement to modify computer code, means that a majority of applied practitioners may struggle to use AI models in any capacity other than standardised "plug and play" packages (Bullock et al., 2022). However, even if "plug and play" packages are made available to applied practitioners, current sports injury models' high likelihood of bias (Bullock et al., 2022) run a high risk of incorrect application. In such high risk situations, it has been shown that individuals tend to rely on their own judgement and avoid applying these high risk methods, further widening the researcher-practitioner gap (Jøsang & Presti, 2004; Papenmeier et al., 2022). Therefore, in addition to producing accurate injury prediction models, another key barrier may be to overcome the researcher-practitioner gap.

The utilisation of AI-based analyses in injury prediction studies is often hindered by limited data inclusion, restricting analysis to a narrow scope of variables. For instance, some studies only incorporate physical performance metrics (Rommers et al., 2020), perhaps constraining predictive accuracy. However, the potential for heightened precision remains, suggesting an opportunity for enhancement through integrating more extensive datasets (Verhagen & Bolling, 2015). By refining the focus of injury prediction using advanced AI methodologies, such as targeting specific injury types prevalent within distinct athletic cohorts—such as hamstring strains in elite football or anterior cruciate ligament injuries in female athletes—the applicability of these models to real-world practice can be improved (Rommers et al., 2020; Van Eetvelde et al., 2021). This may provide practitioners with more robust datasets, enabling the implementation of more effective and targeted injury prevention strategies.

That said, to create more accurate prediction models, reduce bias, promote practitioner uptake, and reduce the researcher-practitioner gap, theoretically driven variables of injury risk factors still require prioritisation when deciding on input features during preprocessing stages of AI analyses. To illustrate, a strong relationship exists between the amount of ice cream sold and shark attack incidences, and it may even be possible to predict the number of shark attacks that will occur based on the number of ice creams sold. However, in reality, no amount of regulating ice cream sales will have an effect on the number of shark attacks; ice cream sales are epiphenomenal to shark attacks and is likely a byproduct of another process, such as warmer weather resulting in more demand for ice cream and people visiting the beach. Regulating the waters with more coastal surveillance and warnings for surfers is likely to be more effective in reducing the number of shark attacks. The point is, utilising variables that are theoretically linked to sports injury will reduce the likelihood of erroneous discoveries, which would affect the interpretability and reliability of the models.

5.6 Conclusion

AI-based approaches to sports injury prediction provide many opportunities to advance the field. Firstly, it has the capacity to treat sporting injury as the complex phenomenon it appears to be. Secondly, it allows for consideration of the non-linear context surrounding athlete injuries, which previous reductionist statistical approaches were forced to omit. Lastly, it can provide a supplement to practitioner reasoning, to facilitate quicker decisions. However, one should not overlook the challenges of using AI. Training effective AI requires large and representative datasets, which has been a key barrier faced in sports injury research. Additionally, until accurate models become available as "plug and play" solutions, they may be prohibitively complex/novel for applied practitioners to use; thus potentially widening researcher-practitioner gaps. If these challenges are overcome though, AI may one day revolutionise not only sports injury prediction accuracy, but also our understanding of underlying factors and their interaction.

Prediction models may, therefore prompt early intervention and manipulation of variables which are known to have an effect on injury risk however unless the relationship is causal, manipulating certain metrics does not mean that injury risk will be altered (Hernan et al., 2019); therefore, assuming that manipulating certain variables reduces the risk of injury is the equivalent of banning ice cream sales to prevent shark attacks (Impellizzeri et al., 2020). When handling data regarding injury prediction and prevention, identifying the optimal set of risk factors for athletes at greater risk of injury would prove invaluable for coaches, medical practitioners, and for the overall well-being of athletes. Achieving this necessitates a tailored approach to athlete monitoring practices and addressing key performance indicators tailored to the demands of each individual sport. Within the realm of sports, the cost of injury—weighing the costs of medical procedures, rehabilitation, player time loss due to injury, and its impact of team success against the benefits of injury reduction—is pivotal in the decision making process (Gabbett et al., 2016). When utilising AI, more efforts need to be made in relation to understand the relative weight of individual risk factors and injury risk, portraying a picture of the probability of injury rather than classifying an athlete into a high or low risk group (Rossi et al., 2018; Van Eetvelde et al., 2021), which would be of more benefit for sporting practitioners when it comes to making adjustments to training regimes and team selection. Employing an

AI approach to injury management should, therefore, not only be able to identify risk factors but also provide practitioners with actionable thresholds for heightened injury probability, allowing for the implementation of timely prevention strategies with the hope of minimising the cost of injury for both athlete and team.

References

Bahr, R. (2016) Why screening tests to predict injury do not work—and probably never will…: A critical review. *British Journal of Sports Medicine, 50*, 776-780.

BASPO—Bundesamt für Sport. (2001). Volkswirtschaftlicher Nutzen der Gesundheitseffekte der körperlichen Aktivität: erste Schätzungen für die Schweiz. *Schweizer Zeitschrift Für Sportmedizin und Sporttraumatologie, 49*(2), 84–86.

Bekker, S., & Clark, A. M. (2016). Bringing complexity to sports injury prevention research: From simplification to explanation. *British Journal of Sports Medicine, 50*(24), 1489–1490.

Blumer, A., Ehrenfeucht, A., Haussler, D., & Warmuth, M. K. (1987). Occam's Razor. *Information Processing Letters, 24*(6), 377–380.

Bittencourt, N. F., Meeuwisse, W. H., Mendonça, L. D., Nettel-Aguirre, A., Ocarino, J. M., & Fonseca, S. T. (2016). Complex systems approach for sports injuries: Moving from risk factor identification to injury pattern recognition—Narrative review and new concept. *British Journal of Sports Medicine, 50*(21), 1309–1314.

Bullock, G. S., Mylott, J., Hughes, T., Nicholson, K. F., Riley, R. D., & Collins, G. S. (2022). Just how confident can we be in predicting sports injuries? A systematic review of the methodological conduct and performance of existing musculoskeletal injury prediction models in sport. *Sports Medicine, 52*(10), 2469–2482.

Chalmers, D. J., Samaranayaka, A., Gulliver, P., & McNoe, B. (2012). Risk factors for injury in rugby union football in New Zealand: A cohort study. *British Journal of Sports Medicine, 46*(2), 95–102.

Conn, J. M., Annest, J. L., & Gilchrist, J. (2003). Sports and recreation related injury episodes in the US population, 1997–99. *Injury Prevention, 9*(2), 117–123. https://doi.org/10.1136/ip.9.2.117

de Leeuw, A. W., van der Zwaard, S., van Baar, R., & Knobbe, A. (2022). Personalized machine learning approach to injury monitoring in elite volleyball players. *European Journal of Sport Science, 22*(4), 511–520.

Emery, C. A., Meeuwisse, W. H., & McAllister, J. R. B. (2006). Survey of sport participation and sport injury in Calgary and area high schools. *Clinical Journal of Sport Medicine, 16*(1), 20–26. https://doi.org/10.1097/01.jsm.0000184638.72075.b7

Emery, C. A., Rose, M. S., McAllister, J. R., et al. (2007). A prevention strategy to reduce the incidence of injury in high school basketball: A cluster randomized controlled trial. *Clinical Journal of Sport Medicine, 17*, 17–24.

Eime, R. M., Young, J. A., Harvey, J. T., et al. (2013). A systematic review of the psychological and social benefits of participation in sport for children and adolescents: Informing development of a conceptual model of health through sport. *International Journal of Behavioral Nutrition and Physical Activity, 10*, 98. https://doi.org/10.1186/1479-5868-10-98

Finch, C. F., Kemp, J. L., & Clapperton, A. J. (2015). The incidence and burden of hospital-treated sports-related injury in people aged 15+ years in Victoria, Australia, 2004–2010: A future epidemic of osteoarthritis? *Osteoarthritis Cartilage, 23*(7), 1138–1143. https://doi.org/10.1016/j.joca.2015.02.165. PMID: 25749009.

Fonseca, S. T., Souza, T. R., Verhagen, E., Van Emmerik, R., Bittencourt, N. F., Mendonça, L. D., Ocarino, J. M., et al. (2020). Sports injury forecasting and complexity: A synergetic approach. *Sports Medicine, 50*, 1757–1770.

Gabbett, H. T., Windt, J., & Gabbett, T. J. (2016). Cost-benefit analysis underlies training decisions in elite sport. *British Journal of Sports Medicine, 50*(21), 1291–1292.

Galdino de Souza, M., & Wicker, P. (2023). A culture of constraints: How head coach turnovers affect the backroom staff and player development in professional football. *International Journal of Sports Science and Coaching.*

Henriquez, M., Sumner, J., Faherty, M., Sell, T., & Bent, B. (2020). Machine learning to predict lower extremity musculoskeletal injury risk in student athletes. *Frontiers in Sports and Active Living, 2*, 576655.

Hernán, M. A., Hsu, J., & Healy, B. (2019). A second chance to get causal inference right: A classification of data science tasks. *Chance, 32*(1), 42–49.

Herrera, F., Carmona, C. J., González, P., & Del Jesus, M. J. (2011). An overview on subgroup discovery: Foundations and applications. *Knowledge and Information Systems, 29*, 495–525.

Hulme, A., & Finch, C. F. (2015). From monocausality to systems thinking: A complementary and alternative conceptual approach for better understanding the development and prevention of sports injury. *Injury Epidemiology, 2*, 1–12. https://doi.org/10.1186/s40621-015-0064-1

Impellizzeri, F. M., Menaspà, P., Coutts, A. J., Kalkhoven, J., & Menaspà, M. J. (2020). Training load and its role in injury prevention, part I: Back to the future. *Journal of Athletic Training, 55*(9), 885–892.

Jacobsson, J., Timpka, T., Kowalski, J., et al. (2012). Prevalence of musculoskeletal injuries in Swedish elite track and field athletes. *American Journal of Sports Medicine, 40*, 163–169.

Jauhiainen, S., Kauppi, J. P., Leppänen, M., Pasanen, K., Parkkari, J., Vasankari, T., Kannus, P., & Äyrämö, S. (2021) New machine learning approach for detection of injury risk factors in young team sport athletes. *International Journal of Sports Medicine, 42*(2), 175-182. https://doi.org/10.1055/a-1231-5304. Epub 2020 Sep 13. PMID: 32920800.

John, G. H., & Langley, P. (1995). Estimating continuous distributions in Bayesian classifiers. In *Conference on uncertainty in artificial intelligence.*

Jøsang, A., & Presti, S. L. (2004, March). *Analysing the relationship between risk and trust. In International conference on trust management* (pp. 135–145). Springer.

Kanal, L., & Chandrasekaran, B. (1971). On dimensionality and sample size in statistical pattern classification. *Pattern Recognition, 3*(3), 225–234.

Keerthi, S. S., Chapelle, O., & DeCoste, D. (2006). *Building support vector machines with reduced classifier complexity* (p. 23).

Kisser, R., & Bauer, R. (2012). The burden of sports injuries in the European Union. *Austrian Road Safety Board*, 1–94.

Kuhn, T. S. (2012). *The structure of scientific revolutions.* University of Chicago Press.

Lacny, S., Marshall, D. A., Currie, G., et al. (2014). Reality check: The cost–effectiveness of removing body checking from youth ice hockey. *British Journal of Sports Medicine, 48*, 1299–1305.

Lenfant, C. (2003). Shattuck lecture—clinical research to clinical practice—lost in translation? *The New England Journal of Medicine, 349*(9), 868-74. https://doi.org/10.1056/NEJMsa035507. PMID: 12944573.

Lockwood, D. (2021). *Fooled by the winners: How survivor bias deceives us.* Greenleaf Book Group.

Lombard, W. P., Durandt, J. J., Masimla, H., Green, M., & Lambert, M. I. (2015). Changes in body size and physical characteristics of South African under-20 rugby union players over a 13-year period. *The Journal of Strength & Conditioning Research, 29*(4), 980–988.

López-Valenciano, A., Ayala, F., Puerta, J. M., Croix, M. D. S., Vera-García, F., Hernández-Sánchez, S., Myer, G., et al. (2018). A preventive model for muscle injuries: A novel approach based on learning algorithms. *Medicine and Science in Sports and Exercise, 50*(5), 915.

L'heureux, A., Grolinger, K., Elyamany, H. F., & Capretz, M. A. (2017). Machine learning with big data: Challenges and approaches. *IEEE Access, 5*, 7776–7797.

Meeuwisse, W. (1994). Assessing causation in sport injury: A multifactorial model. *Clinical Journal of Sport Medicine, 4*, 66–170.

Meeuwisse, W. H., Tyreman, H., Hagel, B., et al. (2007). A dynamic model of etiology in sport injury: The recursive nature of risk and causation. *Clinical Journal of Sport Medicine, 17*, 215–219. https://doi.org/10.1097/JSM.0b013e3180592a48

Papenmeier, A., Kern, D., Englebienne, G., & Seifert, C. (2022). It's complicated: The relationship between user trust, model accuracy and explanations in AI. *ACM Transactions on Computer-Human Interaction (TOCHI), 29*(4), 1–33.

Pham, Q. V., Nguyen, D. C., Huynh-The, T., Hwang, W. J., & Pathirana, P. N. (2020). Artificial intelligence (AI) and big data for coronavirus (COVID-19) pandemic: A survey on the state-of-the-arts. *IEEE Access, 8*, 130820–130839.

Philippe, P., & Mansi, O. (1998). Nonlinearity in the epidemiology of complex health and disease processes. *Theoretical Medicine and Bioethics, 19*(6), 591–607. https://doi.org/10.1023/a:1009979306346. PMID: 10051792.

Quinlan, J. R. (1993). *Programs for machine learning*. Morgan Kauffmann Publishers.

Rommers, N., Rössler, R., Verhagen, E., Vandecasteele, F., Verstockt, S., Vaeyens, R., Lenoir, M., D'Hondt, E., & Witvrouw, E. (2020). A machine learning approach to assess injury risk in elite youth football players. *Medicine & Science in Sports & Exercise, 52*(8), 1745–1751.

Rossi, A., Pappalardo, L., Cintia, P., Iaia, F. M., Fernàndez, J., & Medina, D. (2018). Effective injury forecasting in soccer with GPS training data and machine learning. *PLoS ONE, 13*(7), e0201264. https://doi.org/10.1371/journal.pone.0201264

Rossi, A., Pappalardo, L., & Cintia, P. (2022). A narrative review for a machine learning application in sports: An example based on injury forecasting in soccer. *Sports, 10*(1), 5. https://doi.org/10.3390/sports10010005

Ruddy, J. D., Shield, A. J., Maniar, N., Williams, M. D., Duhig, S. J., Timmins, R. G., Opar, D. A., et al. (2018). Predictive modeling of hamstring strain injuries in elite Australian footballers. *Medicine & Science in Sports & Exercise, 50*(5), 906–914.

Shmueli, G. (2010) To Explain or To Predict?. Statistical Science, Available at SSRN: https://ssrn.com/abstract=1351252 or https://doi.org/10.2139/ssrn.1351252

Sigurdson, H., & Chan, J. H. (2021). Machine learning applications to sports injury: A review. *icSPORTS*, 157–168.

Smith, A. M. (1996). Psychological impact of injuries in athletes. *Sports Medicine, 22*, 391–405. https://doi.org/10.2165/00007256-199622060-00006

Tee, J. C., McLaren, S. J., & Jones, B. (2020). Sports injury prevention is complex: We need to invest in better processes, not singular solutions. *Sports Medicine, 50*(4), 689–702.

Van Eetvelde, H., Mendonça, L. D., Ley, C., Seil, R., & Tischer, T. (2021). Machine learning methods in sport injury prediction and prevention: A systematic review. *Journal of Experimental Orthopaedics, 8*, 1–15.

Van Mechelen, W., Hlobil, H., & Kemper, H. (1992). Incidence, severity, etiology and prevention of sports injuries—A review of concepts. *Sports Medicine, 14*, 82–99.

Vicente-Saez, R., & Martinez-Fuentes, C. (2018). Open Science now: A systematic literature review for an integrated definition. *Journal of Business Research, 88*, 428–436.

Verhagen, E., & Bolling, C. (2015) Protecting the health of the @hlete: How online technology may aid our common goal to prevent injury and illness in sport. *British Journal of Sports Medicine, 49*, 1174-1178.

Weiß, O. (2000). Sport und Gesundheit: Die Auswirkungen des Sports auf die Gesundheit - Eine sozio

Wolff, R. F., Moons, K. G., Riley, R. D., Whiting, P. F., Westwood, M., Collins, G. S., Reitsma, J. B., Kleijnen, J., Mallett, S., & PROBAST Group. (2019). PROBAST: a tool to assess the risk of bias and applicability of prediction model studies. *Annals of Internal Medicine, 170*(1), 51–58.

Wu, T., He, S., Liu, J., Sun, S., Liu, K., Han, Q. L., & Tang, Y. (2023). A brief overview of ChatGPT: The history, status quo and potential future development. *IEEE/CAA Journal of Automatica Sinica, 10*(5), 1122–1136.

Zhuang, Y. T., Wu, F., Chen, C., & Pan, Y. H. (2017). Challenges and opportunities: From big data to knowledge in AI 2.0. *Frontiers of Information Technology & Electronic Engineering, 18*, 3–14.

Chapter 6
Generative Artificial Intelligence in Anti-doping Analysis in Sports

Maxx Richard Rahman and Wolfgang Maass

Abstract Doping in sports involves the abuse of prohibited substances to enhance performance in the sporting event. Blood doping, a prevalent method, allows the increase in red blood cell count to improve aerobic capacity, often through blood transfusions or synthetic Erythropoietin (rhEPO). Current indirect detection methods require a large amount of data for performing analysis. In this paper, we study the use of generative modelling for generating synthetic blood sample data to improve anti-doping analysis in sports. We performed experiment on the blood samples collected during the clinical trial. The dataset comprised haematological parameters from real blood samples, which were analyzed to understand the baseline characteristics. The Generative Adversarial Network (GAN) is used to understand the complexity and variability of real blood sample data. Results demonstrated that the model could successfully generate synthetic samples that closely resembled real samples, indicating its potential for augmenting datasets used in doping detection. This approach not only enhances the robustness of indirect methods of doping detection by providing a larger dataset for analysis but also addresses ethical concerns related to privacy and consent in using athletes' biological data.

Keywords Blood Doping · rhEPO · GANs · Sports

6.1 Introduction

Doping in sports means the use of banned/prohibited substances or methods by athletes to improve their performance (Vlad et al., 2018). This unethical practice subverts fair competition and poses significant health risks. The history of doping is as early as 1886, when substances such as cocaine, caffeine, and strychnine were used, although they were not illegal at the time, to enhance performance (Holt et al., 2009). This period was the starting point of performance-enhancing practices, which have developed into a complex set of doping techniques, including anabolic steroids,

M. R. Rahman (✉) · W. Maass
Saarland University, Saarbrücken, Germany
e-mail: m.rahman@iss.uni-saarland.de

C. Dindorf et al. (eds.), *Artificial Intelligence in Sports, Movement, and Health*,
https://doi.org/10.1007/978-3-031-67256-9_6

blood doping, human growth hormone, and others. One of the most prominent cases in cycling is that of Lance Armstrong, who was suspended because of doping accusations and later confessed to the use of the performance-enhancing drug Erythropoietin (EPO) (Heuberger et al., 2013). Armstrong's case brought a lot of focus on how widespread the problem of doping was in professional cycling and other sports.

Blood doping is one of the most common forms of doping, which means increasing the number of red blood cells in the bloodstream, improving the athlete's aerobic capacity and endurance (Plumb et al., 2016). This can be done by blood transfusions, the use of certain drugs, or other approaches aimed at increasing the number of red blood cells (Goodnough & Panigrahi, 2017). Blood doping is especially seen among endurance athletes, such as cyclists, whose performance can be remarkably enhanced by the increased oxygen delivery to their muscles.

Recombinant human Erythropoietin (rhEPO) is a synthesized form of a natural hormone that is responsible for the production of red blood cells (Bunn, 2013). The use of rhEPO in sports is also known as "EPO doping", which has become a major issue because it can help improve performance of the athlete. The administration of rhEPO enables athletes to increase their red blood cell mass without the need for blood transfusions, thus making the procedure a more covert way of doping (Robinson et al., 2006). Nevertheless, using rhEPO may be associated with cardiovascular risks, such as hypertension and thrombosis, which create serious health issues to athletes (Santhanam et al., 2010). The detection of blood doping has been a challenge for World Anti-Doping Agency (WADA) and the associated laboratories. In 2009, they developed the Athlete Biological Passport, which involves the monitoring of selected biological markers over time and indirectly detecting the effects of blood doping by observing the variations in an athlete's biological markers, which may suggest manipulation (WADA, 2022).

Current detection techniques include both direct testing for the presence of prohibited substances in blood or urine samples and indirect methods that may provide the indication of doping, such as changes in haematological parameters. Manfredini et al. (2011) proposed a statistical score that included several blood parameters and emphasized variations from their normal levels. Sharpe et al. (2006) used a single previous sample to determine the baseline values for an athlete. Parisotto et al. (2001) looked at how different statistical models, namely the ON and OFF models, fared in their analysis according to specific possible parameters. Hence, the use of statistics and Machine Learning (ML) techniques to deal with doping has been the subject of different studies. Similarly, Kelly et al. (2019) use ML algorithms to discover doping risks among 791 UFC athletes through their performance data, with a high sensitivity rate of 44%. Sottas et al. (2006) developed the Abnormal Blood Profile Score (ABPS), a testing strategy that utilizes statistical classifications of indirect biomarkers. The ABPS calculation, which used both Support Vector Machine and Naive Bayes algorithms, reached a sensitivity of 45% and a specificity of 100%. Rahman et al. (2022) also showed how different ML approaches could be useful to identify the presence of the rhEPO in the blood samples. Therefore, this study is the current state-of-the-art method and could be used as a benchmark for future studies.

Despite these advancements, one of the significant limitations is the difficulty in gathering enough data for effective ML analysis.

Therefore, in this paper, we will discuss the potential uses of generative modelling in doping analysis in the sport. This research work focuses on whether generative algorithms can help eliminate the constraints of limited data and positively impact the doping detection. Thus, we apply a Generative Adversarial Network to generate blood samples that can be further used to train ML algorithms to detect and identify the presence of rhEPO in blood samples to improve the detection of blood doping.

6.2 Generative Modelling

6.2.1 Haematological Profile of Blood Sample

The haematological profile of the blood sample comprises a set of crucial blood parameters that exhibit significant variations due to rhEPO intake (Krumm & Faiss, 2021). It helps in understanding the size and important characteristics of each circulating blood cell. Table 6.1 shows all the important parameters with the description.

The significance of the OFF-HR parameter becomes evident through an example. Imagine an athlete using small doses of rhEPO. While this may not significantly elevate hemoglobin levels, reticulocytes are likely to respond markedly, impacting the OFF-HR score. Conversely, an athlete taking substantial rhEPO doses might maintain constant hemoglobin levels through plasma expansion, evading detection. However, infusing a blood bag would decrease reticulocytes, triggering the OFF-HR. Thus, the OFF-HR serves as a crucial indicator of erythropoiesis acceleration or deceleration.

6.2.2 Requirements for Synthesizing Haematological Profile

There are several requirements for the generation of haematological profiles due to their longitudinal nature (Mosquera et al., 2023). To begin with, we outline a set of prerequisites necessary for synthesizing longitudinal datasets. By doing so, we aim to define specific criteria for our generative algorithm. The goal is to ensure the generated samples' authenticity and the generative models' applicability to actual data scenarios.

(1) **Temporal Nature of the Data**: The haematological profile consists of longitudinal elements, which means that it tracks the same athlete over time. This longitudinal element involves the collection of multiple samples from each athlete at different times.

Table 6.1 Description of all the haematological parameters in blood sample

Parameter	Description
Haemoglobin concentration (HB)	The amount of hemoglobin in the blood, measured in grams per liter (g/L)
Haematocrit (HCT)	The proportion of blood volume occupied by red blood cells
Reticulocytes percentage (RET%)	The percentage of immature red blood cells (reticulocytes) in the blood
Reticulocytes count (RET#)	The absolute number of reticulocytes per microliter of blood
Reticulocytes haemoglobin (RET-HB)	The hemoglobin content within reticulocytes
Mean corpuscular volume (MCV)	The average volume of red blood cells
Mean corpuscular haemoglobin mass (MCH)	The average mass of hemoglobin in red blood cells
Mean corpuscular haemoglobin concentration (MCHC)	The concentration of hemoglobin in red blood cells
Red blood cell count (RBC)	The total number of red blood cells
Red blood cell distribution width—standard deviation (RDW-SD)	A measure of the variation in red blood cell size
Red blood cell distribution width—coefficient of variation (RDW-CV)	Another indicator of red blood cell size variability
White blood cell count (WBC)	The total number of white blood cells
Immature reticulocyte fraction (IRF)	The proportion of immature reticulocytes
Low fluorescence reticulocyte fraction (LFR)	The fraction of reticulocytes with low fluorescence
Medium fluorescence reticulocyte fraction (MFR)	The fraction of reticulocytes with medium fluorescence
High fluorescence reticulocyte fraction (HFR)	The fraction of reticulocytes with high fluorescence
OFF-HR score	The relationship between reticulocytes and hemoglobin. Calculated using the expression: $\text{OFF} - \text{HR} = \text{HB}(g/L) - 60\sqrt{\text{RET\%}}$

(2) **Variability in Profile Sequence Length**: The variation in the number of samples per athlete is highly dependent on the athlete's career length or experience level. The younger or newer athletes usually have fewer samples whereas the more experienced athletes who have been active for a long time and therefore have collected many more samples. This difference in sequence length needs consideration for analysis the data.

(3) **Diversity of Data Types**: The longitudinal dataset is heterogeneous in nature, which means that it consists of different types of data types. Specifically, it includes:

a. **Categorical or discrete features**, which are data that can be divided into different categories without any inherent order (e.g., gender, sample collection).
b. **Continuous features** which are numeric and can take any value within a range, representing measurements or quantities (e.g., concentration level of different haematological parameters).

(4) **Presence of Outliers and Anomalies**: The dataset contains outliers that are values which are differ from the reference ranges. They can be crucial for analyses, and can allow to identify exceptional cases, errors in data collection or unique characteristics that might be important for the analysis.
(5) **Data Sparsity Due to Missing Values**: It is quite usual for the dataset to contain a lot of missing values that result in sparsity. This implies that not all haematological parameters are available for all the samples.

6.2.3 Generative Adversarial Networks (GANs)

Generative models learn to understand and replicate the underlying distribution of a given dataset, allowing them to produce new samples that could plausibly come from the same distribution as the original data. This approach is particularly powerful in many fields, such as image and voice generation, where models like Generative Adversarial Networks (GANs) (Goodfellow et al., 2014) and Variational Autoencoders (VAEs) (Kingma & Welling, 2014) have shown remarkable ability to produce high-quality, realistic outputs. In this study, we used GANs to generate blood samples based on the collected clinical samples.

In this section, we discuss the concept and architecture of GANs. A basic GAN framework includes an input vector along with two main components: a generator and a discriminator, both of which are typically realized using deep neural networks. The concept relies on a predetermined distribution, $P_{data}(x)$, which is assumed to represent the data distribution of a training sample x. Identifying this distribution accurately is challenging. Conventional approaches often assume that $P_{data}(x)$ adheres to a Gaussian mixture model. However, these approaches can falter with complex models, leading to unsatisfactory outcomes. Consequently, neural networks are suggested to define the distribution. The generator, parameterized by G, takes a random variable z from a prior distribution and transforms it via the neural network into a pseudo-sample distribution, denoted as $G(z)$, with its data distribution labeled as $P_G(z)$. The variable z typically originates from Gaussian noise, representing a stochastic variable in a latent space. Leveraging G, the generator can generate a straightforward input distribution into a variety of intricate distributions. The goal is for the $P_G(x)$ generated by the generator is to closely mimic the actual data distribution $P_{data}(x)$. Therefore, the generator's objective is to optimize and find an ideal G^*.

$$G^* = \arg\min\left[Diff(P_G, P_{data})\right]$$

The next question is to identify the difference between the two distributions. Despite the lack of precise knowledge about these distributions, it is possible to draw samples from them. To address this, we have a discriminator characterized by the parameter D. In the training phase, the discriminator is expected to output a value of 1 for real samples x, and shift to 0 for generated samples. Goodfellow et al. (2014) used binary cross entropy function, which is commonly used for binary classification problems.

$$Loss = -(y \log \hat{y} + (1 - y) \log(1 - \hat{y}))$$

In this context, $\hat{y}$ represents the predicted label by the model and y denotes the actual label of the sample. Each sample under consideration could originate from either the real distribution or the generated distribution. Accordingly, positive examples are associated with P_{data}, and negative examples correspond to P_G. The entire objective function for the discriminator is defined as follows:

$$V(G, D) = E_{x \sim P_{data}}\big[\log D(x)\big] + E_{x \sim P_G}\big[\log(1 - D(x))\big]$$

Integrating these equations give the foundational GAN's objective function as outlined below:

$$\min \max V(G, D) = \min \max E_{x \sim P_{data}}\big[\log D(x)\big] + E_{x \sim P_G}\big[\log(1 - D(G(z)))\big]$$

The training process of a GAN is essentially a min–max game. The generator aims to fool the discriminator by maximizing the discriminator's output for a synthetic sample. Conversely, the discriminator works to accurately identify real from generated samples, striving to maximize the function $V(G, D)$ for real samples and minimize it for generated ones, creating a minimax scenario. Throughout GAN training, the parameters for the generator and the discriminator are iteratively adjusted. While training the generator, the discriminator's parameters remain constant, and the generated data is fed into the discriminator. The difference between the discriminator's output, $D(G(z))$, and the actual label is calculated, and the generator's parameters are updated based on this error using the backpropagation algorithm. Conversely, during the discriminator's training phase, the generator's parameters are kept constant. The discriminator receives real samples (x) from the real dataset, while the generator gives a generated sample $G(z)$. The error is determined using the discriminator's output and the ground truth labels, and the discriminator's parameters are updated according to this error through the backpropagation algorithm as shown in Fig. 6.1.

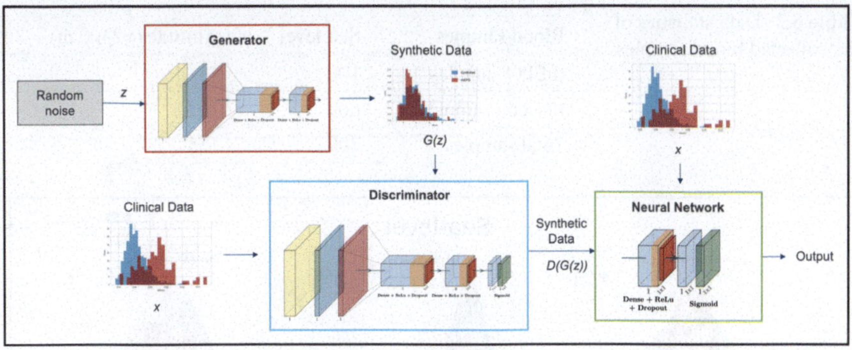

Fig. 6.1 Architecture of GAN for generating blood samples

6.3 Evaluation

6.3.1 Data Description

Collecting health-related data on elite athletes is a difficult task as there are issues like data accessibility and privacy. Therefore, the dataset used in this study is from the clinical experiment, which is well described by Rahman et al. (2022). The clinical trial was performed under real-world conditions and included two groups: one at "sea-level" with 34 participants and another at "altitude" with 39 participants. The experiment was divided into three phases: at baseline (weeks 1–4), intervention (weeks 5–8), and follow-up (weeks 9–12) period. Both groups were at sea-level during the baseline and follow-up. However, during the 4-week intervention period, one group stayed at the sea-level while the other group was at a moderate altitude of 2300 m. This 4-week duration corresponds to the usual regimes of athletic training, in which the altitude training camps are rarely longer than that.

None of the participants were exposed to the performance-enhancing drug throughout the baseline and follow-up phases. However, during the intervention phase, the participants were given 11 injections, one after another, every two days. For the sea-level group, 25 individuals were given rhEPO injections, and the remaining 9 were given placebos. In the case of the altitude group, 12 patients were injected with rhEPO, and 27 were given placebos. In total, 864 blood samples were collected during the complete study. The data statistics are well described in the Table 6.2. Figure 6.2 shows the distribution of all the haematological parameters of the rhEPO as well as the placebo samples collected at the sea-level.

Table 6.2 Data statistics of the collected blood samples

Blood samples	Sea-level	Altitude (=2300 m)
rhEPO samples	100	48
Placebo samples	609	107
Total samples	709	155

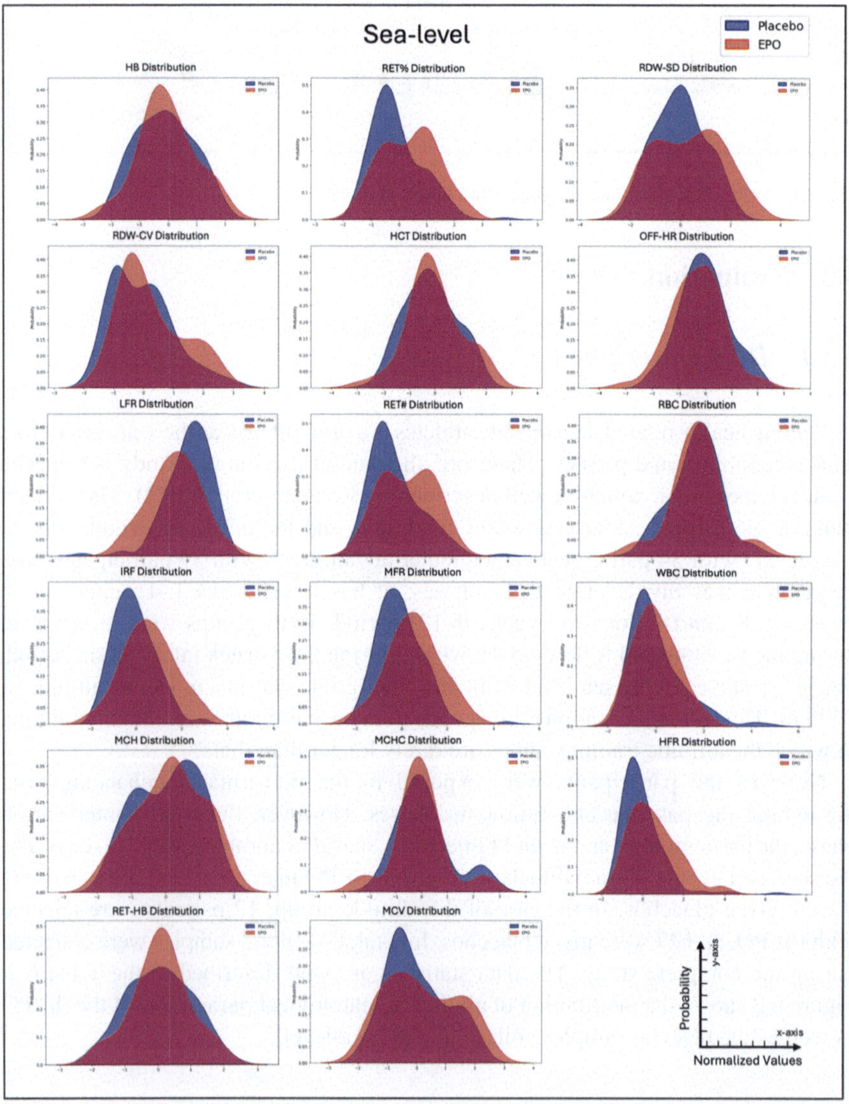

Fig. 6.2 Distribution of all the haematological parameters for rhEPO and Placebo samples collected at sea-level

6.3.2 Performance Metrics

Sample Distribution Comparison

The most basic method for evaluating the utility of generated datasets involves comparing the quantity and distribution of samples generated for each simulated individual against those in the real clinical data. This consists in plotting the number of samples per participant as histograms to observe and compare the average values. Additionally, to assess the distribution of sample types in both real and generated datasets, we calculate the probability distribution for each type of sample within each dataset.

Marginal Distribution Comparison

To evaluate how closely synthetic datasets mimic real clinical samples, we can look at the marginal distributions of individual haematological parameters. This involves analyzing the distribution of each parameter independently to understand how well the synthetic data captures the variability and central tendencies observed in real blood samples. This approach ensures that our comparison of parameter distributions is not skewed by any irrelevant or missing values.

Kolmogorov–Smirnov test

To assess the distribution of the generated blood samples quantitatively, we can apply the two-sample Kolmogorov–Smirnov test (K-S test) to identify the key difference between the real and generated data samples. The K-S test is a well-established method for evaluating whether two datasets are likely to come from the same distribution (Dimitrova et al., 2020). It calculates the maximum discrepancy between the cumulative distribution functions of two populations (one placebo and the other subjected to rhEPO) as follows:

$$D_{a,b} = sup|F_a(x) - F_b(x)|$$

The test's null hypothesis, which assumes the two distributions originate from the same parent distribution, is rejected at a significance level of α if $D_{a,b}$ exceeds a specific threshold determined by the following equation involving the sample sizes of the placebo and rhEPO cohorts.

$$D_{a,b} > \sqrt{-\ln \frac{\alpha}{2} \cdot \frac{1 + \frac{b}{a}}{2b}}$$

where a and b are the number of placebo and rhEPO samples respectively.

6.4 Results

We performed the evaluation on the generated samples by using both qualitative and quantitative measures described in the previous section. Table 6.3 shows the mean and standard deviation of both real and generated samples. The d-value and p-values are calculated using the 2-sample K-S test to quantify the difference between the two distributions. Figure 6.3 shows the distribution of all the haematological parameters for real and generated samples at sea-level. The density plots demonstrate the quantitative analysis, showing that the generated data approximates the real data well in terms of central tendencies and variability. Nonetheless, the nuances captured in the plots highlight the need for further refinement of the data generation algorithms to ensure that the tail of the distribution and the very specific characteristics of the haematological distributions are more accurately generated. This is particularly important for any decision-making process where the accuracy of data simulation could have significant consequences.

Table 6.3 Comparison analysis of the generated data samples with respect to the real blood samples

	Real samples		Generated samples		2 sample K-S test	
	Mean	Std	Mean	Std	d-value	p-value
HB	14.24	1.13	14.09	1.05	0.10	2.1e−03
RET%	1.04	0.39	0.93	0.25	0.15	3.3e-07
RDW-SD	41.63	2.32	41.34	2.22	0.14	9.2e−07
RDW-CV	12.66	0.62	12.58	0.59	0.13	1.2e−05
HCT	41.52	2.98	41.06	2.71	0.11	4.5e−04
OFF-HR	82.00	15.03	83.58	13.62	0.07	5.1e−02
LFR	92.78	3.33	93.71	2.58	0.14	1.8e−06
RET#	0.05	0.02	0.04	0.01	0.16	1.9e−08
RBC	4.67	0.38	4.64	0.37	0.09	4.3e−03
IRF	7.22	3.33	6.29	2.59	0.14	3.7e−06
MFR	6.41	2.77	5.62	2.15	0.14	1.1e−06
WBC	5.65	1.51	5.44	1.5	0.16	2.1e−08
MCH	30.50	1.26	30.42	1.19	0.09	2.9e−03
MCHC	34.28	0.01	34.27	0.83	0.05	2.4e−01
HFR	0.81	0.74	0.67	0.58	0.17	1.0e−09
RET-HB	33.44	1.7	33.92	1.63	0.10	1.0e−03
MCV	88.98	3.08	88.77	2.95	0.05	1.8e−01

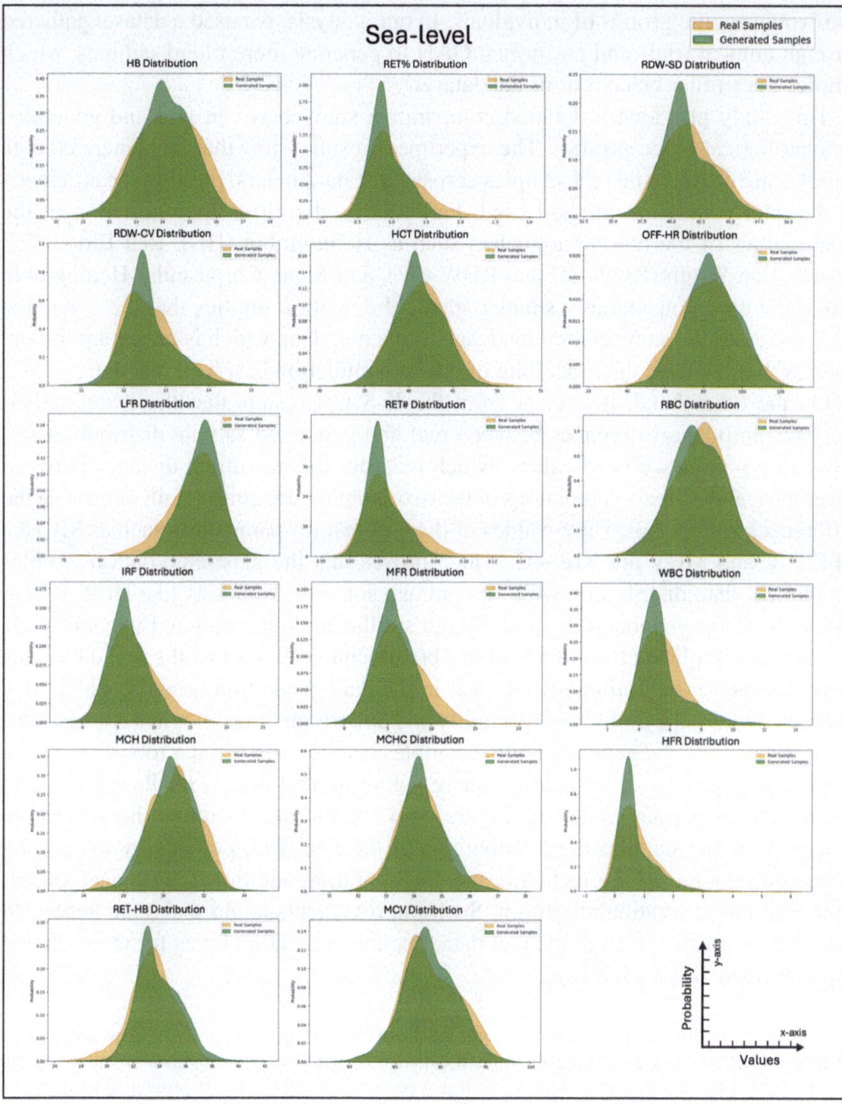

Fig. 6.3 Distribution of all the haematological parameters for real and generated samples for sea-level cohort

6.5 Conclusion

This study aims to explore the potential of generative modelling to improve the detection of blood doping in sports. In the recent past, the application of ML, particularly supervised learning techniques, has been a topic of interest in the context of anti-doping efforts. Such research often relies on data obtained from clinical studies involving specific groups of individuals. In our analysis, we used a dataset gathered through clinical trials and performed GAN to generate more blood samples, which mimics the similar behaviour of the dataset.

This study provided a detailed comparative study between real and generated haematological blood profiles. The experiment results show that the generated data samples are close to the real samples across most parameters, proving the efficiency of the data generation method used. Particularly, the close approximation in the mean values of the blood parameters such as Hemoglobin (HB), Red Blood Cell Distribution Width (RDW-SD and RDW-CV), and Mean Corpuscular Hemoglobin (MCH), with a considerably smaller standard deviation implies that the generated data possesses the same central tendency as the real data, which is important for any process that involves the modelling of data or simulation based on real data.

On the other hand, it is clear from the K-S test results that there are statistically insignificant differences between real and generated sample distributions, as proven by p-values. The d-values, which measure the maximum distance between the empirical distribution functions of the two samples, are quite small, indicating the differences are not big. The p-values of the K-S test for parameters such as MCHC, OFF-HR, and MCV are >1e−02, which proves that the generated data resembles the clinical data distribution well. In contrast, some distributions like HFR, RET#, and WBC had a p-value < 1e−08, though similar in their mean and variability, do not perfectly replicate the complex distribution characteristics of the real data. This could be due to the limitations inherent in the data generation process, which may not fully capture the biological variability and underlying physiological correlations.

In conclusion, the generated blood samples can be considered a robust proxy for real blood sample data for studies where gathering real data is challenging due to insufficient or privacy concerns. Future work should aim to refine the generation process to better capture the distributions of the real data, perhaps by integrating more complex modelling techniques or incorporating additional biological knowledge into the generation algorithm. Such improvements could make the generated data indistinguishable from the real data, opening new boundaries for research and application in doping analysis.

Acknowledgements We thank Prof. Nikolai Baastrup Nordsborg, University of Copenhagen and his research group for conducting the clinical experiment with the participants and collecting the blood samples for this analysis. This work was a part of the EPOPredictII project funded by the World Anti-Doping Agency (WADA).

References

Bunn, H. F. (2013). Erythropoietin. *Cold Spring Harbor Perspectives in Medicine, 3*(3), a011619.

Dimitrova, D. S., Kaishev, V. K., & Tan, S. (2020). Computing the Kolmogorov-Smirnov distribution when the underlying cdf is purely discrete, mixed or continuous. *Journal of Statistical Software, 95*(10), 1–42.

Goodfellow, I., Pouget-Abadie, J., Mirza, M., Xu, B., Warde-Farley, D., Ozair, S., Courville, A., & Bengio, Y. (2014). Generative adversarial nets. In *Advances in neural information processing systems* (pp. 2672–2680).

Goodnough, L. T., & Panigrahi, A. K. (2017). Blood transfusion therapy. *The Medical Clinics of North America, 101*(2), 431–447.

Heuberger, J. A., Cohen Tervaert, J. M., Schepers, F. M., Vliegenthart, A. D., Rotmans, J. I., Daniels, J. M., Burggraaf, J., & Cohen, A. F. (2013). Erythropoietin doping in cycling: Lack of evidence for efficacy and a negative risk-benefit. *British Journal of Clinical Pharmacology, 75*(6), 1406–1421.

Holt, R. I., Erotokritou-Mulligan, I., & Sönksen, P. H. (2009). The history of doping and growth hormone abuse in sport. *Growth Hormone & IGF Research: Official Journal of the Growth Hormone Research Society and the International IGF Research Society, 19*(4), 320–326.

Kelly, T., Beharry, A., & Fedoruk, M. (2019). Applying machine learning techniques to advance anti-doping. *European Journal of Sports and Exercise Science, 7*(2).

Kingma, D. P. & Welling, M. (2014). Auto-encoding variational Bayes. In *2nd International Conference on Learning Representations, ICLR 2014, Banff, AB, Canada, April 14–16, 2014, Conference Track Proceedings.*

Krumm, B., & Faiss, R. (2021). Factors confounding the athlete biological passport: A systematic narrative review. *Sports Medicine—Open, 7*(1), 65.

Manfredini, F., Malagoni, A. M., Litmanen, H., Zhukovskaja, L., Jeannier, P., Follo, D., Felisatti, M., Besseberg, A., Geistlinger, M., Bayer, P., & Carrabre, J. (2011). Performance and blood monitoring in sports: The artificial intelligence evoking target testing in antidoping (AR.I.E.T.T.A.) project. *The Journal of Sports Medicine and Physical Fitness, 51*(1), 153–159.

Mosquera, L., El Emam, K., Ding, L., et al. (2023). A method for generating synthetic longitudinal health data. *BMC Medical Research Methodology, 23*, 67.

Parisotto, R., Wu, M., Ashenden, M. J., Emslie, K. R., Gore, C. J., Howe, C., Kazlauskas, R., Sharpe, K., Trout, G. J., Xie, M., & Hahn, A. G. (2001). Detection of recombinant human erythropoietin abuse in athletes utilizing markers of altered erythropoiesis. *Haematologica, 86*(2), 128–137.

Plumb, J. O. M., Otto, J. M., & Grocott, M. P. W. (2016). 'Blood doping' from Armstrong to prehabilitation: Manipulation of blood to improve performance in athletes and physiological reserve in patients. *Extrem Physiol Med, 5*, 5.

Rahman, M.R., Bejder, J., Bonne, T. C., Andersen, A. B., Huertas, J.R., Aikin, R., Nordsborg, N. B., & Maass, W. (2022). Detection of erythropoietin in blood to uncover doping in sports using machine learning. In *Proceedings of the IEEE International Conference on Digital Health (ICDH)* (pp. 193–201).

Robinson, N., Giraud, S., Saudan, C., Baume, N., Avois, L., Mangin, P., & Saugy, M. (2006). Erythropoietin and blood doping. *British Journal of Sports Medicine, 40*(Suppl 1), i30–i34.

Santhanam, A. V., d'Uscio, L. V., & Katusic, Z. S. (2010). Cardiovascular effects of erythropoietin an update. *Advances in Pharmacology (San Diego, Calif.), 60*, 257–285.

Sharpe, K., Ashenden, M. J., & Schumacher, Y. O. (2006). A third generation approach to detect erythropoietin abuse in athletes. *Haematologica, 91*(3), 356–363.

Sottas, P.-E., Robinson, N., Giraud, S., Taroni, F., Kamber, M., Mangin, P., & Saugy, M. (2006). Statistical classification of abnormal blood profiles in athletes. *The International Journal of Biostatistics, 2*(1).

Vlad, R. A., Hancu, G., Popescu, G. C., & Lungu, I. A. (2018). Doping in sports, a never-ending story? *Advanced Pharmaceutical Bulletin, 8*(4), 529–534.

WADA. (2022). *Athlete biological passport*. https://www.wada-ama.org/en/athlete-biological-passport. Last accessed March 1, 2024.

Part III
Human-Computer Interaction

Chapter 7
A Brief Review of Artificial Intelligence for Sport Informatics in the Scope of Human–Computer Interaction

Marco Speicher and Patrick Berndt

Abstract This chapter delineates the evolving landscape at the intersection of Artificial Intelligence (AI), sports, movement, and health, emphasizing the pivotal role of Human–Computer Interaction (HCI). Highlighting the surge in AI integration within sports, movement analysis, and health management, we want to underscore its transformative impact on performance analysis, injury prevention, and personalized healthcare interventions. By elucidating the progression from rudimentary applications to sophisticated data-driven analyses, HCI has an indispensable role in crafting user-centric interfaces and experiences tailored to individuals' needs and preferences. Therefore, we provide a brief overview of AI's influence on athletic performance, injury management, and healthcare, advocating for human-centered design (HCD) principles to optimize user engagement and outcomes in this dynamic domain.

Keywords Artificial Intelligence · Computer Science in Sports · Human-Centered Design · Human-Computer Interaction · Human-Centered AI

7.1 Introduction

The convergence of Artificial Intelligence (AI) and the domains of sports, movement, and health have led to a new era of innovation and possibilities, reshaping the landscape of Human-Computer Interaction (HCI). This brief review navigates the multifaceted intersection of AI and HCI, shedding light on emerging trends that impact the way individuals engage with technology in the pursuit of fitness, sports excellence, and overall wellbeing.

M. Speicher (✉) · P. Berndt
Deutsche Hochschule für Prävention und Gesundheitsmanagement (DHfPG), Saarbrücken, Germany
e-mail: m-speicher@dhfpg-bsa.de

C. Dindorf et al. (eds.), *Artificial Intelligence in Sports, Movement, and Health*,
https://doi.org/10.1007/978-3-031-67256-9_7

In recent years, the integration of AI into sports, movement analysis, and health management has surged, fueled by advancements in Machine Learning (ML) algorithms, sensor technology, and data analytics (Teufl et al., 2021). From the analysis of biomechanical data to the prediction of injury risks and the optimization of training regimens, AI is transforming how athletes, coaches, and healthcare professionals approach performance enhancement and injury management (Bates et al., 2023). Moreover, the proliferation of wearable devices, smart sensors, as well as mobile health and exercise applications has facilitated the collection of vast amounts of data on individual movement patterns, physiological metrics, and lifestyle behaviors, providing valuable insights for personalized health and sports performance monitoring, exercise prescription and intervention strategies (Oyebode et al., 2022; Phatak et al., 2021).

The development of AI in the field of sports and health informatics is characterized by the path from rudimentary applications to highly developed, data-driven analyses. Central to this evolution is the crucial role of HCI, a facet that has grown essentially as human-centered technologies and interfaces have settled in the landscape of athletic performance and health management. HCI encompasses the design, evaluation, and optimization of user interfaces, interactive systems, and digital experiences tailored to the needs, preferences, and capabilities of individuals (Dix, 2003). In the context of sports and health AI applications, effective HCI is essential for ensuring seamless interaction, intuitive user experiences, valid data collection, and meaningful engagement with technology-driven solutions. By integrating principles of Human-Centered Design (HCD), usability engineering, and User Experience (UX) research, HCI professionals strive to create AI-powered applications that empower users to make informed decisions, optimize recovery and athletic performance, and enhance their overall health, fitness, and wellbeing (Blandford, 2019).

This review aims to provide a concise understanding of the growing intersection between AI, sports, movement, and health. We have explored how AI technologies are transforming various facets of athletic performance, injury prevention, rehabilitation, and personalized healthcare. Additionally, we want to underscore the critical role of HCI in facilitating effective communication and collaboration between humans and AI systems in this dynamic domain. The scope encompasses key applications, trends, and implications of AI in sports, movement, and health while emphasizing the need for HCD and seamless integration of technology to optimize outcomes and experiences for stakeholders across diverse disciplines.

7.2 Artificial Intelligence Applications in Sports Informatics

AI applications in sports informatics take center stage, with a focus on analytics, performance analysis, exercise prescription and strategic optimization. We briefly present the benefits of AI and highlight its role in designing not only results, but also improving health, performance and injury prevention. This is followed by an overview of AI applications in sports analysis in order to be able to discuss the role of HCI in the sports, fitness and health sector in more detail with regard to AI.

7.2.1 *Overview of Artificial Intelligence Applications in Sports Analytics*

Sports analytics has seen a fundamental shift with the integration of AI technologies, revolutionizing the way in which coaches and athletes analyze and interpret data. AI applications in sports analytics include a variety of techniques and methods that aim to extract actionable insights from complex data sets. The quantitative analysis of sports has grown initially through non-academic work (Kubatko et al., 2007) and has received extensive academic interest in the past decade. This section provides an overview of contemporary AI applications in scientific sports analytics and highlights their importance for improving performance, optimizing strategies, and driving innovation in the sports industry.

7.2.1.1 Data Processing and Pattern Recognition

The core of AI-powered sports analytics is the ability to process large amounts of data with high speed and accuracy. ML algorithms, including Deep Learning (DL) models, excel at recognizing patterns and extracting meaningful insights from various data sources such as training statistics, recordings, and sensor data.

Topics such as data processing and pattern recognition are particularly fundamental components of AI-powered sports analytics, facilitating the extraction of actionable insights from complex data sets (Biró et al., 2023). When analyzing complex data sets, the five V's of big data should be taken into account: volume, velocity, variety, veracity, and value (George et al., 2016). In the field of sports, where data volumes continue to grow rapidly, and the pace of data generation shows no signs of slowing down, the application of advanced ML algorithms is central to uncovering meaningful patterns and trends. Moreover, the variety of data sources, including game footage, player statistics, and sensor data, presents both challenges and opportunities for analysis. Through the use of AI-powered systems, sports organizations can harness the value of this diverse data landscape, leveraging it to gain valuable insights into player performance and team strategies. Additionally, the veracity of data, ensuring its accuracy and reliability, is paramount in the development and deployment of ML models for sports analytics. Finally, velocity is represented by the ability to process data in real-time, which allows for timely decision-making and adaptive strategies during live games and training sessions, further emphasizing the significance of advanced algorithms in the modern sports landscape. By analyzing historical performance data and identifying correlations between variables, AI systems can uncover hidden patterns and trends that may elude human observation, providing valuable insights into athlete behavior, training data dynamics, and team strategies (Novatchkov & Baca, 2013).

Techniques such as DL, Convolutional Neural Networks (CNNs), and Recurrent Neural Networks (RNNs) are characterized by the detection of complex patterns in various data sources. CNNs, for example, have been successfully used in the analysis of sports videos and have enabled the automatic recognition of player actions and events in soccer matches (Jiang et al., 2016). In addition, RNNs have demonstrated their effectiveness in modeling temporal dependencies in sequential sports data, such as player trajectories and match sequences (Lucey et al., 2014).

7.2.1.2 Predictive Modeling and Performance Forecasting

The advent of wearable sensors and computer vision technology has revolutionized athlete tracking and movement analysis in sports. AI algorithms can process real-time data streams from GPS trackers, accelerometers, and video feeds to monitor athletes' movements, quantify performance metrics, and identify areas for improvement. Through techniques such as pose estimation and motion capture, AI systems can reconstruct player trajectories, measure biomechanical parameters, and assess movement efficiency, providing coaches and trainers with actionable feedback for optimizing training regimens and preventing injuries (Claudino et al., 2019).

For example, researchers demonstrated the effectiveness of ML algorithms in predicting game outcomes and player performance in basketball based on factors such as player statistics, team dynamics, and situational variables (Kubatko et al., 2007). They used Support Vector Machine (SVM) considering both classifier performance and the complexity of the dataset. The resulting model was developed based on a tracking dataset of players and ball trajectories in 32,377 possessions from nearly 630 basketball games in the 2012/13 NBA season. Furthermore, the analysis of basketball data to gain competitive advantages is of interest to the clubs and is linked to the financial success of a team (Demenius & Kreivytė, 2017).

AI-powered predictive models enable organizations in sports to anticipate outcomes, evaluate athletes' potential, and predict performance metrics with higher accuracy. By using historical data and statistical algorithms, predictive analytics tools can make forecasts for various scenarios, including at sporting events, such as results, injuries, and team dynamics (Molavian et al., 2023). These insights enable coaches and managers to make informed decisions regarding player selection, match tactics, and resource allocation to maximize their team's competitive advantage and performance results.

Similarly, a recent work has highlighted the potential of predictive modeling techniques in predicting match outcomes in soccer, using complex datasets that include player biometrics, match conditions and tactical strategies (Bunker & Susnjak, 2022). By leveraging these predictive insights, sports teams can make informed decisions regarding player selection, match tactics, and resource allocation, ultimately maximizing their competitive advantage and on-field performance outcomes.

By analyzing game footage, scouting reports, and statistical data, AI systems can identify recurring patterns, exploit opponent weaknesses, and recommend strategic adjustments tailored to specific game situations (Pavitt et al., 2021). Whether through automated play recommendation systems or interactive decision support tools, AI empowers coaches and players to adapt their strategies dynamically, maximize their team's strengths, and outmaneuver their opponents on the field.

7.2.1.3 Using Wearable Technology for Fitness Training

In addition to the individualized application of current findings for training control, the development, research, and application of new technical possibilities are also becoming increasingly important for modern strength and fitness training. Many individuals struggle to maintain or increase their exercise routines, leading to suboptimal activity levels. However, research indicates that automatically tracking exercise, especially through pedometry, can significantly boost motivation and encourage physical activity (Pelletier et al., 2021). This underscores the importance of leveraging technology to facilitate and sustain healthy lifestyles.

Although the implementation of emerging technologies, such as fitness wearables, presents trainers and athletes with the challenge of integrating these tools and methods into training management in a meaningful way, in most cases, it enables more precise load control or more comprehensive monitoring of recovery and performance parameters (Pizzo et al., 2021). Such technical aids are usually based on compact sensor systems that are either worn on the body or attached to training equipment to record, process, and transmit relevant health or performance-related parameters to other devices. Fitness wearables and other sensor-based aids are used in the context of sports training not only to test the actual performance level or to check performance development but also to record the health and regeneration status, to monitor the training load and individual stress within a training session and to automatically record movements (Passos et al., 2021).

A special category of these wearable sensor systems uses so-called inertial measurement units (IMU) to record translational and rotational accelerations in multi-dimensional space. A systematic review of the use of wearable inertial sensor units showed that such devices are used in sport, particularly to record athletic or physical performance, physical activity and sport motor requirements, as well as to analyze the quality of movement in competitive and high-performance sport (Camomilla et al., 2018). In the context of resistance training, these devices are primarily used to record the movement trajectory and velocity of free weights, such as barbells, which enables, among other things, the monitoring of movement technique and the velocity-based control of load intensity and duration (Weakley et al., 2021). Most inertial sensor systems available on the market for recording barbell speed are considered valid and reliable (Clemente et al., 2021).

In the context of resistance training, the use of this sensor technology to measure velocity has led to the establishment of a new approach to exercise prescription known as "velocity-based training". In contrast to the traditional load-based approach, in which the intensity is controlled by the amount of load and the duration by the number of repetitions, the velocity-based approach uses the velocity of the moving load or the extent of its reduction over several repetitions within a training set as the central prescription variable (Weakley et al., 2021).

Overall, the increasing interest in wearables for sports and fitness emphases the need for design knowledge to shape future designs in this area. To address this, researchers presented a design space of wearables for sports and fitness practices, drawing from a survey of previous research (Turmo Vidal et al., 2021). They identified core design decisions related to wearability, technology design, and wearable use in practice, considering the goals of introducing technology, the balance between pre-designed features and user appropriation, and the social dynamics of the practice. By characterizing prior work within this design space, the authors identified trends and opportunities for design in wearables for sports and fitness.

7.2.2 *Examples of Successful Artificial Intelligence Implementations in Professional Sports*

The following non-academic examples demonstrate the significant impact of AI implementations in professional sports, ranging from player performance monitoring and injury prevention to fan engagement and data-driven decision-making. As AI technologies continue to evolve, we can expect further innovations and advancements that will reshape the landscape of sports analytics and enhance the overall sports experience for athletes, teams, and fans alike.

7.2.2.1 Catapult Sports in Soccer

Catapult Sports (https://www.catapult.com) is a company that specializes in wearable technology designed to monitor athlete performance in various sports, including soccer. Professional soccer teams have increasingly adopted Catapult's wearable devices to track player movements, physical exertion, and injury risks during training sessions and matches. By leveraging AI algorithms, Catapult's technology processes data collected from these wearables to provide coaches and sports scientists with actionable insights into player performance and conditioning. For instance, AI-powered analytics can identify patterns in player movement, assess fatigue levels, and recommend personalized training programs to optimize performance and minimize injury risks (Barrett, 2017). Several soccer clubs, including English Premier League teams and international squads, have reported significant improvements in player fitness, tactical decision-making, and injury prevention because of implementing Catapult's AI-driven sports analytics solutions.

7.2.2.2 HomeCourt for Basketball Analytics

HomeCourt (https://www.homecourt.ai) is an AI-powered mobile application designed to revolutionize basketball training and skill development. Leveraging computer vision and ML algorithms, HomeCourt analyzes basketball players' movements and shooting techniques using the camera of a smartphone or tablet. The app tracks key metrics such as shot accuracy, release angle, and shooting arc in real-time, providing instant feedback and personalized coaching tips to help players improve their skills. With its AI-driven analysis capabilities, HomeCourt enables players to track their progress, identify areas for improvement, and compete with friends and teammates in skill challenges and drills. The app's intuitive interface and gamified features make basketball training more engaging and accessible to players of all skill levels, from amateur enthusiasts to professional athletes. HomeCourt has garnered widespread acclaim within the basketball community and has been endorsed by top players and coaches for its innovative approach to skill development and performance optimization. As a result, HomeCourt represents a groundbreaking example of how AI technology is transforming sports training and empowering athletes to reach their full potential on the court.

7.2.2.3 Enduco for Endurance Training

Endurance training is a critical component of athletic development, particularly for endurance athletes such as cyclists, runners, and triathletes. To optimize performance and achieve peak fitness levels, athletes require tailored training plans, personalized coaching, and effective performance tracking tools. Enduco (https://enduco.app), a leading platform for endurance training, offers comprehensive solutions designed to meet the unique needs of endurance athletes. Enduco has emerged as a valuable asset for endurance athletes, offering a comprehensive suite of tools and resources to optimize training, track performance, and achieve peak athletic performance. By leveraging Enduco's capabilities, athletes can unlock their full potential, push their limits, and reach new heights in their endurance pursuits. The key takeaways can be summarized as follows: (1) Personalized training plans tailored to individual needs can optimize performance, (2) real-time performance tracking and analysis are essential for informed decision-making, (3) seamless coach collaboration fosters effective communication and training strategies, and (4) motivation and accountability are crucial factors in achieving endurance training goals. By embracing innovative solutions like Enduco, athletes can embark on a journey of continuous improvement, resilience, and success in their endurance endeavors.

7.2.2.4 Enode for Strength Training

Enode (https://enode.ai) has revolutionized strength training in professional sports through its innovative AI-driven approach. By integrating advanced algorithms and data analytics, Enode provides personalized training programs tailored to individual athletes' needs, optimizing performance and minimizing the risk of injury. Utilizing an in-house IMU, the technology records biomechanical data and visualizes it in the app in real-time. Their velocity-based training approach allows for precise monitoring and adjustment of training protocols based on velocity metrics, enhancing strength, power, and endurance. Professional sports teams worldwide rely on Enode's platform to maximize their athletes' potential and maintain peak physical condition throughout the rigorous season.

7.3 HCI in Sports and Health Artificial Intelligence

A critical facet of this survey is the examination of HCI within the context of AI applications in sports and health. The seamless integration of AI technologies into user experiences is essential for their effective adoption. With this survey, we want to shed light on design considerations, challenges, and solutions in ensuring that AI enhances rather than hinders the interaction between humans and technology in the pursuit of fitness and well-being.

7.3.1 Evolution of HCI in Sports, Health and Fitness

The fitness sector is a sub-sector of the sports and health industry that often goes unnoticed. The fitness industry has undergone a remarkable transformation with the advent of technology, particularly in the realm of HCI. Historically, fitness enthusiasts relied on conventional methods for tracking progress and monitoring performance, such as pen-and-paper logs and manual calculations. However, the integration of digital technologies, wearable devices, and AI-powered applications has revolutionized how individuals engage with fitness and health activities (Cooper et al., 2018).

In the early stages, HCI in the fitness industry primarily focused on digitizing traditional workout routines and providing basic tracking capabilities. Simple interfaces and rudimentary feedback mechanisms laid the groundwork for more sophisticated applications that catered to the evolving needs and expectations of users. As technology advanced, HCI principles began to play a more prominent role in the design and development of fitness-oriented software and hardware (Chatterjee et al., 2022).

The emergence of AI-driven analytics and personalized coaching platforms marked a significant turning point in the evolution of HCI in the fitness industry. These platforms leverage ML algorithms to analyze user data, generate actionable insights, and deliver tailored recommendations for optimizing performance and achieving fitness goals. By harnessing the power of AI, HCI practitioners have been able to create immersive and adaptive experiences that resonate with users on a deeper level (Palumbo et al., 2020).

As HCI continues to evolve in the fitness industry, there is a growing emphasis on inclusivity, accessibility, and User-Centered Design (UCD). Developers are striving to create inclusive experiences that cater to diverse demographics and accommodate varying levels of physical ability and technological literacy. Additionally, ensuring seamless integration with existing hardware and software ecosystems remains a key priority, as interoperability and compatibility issues can hinder user adoption and satisfaction.

In conclusion, the evolution of HCI in fitness, sports and health reflects a dynamic interplay between technological innovation, UX design, and evolving consumer expectations. By embracing HCD principles and leveraging cutting-edge technologies, HCI practitioners are driving forward the next frontier of fitness, sports, and health innovation, empowering individuals more efficiently to lead healthier, more active lifestyles.

7.3.2 Importance of Seamless Interaction Between Humans and Artificial Intelligence Systems

AI-driven applications can personalize user experiences based on individual preferences, behaviors, and performance metrics. This personalization should enhance engagement and effectiveness by tailoring recommendations, feedback, and for example training programs to the specific needs and goals of users. HCI methods prioritize understanding the needs, preferences, and behaviors of users to inform the design process (Dix, 2003). User research, personas, and user journeys help identify user requirements and pain points, ensuring that the applications address real-world challenges effectively. Moreover, UI/UX design focuses on creating interfaces that are intuitive, visually appealing, and easy to navigate. Clear navigation, logical information architecture, and consistent visual elements enhance usability and accessibility, enabling users to interact with the applications effortlessly.

However, there is limited understanding of how individuals interact with personalized predictions. To address this, a smartphone app called GlucOracle generates personalized forecasts for post-meal blood glucose levels using self-tracking data from individuals with type 2 diabetes (Desai et al., 2019). The app was pilot tested with two populations: an online diabetes community and a low socio-economic status community. Individuals from both groups found the personalized glucose forecasts useful for adjusting immediate meal options and planning future meals. The study also highlighted new questions regarding the appropriate timing, format, and focus of forecasts, and suggested new research directions for personalized predictions in health.

Consumer-facing health technologies, particularly AI-based symptom checkers (AISCs), emerge in everyday healthcare practice. AISCs gather symptom information from users and offer medical suggestions and potential diagnoses, a role traditionally associated with healthcare professionals such as physicians and expert patients. This development raises questions about how AISCs influence and transform the concept of medical authority in individuals' healthcare practices. To explore this, a recent study conducted interviews with thirty AISC users, examining how users perceive the medical authority of AISCs based on factors like automated decisions, interaction design patterns, connections to established medical authorities, and comparisons with other health technologies (You et al., 2021). The findings shed light on the utilization of AISCs in healthcare delivery, the transformation of traditional notions of medical authority by AI, and implications for designing AI-enabled health technologies.

In general, AI algorithms enable applications to process large volumes of complex data quickly and accurately. In clinical settings, algorithms often have to work with incomplete patient data and incompletely documented disease progressions (Schmidt et al., 2015). In sports analytics, AI processes data from various sources, such as player statistics, game footage, and sensor data, to derive actionable insights and predictions.

AI techniques such as ML and DL enable the identification of patterns, trends, and correlations within the data. This allows for predictive modeling in sports analytics, such as forecasting match outcomes, player performance, and injury risks. Despite the promise of DL algorithms to enhance workflows and outcomes, their real-world efficacy remains to be fully demonstrated. A recent study emphasizes the importance of conducting human-centered evaluative research alongside prospective evaluations of model accuracy to better understand and optimize the integration of AI technologies into health settings (Beede et al., 2020).

Specifically, the focus in medical image retrieval systems for aiding medical decision-making processes using ML is on retrieving visually similar medical images from past cases to assist in diagnosing new patients. However, no algorithm can perfectly match an expert's notion of similarity for every case, potentially leading to irrelevant results for a doctor's specific diagnostic needs (Cai et al., 2019). Therefore, one major requirement when searching for similar images retrieved by a DL algorithm is to empower users to adjust the search algorithm dynamically, emphasizing the types of similarity most crucial at different moments. Furthermore, users adopt new strategies by repurposing these tools to test the underlying algorithm and differentiate ML errors from their own mistakes. These insights could inform the development of future human-ML collaborative systems for expert decision-making in fitness, sports and health contexts.

HCI methods emphasize providing timely and meaningful feedback to users to guide their interactions and facilitate learning. Visual feedback, progress indicators, and notifications keep users informed about their actions, progress, and achievements, fostering motivation and engagement. Interaction design ensures that the user journey within the application is seamless and coherent. Well-designed interaction patterns, gestures, and transitions enhance the flow of interaction, minimizing cognitive load and friction points, and maximizing user satisfaction and retention.

7.3.3 The Role of HCD in the Interaction Design Process

HCD is an approach to creating products, services, and systems that focuses on understanding the needs, behaviors, and preferences of the people who will use them. It involves actively involving end-users in the design process, empathizing with their experiences, and iterating on designs based on their feedback. HCD aims to ensure that the final product meets the users' needs effectively and provides a positive and intuitive user experience.

7.3.3.1 Human-Centered Design and Human-Centered Artificial Intelligence

In the context of AI-powered applications for sports and health, HCD is particularly crucial for several reasons. First and foremost, these applications deal with sensitive and personal aspects of individuals' lives, such as their physical health, fitness goals, and performance metrics. By prioritizing HCD principles, developers can create applications that are sensitive to users' privacy concerns, preferences, and comfort levels with technology.

Furthermore, the effectiveness of sports and health applications relies heavily on user engagement and adherence to the recommended activities or interventions. By involving users in the design process and incorporating their feedback, developers can create applications that are intuitive, motivating, and enjoyable to use. This, in turn, could increase user engagement and improve outcomes related to health and wellness.

Concerns are growing regarding the values embedded in AI systems, their decision-making processes, and their social consequences, especially in everyday applications such as spam filtering, credit scoring, and search engines. The inscrutability of AI models, embedded biases, privacy issues, and environmental costs are significant considerations. The term "human-centered AI" (HCAI) is gaining traction, reflecting a desire for AI to serve people amidst concerns about potential exploitation and manipulation. However, the definition of HCAI varies widely, encompassing different perspectives on the role of humans in AI systems. By examining peer-reviewed articles, a recent review paper seeks to identify trends, gaps, and opportunities in HCAI research, providing a foundation for further exploration in this field (Capel & Brereton, 2023). They present a historical overview of HCAI and describe the methodology used to review papers, culminating in a map of the current state of HCAI research. This map aids in visualizing relationships between different approaches, methods, and tools in the field and underlines the complexity of designing and evaluating AI. Their approach includes Ethical AI, Explainable and Interpretable AI, and Humans Teaming with AI, and combines those fields with an Human-centered Approach to design and evaluate AI.

While User-Centered Design (UCD) is undoubtedly valuable for creating products and systems tailored to the needs and preferences of users, HCD offers a broader and more holistic approach that considers the entire spectrum of human experiences, capabilities, and contexts (Dix, 2003). HCD is considered as the right choice for future developments of AI-driven applications in fitness, sports, and health.

HCD extends beyond individual users to encompass diverse stakeholders, including caregivers, family members, communities, and the society as a whole. By considering the broader human ecosystem, HCD ensures that technological solutions are inclusive, equitable, and responsive to the needs of all individuals, regardless of age, ability, background, or circumstance.

- HCD places a strong emphasis on empathy, understanding, and advocacy for users' voices and experiences. By engaging users as co-creators and partners in the design process, HCD empowers individuals to actively participate in shaping the technologies that impact their lives, fostering a sense of ownership, trust, and empowerment.
- By prioritizing human needs, values, and well-being, HCD creates opportunities for long-term value creation and positive social impact. By designing with empathy and foresight, HCD practitioners can develop solutions that not only address immediate challenges but also contribute to meaningful improvements in quality of life, health outcomes, and societal well-being over time.

In summary, while UCD is an important aspect of HCD, the latter offers a more comprehensive and inclusive approach that considers the broader human experience, societal impacts, and ethical dimensions of technology design and implementation. As we navigate an increasingly complex and interconnected world, HCD serves as a guiding framework for creating technologies that are not only useful and usable but also ethical, equitable, and empowering for all individuals and communities.

7.3.3.2 Brief Outline of HCD from the HCI Community Regarding Sports, Fitness and Health

The HCD framework is an approach to designing products, services, and systems that prioritizes understanding the needs, behaviors, and preferences of the people who will use them. It involves iterative processes of observation, ideation, prototyping, and testing, with a focus on empathizing with users and incorporating their feedback throughout the design process.

In the context of health and sports software and hardware, the HCD framework is used to develop solutions that are tailored to the unique requirements of users in these domains. This includes considerations such as usability, accessibility, motivation, and engagement, as well as integration with existing workflows and technologies in healthcare and sports settings.

Researchers and practitioners in HCI have explored various applications of HCD in health and sports technology. While specific studies and papers from high impact conferences vary from year to year, there have been numerous contributions that address HCD principles and methodologies in these domains. Some noteworthy examples of topics related to HCD in health and sports technology that have been presented in the last decade include:

- **UCD of Fitness Trackers**: Studies focusing on the design and evaluation of fitness trackers and wearables, considering factors such as user preferences, motivation, and usability.
- **Interactive Systems for Physical Rehabilitation**: Research on the development of interactive systems and applications to support physical rehabilitation and therapy, with a focus on user engagement and adherence to treatment protocols.
- **Mobile Health Applications**: Investigations into the design and usability of mobile health applications for chronic disease management, medication adherence, and behavior change interventions.
- **Accessible and Inclusive Design**: Efforts to make health and sports technologies more accessible to users with disabilities, including studies on inclusive design practices and the development of assistive technologies.
- **Gamification and Behavior Change**: Exploration of gamification strategies and behavior change techniques to promote healthy lifestyles and facilitate adherence to exercise and wellness programs.

The HCI community has consistently demonstrated interest in applying human-centered design principles to address challenges and opportunities in health and sports technology. Researchers and practitioners continue to explore innovative approaches to designing interactive systems and interfaces that enhance user experiences and improve outcomes in these domains.

7.3.4 *Challenges and Solutions in Ensuring Effective HCI in Artificial Intelligence-Powered Applications*

By considering the human factors throughout the design and development process, sports and health applications can be tailored to meet the unique needs and preferences of users, ultimately leading to more effective and impactful solutions for promoting health. Nonetheless, ensuring effective HCI for AI-powered software and hardware in the context of fitness, sports, and health presents several challenges.

AI algorithms often operate as "black boxes", making it difficult for users to understand how decisions are made. In the context of health and sports, users may be hesitant to trust AI recommendations without insight into the underlying rationale. Assessments can be contentious, leading to expert disagreement. This raises the question of how AI assistants should be designed to handle the classification of ambiguous cases. Explanations containing irrelevant arguments could reduce experts' accuracy in correcting AI-suggested labels, potentially dropping below 50% (Schaekermann et al., 2020). These observations underscore the importance of clarity and relevance in AI-generated explanations for enhancing experts' decision-making processes.

Despite the widespread use of AI applications, the general public often lacks the understanding of how black-box algorithms operate and how to address biases effectively. Therefore, researchers have addressed these challenges through various approaches and methodologies. They provided insights into the importance of Explainable AI (XAI) in healthcare and discussed potential ethical concerns related to the lack of transparency in AI-powered systems (Yuan et al., 2023). Researchers have formulated 18 human-AI interaction guidelines (Amershi et al., 2019), like "Make clear what the system can do". The User Interface (UI) should help the user to understand what the AI system is capable of doing. An example of the application of this policy would be an activity tracker where all the metrics it tracks should be displayed and explained at the same time.

Despite existing strategies, translating research findings into practical design applications is a key challenge for effective solutions. For example, there are several challenges and opportunities in integrating insights from personal health informatics research into the design of applications for health, everyday life, or collaboration with clinicians. Researchers tested a prototype set of design cards through interviews with student designers and health-focused professional designers/researchers, revealing various tensions, barriers, and needs in designing health-related technologies (Kirchner et al., 2021). The findings emphasize the importance of supporting designers in addressing knowledge gaps, advocating for user needs, and integrating evidence-based approaches in health-related design projects.

Ideally, those systems should be able to personalize recommendations and adapt to individual user needs and preferences. However, designing algorithms that accurately capture user preferences while avoiding biases and ensuring data privacy can be challenging. Furthermore, providing meaningful feedback to users is crucial for fostering trust in AI-powered systems. Feedback mechanisms must strike a balance between being informative and not overwhelming users with unnecessary information. A recent paper examined the role of personalization in adaptive and persuasive systems for health and wellness. In this work, they presented strategies for designing personalized interventions that effectively motivate behavior change (Oyebode et al., 2022).

One of the most important and equally most difficult challenges to ensure is data privacy and security. Health and fitness data are highly sensitive, and users expect strict privacy protections. Designing AI-powered systems that collect, store, and analyze data while maintaining user privacy and complying with regulations presents significant challenges. Researchers explored privacy concerns in mobile technology for personal healthcare (Avancha et al., 2012). They discussed privacy-preserving techniques and design strategies for ensuring the security of user data in health-related applications.

Overall, HCD is important for AI-powered applications in sports and health contexts because it helps ensure that the technology is not only technically robust but also genuinely useful, usable, and valuable to the people it is intended to serve. These challenges should not be disregarded, as otherwise, both the UX and the effectiveness of the system could suffer. In summary, by addressing challenges related to interpretability, personalization, feedback, privacy, and user engagement, researchers can create more effective and user-friendly systems that promote health and effective training.

7.4 Conclusion and Future Work

In conclusion, this survey summarizes the transformative impact of AI on sports, exercise, and health informatics and highlights its profound influence through concepts from HCI. We can only speculate about the future of these advances. However, an increasingly dynamic landscape indicates that new innovations combining AI and HCI must continually redefine the boundaries of what is achievable in the realm of human performance, health and wellbeing.

The success of AI applications in sports depends on the synergy between AI capabilities and HCI methods. While AI enables advanced data analysis, prediction, and personalization, HCI methods ensure that the applications are user-centered, intuitive, engaging, and easy to use. The effective integration of AI and HCI principles results in applications that not only leverage the power of data-driven insights but also deliver superior user experiences that drive adoption, retention, and satisfaction.

While designers commonly encounter challenges when working with AI, particularly in the realms of sports, fitness, and health, these difficulties are not solely due to AI's algorithmic complexity and unpredictable behaviors. Given the multifaceted nature of these domains, there is a pressing need for increased collaboration between researchers in the fields of AI, HCI, sports science, exercise physiology, and healthcare. By fostering interdisciplinary partnerships, new conceptual frameworks can be developed to address human interactions with AI technologies within the context of sports training, fitness tracking, and healthcare management. This collaborative approach not only enhances the understanding of how AI can effectively support human performance and wellbeing but also promotes the integration of diverse perspectives and expertise, ultimately leading to more holistic and user-centric solutions in the sport, fitness, and health sectors. This collaboration is crucial for guiding more coherent interface designs and reflecting the relationships between user intentions and inferred models. The aim is to create a map of HCAI research that informs researchers about the breadth of ongoing studies, identifies gaps in research formulation, highlights areas for strengthening teams and projects, and encourages the exploration of new HCAI constructs and methodologies. Ultimately, the goal is to foster interdisciplinary efforts that enhance the understanding and application of HCAI principles in research and practice.

In the realm of HCI, the integration of AI presents a paradigm shift in how individuals interact with technology to achieve their health and fitness goals. HCI professionals play a pivotal role in designing intuitive user interfaces, interactive systems, and digital experiences that seamlessly integrate AI capabilities while prioritizing user needs, preferences, and capabilities. Through HCD principles and usability engineering, HCI fosters meaningful engagement with AI-driven solutions, empowering users to make informed decisions, enhance performance, and optimize their health outcomes.

Finally, the convergence of AI, sports, movement, and health informatics holds immense promise for transforming the way we approach fitness, sports excellence, and healthcare delivery. As AI continues to advance, its impact on HCI will be profound, reshaping the landscape of technology-mediated experiences and interactions in pursuit of improved human performance and wellbeing. Embracing the principles of HCD and the seamless integration of AI technologies is crucial to unlocking the full potential of this transformative synergy.

References

Amershi, S., Weld, D., Vorvoreanu, M., Fourney, A., Nushi, B., Collisson, P., Suh, J., Iqbal, S., Bennett, P., Inkpen, K., Teevan, J., Kikin-Gil, R., & Horvitz, E. (2019). Guidelines for human-AI interaction. In *Proceedings of the 2019 CHI Conference on Human Factors in Computing Systems* (pp. 1–13). Association for Computing Machinery.

Avancha, S., Baxi, A., & Kotz, D. (2012). Privacy in mobile technology for personal healthcare. *ACM Computing Surveys (CSUR), 45*(1), 1–54.

Barrett, S. (2017). Monitoring elite soccer players' external loads using real-time data. *International Journal of Sports Physiology and Performance, 12*(10), 1285–1287.

Bates, N. A., Huffman, A., Goodyear, E., Nagai, T., Rigamonti, L., Breuer, L., Holmes, B. D., & Schilaty, N. D. (2023). Physical clinical care and artificial-intelligence-guided core resistance training improve endurance and patient-reported outcomes in subjects with lower back pain. *Clinical Biomechanics (bristol, Avon), 103*, 105902. https://doi.org/10.1016/j.clinbiomech.2023.105902

Beede, E., Baylor, E., Hersch, F., Iurchenko, A., Wilcox, L., Ruamviboonsuk, P., & Vardoulakis, L. M. (2020). A human-centered evaluation of a deep learning system deployed in clinics for the detection of diabetic retinopathy. In *Proceedings of the 2020 CHI Conference on Human Factors in Computing Systems* (pp. 1–12). Presented at the, Honolulu, HI, USA. https://doi.org/10.1145/3313831.3376718

Biró, A., Cuesta-Vargas, A. I., & Szilágyi, L. (2023). AI-assisted fatigue and stamina control for performance sports on IMU-generated multivariate times series datasets. *Sensors (basel, Switzerland), 24*(1), 132. https://doi.org/10.3390/s24010132

Blandford, A. (2019). HCI for health and wellbeing: Challenges and opportunities. *International Journal of Human-Computer Studies, 131*, 41–51.

Bunker, R., & Susnjak, T. (2022). The application of machine learning techniques for predicting match results in team sport: A review. *Journal of Artificial Intelligence Research, 73*, 1285–1322.

Cai, C., Reif, E., Hegde, N., Hipp, J., Kim, B., Smilkov, D., Wattenberg, M., Viegas, F., Corrado, G., Stumpe, M., & Terry, M. (2019). Human-centered tools for coping with imperfect algorithms during medical decision-making. In *Proceedings of the 2019 CHI Conference on Human Factors in Computing Systems* (pp. 1–14). Association for Computing Machinery.

Camomilla, V., Bergamini, E., Fantozzi, S. & Vannozzi, G. (2018). Trends supporting the in-field use of wearable inertial sensors for sport performance evaluation: A systematic review. *Sensors (Basel, Switzerland), 18*(3). https://doi.org/10.3390/s18030873

Capel, T., & Brereton, M. (2023). What is human-centered about human-centered AI? A map of the research landscape. In *Proceedings of the 2023 CHI Conference on Human Factors in Computing Systems*. Association for Computing Machinery.

Chatterjee, A., Prinz, A., Gerdes, M., Martinez, S., Pahari, N., & Meena, Y. K. (2022). ProHealth eCoach: User-centered design and development of an eCoach app to promote healthy lifestyle with personalized activity recommendations. *BMC Health Services Research, 22*(1), 1120.

Claudino, J. G., Capanema, D. O., de Souza, T. V., Serrão, J. C., Machado Pereira, A. C., & Nassis, G. P. (2019). Current Approaches to the use of artificial intelligence for injury risk assessment and performance prediction in team sports: A systematic review. *Sports Medicine—Open, 5*(1), 28. https://doi.org/10.1186/s40798-019-0202-3

Clemente, F. M., Akyildiz, Z., Pino-Ortega, J. & Rico-González, M. (2021). Validity and reliability of the inertial measurement unit for barbell velocity assessments: A systematic review. *Sensors (Basel, Switzerland), 21*(7). https://doi.org/10.3390/s21072511

Cooper, C., Gross, A., Brinkman, C., Pope, R., Allen, K., Hastings, S., Bogen, B. E., & Goode, A. P. (2018). The impact of wearable motion sensing technology on physical activity in older adults. *Experimental Gerontology, 112*, 9–19.

Demenius, J., & Kreivytė, R. (2017). The benefits of advanced data analytics in basketball: Approach of managers and coaches of lithuanian basketball league teams. *Baltic Journal of Sport and Health Sciences, 1*(104).

Desai, P., Mitchell, E., Hwang, M., Levine, M., Albers, D., & Mamykina, L. (2019). Personal health oracle: Explorations of personalized predictions in diabetes self-management. In *Proceedings of the 2019 CHI Conference on Human Factors in Computing Systems* (pp. 1–13). Association for Computing Machinery.

Dix, A. (2003). *Human-computer interaction*. Pearson Education.

George, G., Osinga, E. C., Lavie, D., & Scott, B. A. (2016). Big data and data science methods for management research. *Academy of Management Journal, 59*(5), 1493–1507.

Jiang, H., Lu, Y., & Xue, J. (2016, November). Automatic soccer video event detection based on a deep neural network combined cnn and rnn. In *2016 IEEE 28th International Conference on Tools with Artificial Intelligence (ICTAI)* (pp. 490–494). IEEE.

Kirchner, S., Schroeder, J., Fogarty, J., & Munson, S. (2021). "They don't always think about that": Translational needs in the design of personal health informatics applications. In *Proceedings of the 2021 CHI Conference on Human Factors in Computing Systems*. Association for Computing Machinery.

Kubatko, J., Oliver, D., Pelton, K., & Rosenbaum, D. T. (2007). A starting point for analyzing basketball statistics. *Journal of Quantitative Analysis in Sports, 3*(3).

Lucey, P., Bialkowski, A., Carr, P., & Matthews, I. (2014). Representing and discovering adversarial team behaviors using player roles. In *Proceedings of the IEEE Conference on Computer Vision and Pattern Recognition* (pp. 2679–2686).

Molavian, R., Fatahi, A., Abbasi, H., & Khezri, D. (2023). Artificial intelligence approach in biomechanics of gait and sport: A systematic literature review. *Journal of Biomedical Physics & Engineering, 13*(5), 383–402. https://doi.org/10.31661/jbpe.v0i0.2305-1621

Novatchkov, H., & Baca, A. (2013). Artificial intelligence in sports on the example of weight training. *Journal of sports science & medicine, 12*(1), 27–37.

Oyebode, O., Fowles, J., Steeves, D., & Orji, R. (2022). Machine learning techniques in adaptive and personalized systems for health and wellness. *International Journal of Human–Computer Interaction, 39*(9), 1938–1962. https://doi.org/10.1080/10447318.2022.2089085

Palumbo, F., Crivello, A., Furfari, F., Girolami, M., Mastropietro, A., Manferdelli, G., Röcke, C., Guye, S., Salvá Casanovas, A., Caon, M., Carrino, F., Abou Khaled, O., Mugellini, E., Denna, E., Mauri, M., Ward, D., Subías-Beltrán, P., Orte, S., Candea, C., Candea, G., & Rizzo, G. (2020). "Hi This Is NESTORE, your personal assistant": Design of an Integrated IoT system for a personalized coach for healthy aging. *Frontiers in Digital Health, 2*, 545949.

Passos, J., Lopes, S. I., Clemente, F. M., Moreira, P. M., Rico-González, M., Bezerra, P., Rodrigues, L. P. (2021). Wearables and Internet of Things (IoT) technologies for fitness assessment: A systematic review. *Sensors (Basel, Switzerland), 21*(16). https://doi.org/10.3390/s21165418

Pavitt, J., Braines, D., & Tomsett, R. (2021). Cognitive analysis in sports: Supporting match analysis and scouting through artificial intelligence. *Applied AI Letters, 2*, e21. https://doi.org/10.1002/ail2.21

Pelletier, C., Gagnon, M. P., Alméras, N., Després, J. P., Poirier, P., Tremblay, A., Chabot, C., & Rhéaume, C. (2021). Using an activity tracker to increase motivation for physical activity in patients with type 2 diabetes in primary care: a randomized pilot trial. *mHealth, 7*, 59. https://doi.org/10.21037/mhealth-20-154

Phatak, A. A., Wieland, F. G., Vempala, K., Volkmar, F., & Memmert, D. (2021). Artificial intelligence based body sensor network framework-narrative review: Proposing an end-to-end framework using wearable sensors, real-time location systems and artificial intelligence/machine learning algorithms for data collection, data mining and knowledge discovery in sports and healthcare. *Sports Medicine—Open, 7*(1), 79. https://doi.org/10.1186/s40798-021-00372-0

Pizzo, A. D., Baker, B. J., Jones, G. J., & Funk, D. C. (2021). Sport experience design: Wearable fitness technology in the health and fitness industry. *Journal of Sport Management, 35*(2), 130–143. https://doi.org/10.1123/jsm.2020-0150

Schaekermann, M., Beaton, G., Sanoubari, E., Lim, A., Larson, K., & Law E. (2020). Ambiguity-aware AI assistants for medical data analysis. In *Proceedings of the 2020 CHI Conference on Human Factors in Computing Systems (CHI '20)* (pp. 1–14). Association for Computing Machinery, New York, NY, USA. https://doi.org/10.1145/3313831.3376506

Schmidt, M., Schmidt, S. A. J., Sandegaard, J. L., Ehrenstein, V., Pedersen, L., & Sørensen, H. T. (2015). The Danish National Patient Registry: a review of content, data quality, and research potential. *Clinical Epidemiology*, 449–490.

Teufl, W., Taetz, B., Miezal, M., Dindorf, C., Fröhlich, M., Trinler, U., Hogan, A., & Bleser, G. (2021). Automated detection and explainability of pathological gait patterns using a one-class support vector machine trained on inertial measurement unit based gait data. *Clinical Biomechanics, 89*, 105452. https://doi.org/10.1016/j.clinbiomech.2021.105452

Turmo Vidal, L., Zhu, H., Waern, A., & Márquez Segura, E. (2021). The design space of wearables for sports and fitness practices. In *Proceedings of the 2021 CHI Conference on Human Factors in Computing Systems.* Association for Computing Machinery.

Weakley, J., Mann, B., Banyard, H., McLaren, S., Scott, T., & Garcia-Ramos, A. (2021). Velocity-based training: from theory to application. *Strength & Conditioning Journal, 43*(2), 31–49. https://doi.org/10.1519/SSC.0000000000000560

You, Y., Kou, Y., Ding, X., & Gui, X. (2021). The medical authority of AI: A study of AI-enabled consumer-facing health technology. In *Proceedings of the 2021 CHI Conference on Human Factors in Computing Systems.* Association for Computing Machinery.

Yuan, C., Bi, N., Lin, Y. F., & Tseng, Y.H. (2023). Contextualizing user perceptions about biases for human-centered explainable artificial intelligence. In *Proceedings of the 2023 CHI Conference on Human Factors in Computing Systems.* Association for Computing Machinery.

Chapter 8
Transferring Lessons Learned from Uncertainty-Aware Visual Analytics in Clinical Data to Predictive Sporting Applications

Christina Gillmann

Abstract The application of uncertainty-aware visualization techniques in Machine Learning (ML) predictions has proven to be invaluable in the realm of clinical data. This article delves into the prospect of transferring these lessons to sporting applications. By scrutinizing the insights derived from uncertainty-aware visualization in clinical data, our goal is to harness the potential of these techniques and apply them to augment the analysis and interpretation of ML predictions in sports. The article underscores the significance of comprehending and visually representing uncertainty in sporting data, elucidating various visualization methods, including error bars, heatmaps, probability distributions, ensemble methods, and sensitivity analysis. Through this exploration, we illustrate how uncertainty-aware visualization can contribute to enhancing the reliability and decision-making processes associated with ML predictions in sports. Drawing upon the knowledge acquired from uncertainty-aware visualization in clinical data, we can lay the groundwork for more resilient and informed applications of ML in the sporting domain.

Keywords Uncertainty-Aware Visual Analytics · Transferability · Predictive Sports Applications

8.1 Introduction to Data-Driven Methods

Visual analytics has proven to be a successful concept in various applications, such as biology (Maack et al., 2021), environmental sciences (Raith et al., 2021), and mechanical engineering (Kretzschmar et al., 2020). The benefits of this technique have been explicitly demonstrated in Machine Learning (ML) tasks (Gillmann et al., 2021b; Yuan et al., 2020). The concept was introduced by Keim et al. (2008), as depicted in Fig. 8.1b, where data is transformed into hypotheses or visualizations.

C. Gillmann (✉)
Fraunhofer Institute for Applied Information Technology, Sankt Augustin, Germany
e-mail: gillmann@informatik.uni-leipzig.de

C. Dindorf et al. (eds.), *Artificial Intelligence in Sports, Movement, and Health*,
https://doi.org/10.1007/978-3-031-67256-9_8

Furthermore, interaction allows conversion between hypotheses and visualizations. During this process, users can gain new insights into the input dataset, which can be fed back into the dataset component. The concept has been widely used in many fields, with clinical data being one of the most prominent examples.

Unfortunately, the Visual Analytics (VA) process can introduce uncertainty in each of its components. These uncertainty events include missing data, incorrect measurements, model inaccuracy, as well as user uncertainty while interpreting the results produced by the VA cycle. Here, the original cycle by Keim et al. (2008) does not provide a systematic way to include, propagate, and communicate uncertainty throughout the VA cycle. Therefore, the VA cycle has been extended by Maack et al. (2023) to address this issue. In this extension, the cycle by Keim et al. (2008) is augmented by several components and connections. The major changes include uncertainty quantification in each component of the VA cycle, an exchange of all components with uncertainty-aware components, a separation of the feedback loop

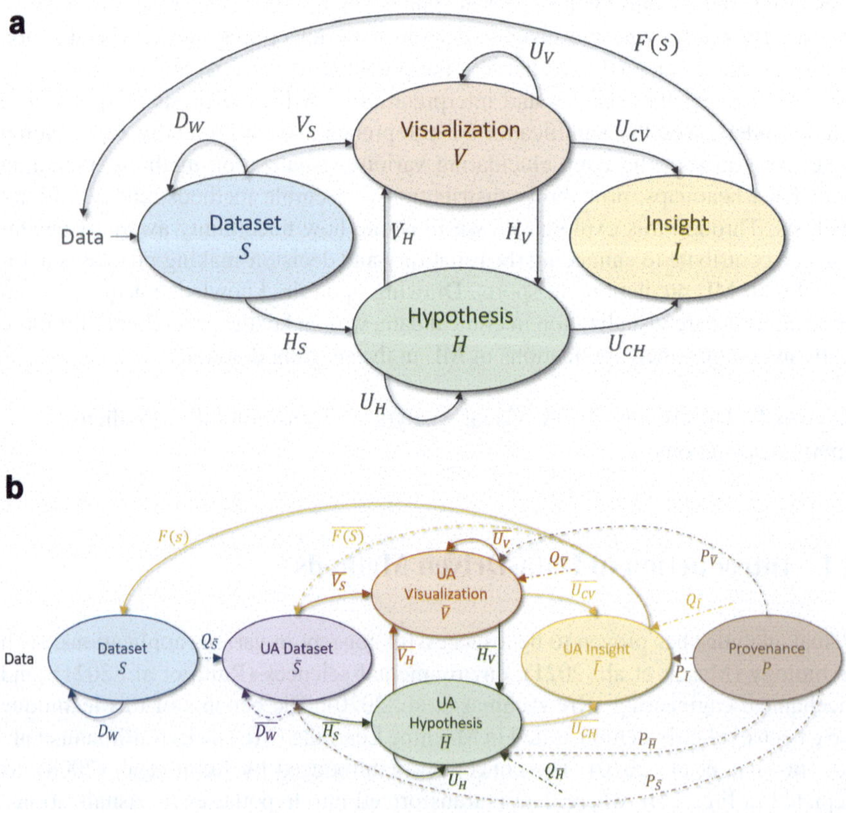

Fig. 8.1 UAVA. **a** Classic visual analytics cycle defined by Keim et al. (2008). **b** Extension to create an UAVA cycle by Gillmann et al.

into uncertainty-aware and regular insight, and a provenance component that keeps track of the uncertainty propagated and accumulated along the VA cycle.

The concept of Uncertainty-Aware Visual Analytics (UAVA) has proven to be a suitable tool for many clinical applications, resulting in a broad set of success stories. These include medical imaging (Gillmann et al., 2021c), clinical health record data (Preim & Lawonn, 2020), and monitoring data (Lourdusamy & Mattam, 2020).

Based on these findings, the question arises of how to transfer this knowledge to predictive sports. Let's consider a scenario where a ML model is trained to predict the location of a knee joint based on video data captured during sports activities, such as basketball. The model aims to track the movement of the knee joint to analyze biomechanics and potentially optimize movements to prevent injuries or improve performance.

Now, imagine a coach using this data for movement optimization, particularly focusing on improving the jumping technique of basketball players to reduce the risk of knee injuries. The coach receives visual representations of the uncertainty associated with the predicted location of the knee joint during various phases of jumping, such as takeoff, flight, and landing. The visual representation of uncertainty provides the coach with insights into the confidence levels of the model predictions. For instance, during takeoff, where the knee joint movements might be more predictable and stable, the uncertainty might be relatively low. However, during the landing phase, where movements can be more dynamic and variable, the uncertainty might be higher. This enables coaches to make more informed decisions regarding movement optimization in sports by understanding the limitations and potential errors associated with the data and predictions.

In this paper, we aim to summarize the success stories of UAVA in clinical data. Building on that, we aim to provide a transfer of this knowledge to predictive sports applications.

We hope that this manuscript inspires researchers in this area to make use of the concept of UAVA, as shown in the example above.

Therefore, this manuscript contributes:

- A summary of UAVA (see Sect. 8.2)
- A collection of success stories of UAVA for clinical data (see Sect. 8.3)
- A guide to approaching predictive sports through UAVA (see Sect. 8.4) including
- A mapping of data types in predictive sports to abstract VA (see Sect. 8.4.2)
- An adapted taxonomy of uncertainty events in VA for predictive sports analysis (see Sect. 8.4.3)
- A workflow to create UAVA cycles for predictive sports analysis (see Sect. 8.4.4).

8.2 Introduction to Data-Driven Methods

In the following, we aim to shed light on the concept of UAVA (see Sect. 8.2). Maack et al. (2023) defined an extension of the VA cycle (see Fig. 8.1b) by Keim et al. (2008) (see Fig. 8.1a), which will serve as a starting point and a goal of the presented consideration. The cycle consists of components (see Sect. 8.2.1) that are connected by operations (see Sect. 8.2.2). Here, novel components and connections, in contrast to the classic VA cycle, are highlighted by a bar over their label. The cycle starts with a dataset S, which shapes the following considerations massively. Therefore, the potential datasets that can be handled in the UAVA cycle will be explained in more detail (see Sect. 8.2.3).

8.2.1 Components of the Uncertainty-Aware Visual Analytics Cycle

There exist 6 major components in the UAVA cycle, that are connected:

Dataset S, is a very general concept that consists of n records $(r_1, r_2, ..., r_n)$, where each record r_i, consists of m observations, variables or attributes $(a_1, a_2,..a_n)$. An attribute a_i is a single entity such as a number or symbol. A Dataset holds a structure that can be syntactic or semantic.

Uncertainty-aware Dataset $\overline{S}$ is resulting from the input dataset S in conjunction with the extracted uncertainty quantification $Q_{\overline{S}}$. It describes the input dataset in conjunction with proper uncertainty quantification.

Hypothesis H, is a supposition or proposed explanation created on the basis of limited evidence as a starting point for further investigation. To achieve this, the null hypothesis is usually utilized. In this case, a hypothesis is formed and tested. Then the hypothesis can either be rejected or failed to be rejected. In conjunction with the null hypothesis, there is also an uncertainty quantification attached to it.

Visualization V, is an uncertainty-aware visual representation that can be interpreted by the user.

Insight I, can be defined as knowledge that is gained during analysis and has to be internalized, synthesized, and related to prior knowledge including the uncertainty related to this insight.

Provenance P. When running a UAVA cycle, uncertainty will propagate and accumulate along with the operations carried out on the VA cycle. This implies the tracking of uncertainty throughout each computational step of the VA cycle, referred to as provenance.

8.2.2 Connections of the Uncertainty-Aware Visual Analytics Cycle

The components of the UAVA cycle are related to each other using the following connections:

- D_W: $S \rightarrow S$, the preprocessing of a dataset
- $\overline{D_W} : \overline{S} \rightarrow \overline{S}$, the preprocessing of an uncertainty-aware dataset
- $\{\overline{Q_S}, \overline{Q_H}, \overline{Q_V}, \overline{Q_I}\} : \{S, H, V, I\} \rightarrow \overline{S}, \overline{H}, \overline{V}, \overline{I}$, the uncertainty quantification for all components of the UAVA cycle
- $\overline{H_{\{S,V\}}} : \{\overline{S}, \overline{V}\} \rightarrow \overline{H}$, the generation of a UA hypothesis from a UA dataset S or visualization V
- $\overline{V_{\{S,H\}}} : \{\overline{S}, \overline{H}\} \rightarrow \overline{V}$, the generation of a UA visualization from dataset S or hypothesis H
- $\overline{U_{\{V,H\}}} : \{\overline{V}, \overline{H}\} \rightarrow \{\overline{V}, \overline{H}\}$, user interaction with the UA visualization V or UA hypothesis H.
- $\overline{U_{\{CV,CH\}}} : \{\overline{V}, \overline{H}\} \rightarrow \overline{I}$, user interaction to generate UA insight I from UA hypothesis H or UA visualization V
- $F(S)$, a feedback loop to insert generated insight I back into the VA cycle
- $\overline{F(S)}$, an uncertainty-aware feedback loop to insert generated uncertainty-aware insight I back into the VA cycle
- $\overline{P_{S,H,V,I}} : \overline{P} \rightarrow \overline{P}$, the generation of Provenance from monitoring the state of $\overline{S}, \overline{H}, \overline{V}, \overline{I}$.

These connections allow a transition between the components and guide through the analytic process.

8.2.3 Datatypes in the Ancertainty-Aware Visual Analytics Process

The UAVA cycle is defined such that it starts with the data that is intended to be analyzed. In the work of Maack et al. (2023), datasets are clearly defined. As we require these definitions in the following considerations, this section provides a short recap on the datatypes and their potential sources of uncertainty.

Geospatial data $\mathbf{S_1}$. This involves geospatial locations or trajectories L, with various attributes A assigned to these domains through a function $f : L \rightarrow A$. Spatial uncertainty and attribute uncertainty (Li et al., 2017) are inherent in such datasets. Spatial uncertainty arises from areas or trajectories that can deviate in shape from the stored data, while attribute uncertainty describes the uncertainty of data attributes themselves. Both uncertainties are illustrated in Fig. 8.2a, demonstrating positional and attribute uncertainty. Analytic models, as outlined by Li et al. (2017), can be employed for uncertainty quantification.

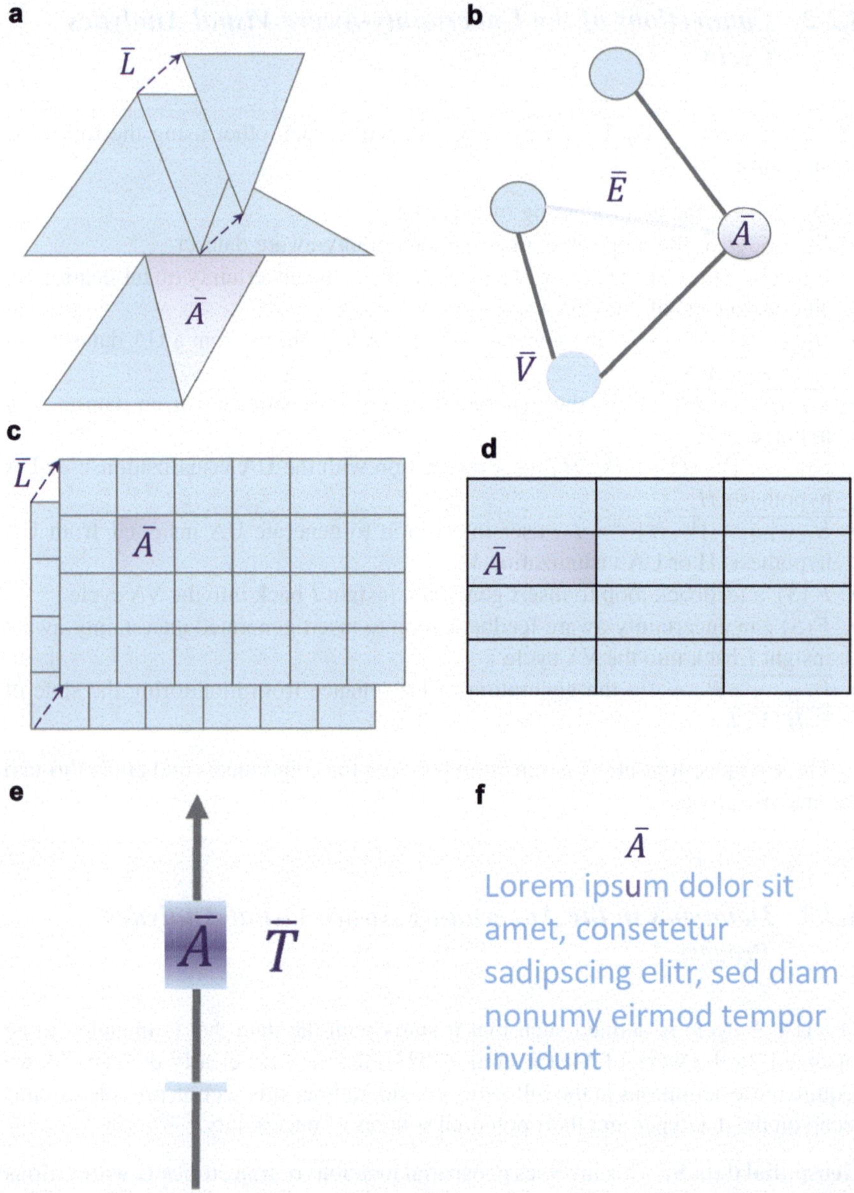

Fig. 8.2 Different types of data and potential sources of uncertainty. Blue figures represent fixed values, whereas purple figures represent uncertainty that can be contained in the data. **a** Spatial data. **b** Graph data. **c** Field data. **d** High-dimensional data. **e** time-dependent data and **f** document data

Graph data S_2. This connects nodes V via links E, forming a graph. Nodes and links can possess various attributes provided by functions $f : V \rightarrow A$ and $g : E \rightarrow A$. Three types of uncertainty (Kassiano et al., 2016) exist in graph data: uncertainty regarding the presence of a node, uncertainty about a link between nodes, and uncertainty related to attributes in nodes or links. The position of visualized nodes is not a fundamental uncertainty but is derived from the graph description or some graph drawing algorithm. Engel et al. (2015) provided uncertainty quantification for graph data, as visually indicated in Fig. 8.2b.

Field data S_3. This data can contain scalars, vectors, and tensors (attributes A), often arranged on a grid defined by positions and neighborhood relations. Two types of uncertainty can occur, as depicted in Fig. 8.2c: uncertainty in positions and uncertainty in attributes defined over P (Hansen et al., 2014). It is important to note that each attribute value may be affected by uncertainty to differing extents. For instance, vector entries can have varying uncertainty depending on their dimension. Potter et al. (Potter et al., 2011) provided a summary of uncertainty quantification for field data.

High-dimensional Data S_4. Defined by a dimension N determining the number of attributes A in one entry, high-dimensional data typically has $N > 10$. Here, only attribute uncertainty needs consideration, as illustrated in Fig. 8.2d.

Temporal Data S_5. This data contains attributes A sorted along a timeline T using a function $f : T \rightarrow A$. Two types of uncertainty arise: time uncertainty and attribute uncertainty (Cheng et al., 2014), as shown in Fig. 8.2e. Each point in time and the attribute attached to it can be affected by uncertainty. Zhen et al. (Hu et al., 2015) demonstrated the quantification of uncertainty in temporal data.

Text/Document Data S_6. This data is in the form of text or documents holding attributes A at specific character positions P, given by the function $f : P \rightarrow A$. Two types of uncertainty can arise, as shown in Fig. 8.2f: Document uncertainty and attribute uncertainty (Kerdjoudj and Curé, 2015). Each document can have an overall uncertainty, and all of its entries can be affected by uncertainty (Kerdjoudj and Curé, 2015) provided quantification of uncertainty in textual data.

8.3 Uncertainty-Aware Visual Analytics and Clinical Data - Examples

In this section, we will introduce various types of clinical data and provide an overview of their potential sources of uncertainty. Clinical data in healthcare encompasses a diverse array of information related to patients, including details about their medical conditions, treatments, outcomes, and personal information. These data

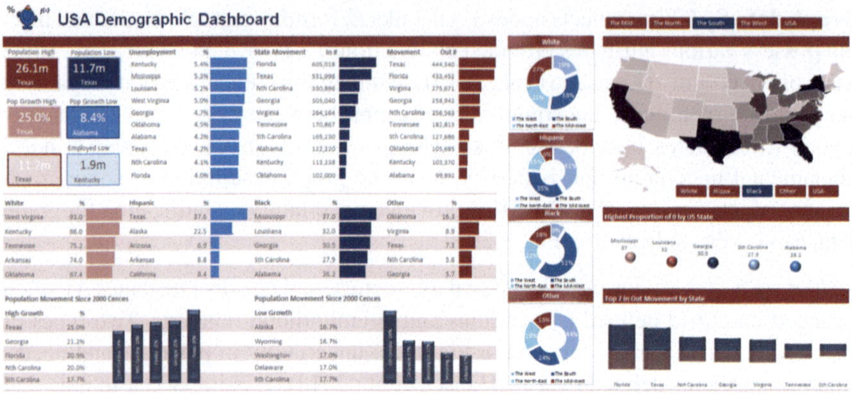

Fig. 8.3 UAVA for demographic data in the U.S (Small, 2023). Demographics data is aggregated and displayed as single values for complete cohorts

types play a crucial role in diagnosis, treatment, research, and healthcare management. Additionally, we will illustrate how UAVA can effectively handle this type of data, with a specific focus on predictive tasks.

8.3.1 Patient Demographics

Patient demographics encompass basic information such as name, age, gender, address, contact details, and insurance information, categorizing this type of data as high-dimensional. Regarding uncertainty, the values stored in patient demographics data are susceptible to uncertainties. This may manifest as outdated, missing, or ambiguous information, often arising from patients providing incomplete or outdated details.

An illustrative example is presented in Fig. 8.3 and is available on the SmallMan website (Small, 2023). The dashboard provides an overview of demographic data, aggregated to offer insights into the entire cohort. Standard deviations are often included to provide additional context. Such dashboards are vital in predictive demographic analysis, offering insights into potential developments, a critical consideration in clinic capacity planning.

8.3.2 Patient Monitoring

Patient monitoring encompasses a broad range of data, including electrocardiograms (ECG or EKG), fetal monitoring during childbirth, telemetry data for intensive care units, as well as single time-step data like vital signs and laboratory results.

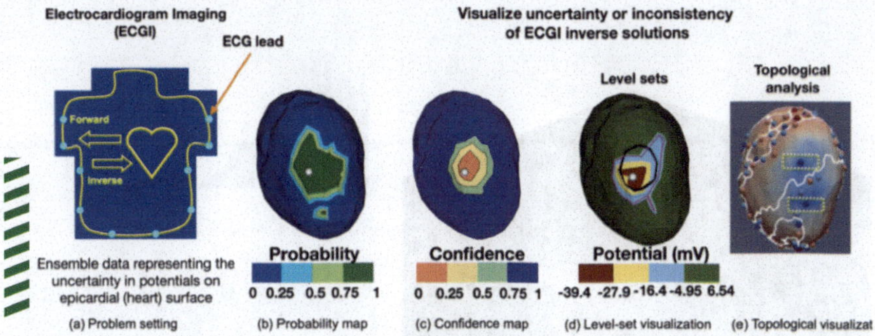

Fig. 8.4 Example for UAVA for ECGI monitoring by Athawale et al. (2019)

Vital signs data includes measurements such as blood pressure, heart rate, respiratory rate, and body temperature, offering valuable insights into a patient's overall health. Laboratory data comprises various diagnostic tests, providing biochemical and hematological information. This type of data is generally considered time dependent.

In terms of uncertainty, patient monitoring can be affected by incorrect or missing values, and the precise time considered may also be imprecise. Figure 8.4 demonstrates an example of Electrocardiographic Imaging (ECGI) developed by Athawale and Johnson (2019). ECGI captures voltages responding to changes in the heart's electrical activity, offering noninvasive insights into arrhythmia sources. While the ECG swiftly provides information on abnormal rhythms, it lacks detailed spatial information about the heart's electrical impulses. Monte Carlo simulations are employed to explore different arrhythmia positions, with various visualizations providing information on probability, confidence, and potential captured in the simulations. These simulations stand as a prominent example of ML based on clinical data.

8.3.3 Imaging Data

In the realm of medicine, medical imaging serves as a crucial technique for generating visual representations of the body's interior, facilitating clinical analysis and medical interventions. These images offer valuable insights into the structure and function of organs, tissues, and internal structures, contributing to the diagnosis, treatment planning, and monitoring of diverse medical conditions. Medical imaging plays an indispensable role in modern healthcare, enabling healthcare professionals to visualize and comprehend the internal aspects of the human body without resorting to invasive procedures. X-rays, MRIs, CT scans, ultrasounds, and other imaging studies constitute medical imaging data, instrumental in diagnosing and monitoring various medical conditions.

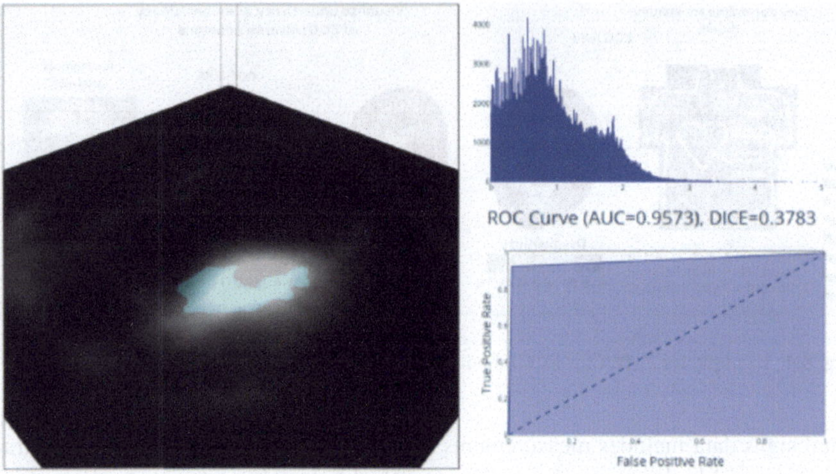

Fig. 8.5 UAVA for brain lesion prediction as shown by Gillmann et al. (2021a). **a** Predicted lesion mapped into a selected brain region. **b** Histogramm of probabilities that brain region is affected by a lesion. **c** ROC for the prediction of a specific patient

Concerning medical imaging, uncertainties may stem from two primary sources. Firstly, the overall position of the image might be influenced by uncertainty. Secondly, the values encapsulated within the image can also be subject to uncertainty.

Figure 8.5 exemplifies the utilization of UAVA for medical images (Gillmann et al., 2021a). In this case, brain lesions occurring during a stroke are examined using over 400 acute stroke images to train a neural network predicting the resulting lesion (Welle et al., 2023). Given the complexity and numerous settings of the network (Nieradzik et al., 2021), UAVA was employed to unravel its mechanisms. The visualization encompasses different modes. First, the network's predictions were overlaid on a selected brain region. Subsequently, a histogram captured the distribution of probabilities indicating the affected area. Lastly, a Receiver-Operator-Curve was presented graphically. This example demonstrates how UAVA assists decision-makers in comprehending ML models.

8.3.4 Written Medical Records

Medical records are diverse, serving as comprehensive documentation for various medical conditions and procedures through textual information. These records encompass medication records, procedure and surgery records, diagnosis and clinical notes, and treatment plans. Medication records, crucial for tracking patient treatment plans and potential drug interactions, include details such as dosage, frequency, and treatment duration. Procedure and surgery records provide information on surgical procedures, including the date, surgeon, type of surgery, and post-operative care.

Physicians' notes and diagnostics contain essential information about a patient's condition, including symptoms, observations, and clinical assessments. Finally, treatment plans document prescribed medications, therapies, and interventions tailored to address a patient's specific condition.

Examining the significance of written medical reports, Reiner (2017) delved into the uncertainties associated with these records. Uncertainties may arise from inaccuracies in the recorded occurrences. Additionally, clinicians might express uncertainties regarding the diagnosis or measurements they report.

8.3.5 Molecular Data

Molecular protein data encompasses detailed information about the structure, function, and interactions of proteins at the molecular level. This dataset includes crucial details such as amino acid sequences, three-dimensional structures, and post-translational modifications, offering valuable insights into the underlying mechanisms governing cellular processes. Analyzing molecular protein data is indispensable for unraveling biological functions, understanding disease mechanisms, and developing targeted therapeutic interventions in medicine. Uncertainty events in this context may manifest as positional uncertainty for specific atoms or values associated with these atoms.

An illustration of uncertainty-aware molecular visualization is presented by Maack et al. (2021) in Fig. 8.6. Considering the dynamic nature of molecules in space, the resulting surfaces computed based on atom positions and sizes may vary. To address this variability, Maack et al. developed a VA tool that offers indicators depicting how the surface of a protein may fluctuate through uncertainty-aware geometry visualization (Gillmann et al., 2018). Examining the protein surface is critical in drug development, and this example showcases how UAVA can enhance this process.

8.3.6 Network Data

Biological network data comprises interconnected sets of biological entities, such as genes, proteins, or metabolites, along with the relationships or interactions between them. These networks serve as representations of intricate systems within living organisms, delineating the complex web of molecular connections that govern various biological processes. Analyzing biological network data facilitates the exploration of cellular functions, identification of key regulatory elements, and insights into the dynamic relationships shaping biological systems, providing valuable information for fields like systems biology and bioinformatics.

Regarding uncertainty, Conroy et al. (2024) addressed uncertainty in network data, acknowledging that while their article is based on historical network data, the sources of uncertainty remain consistent when considering clinical data. Uncertainty

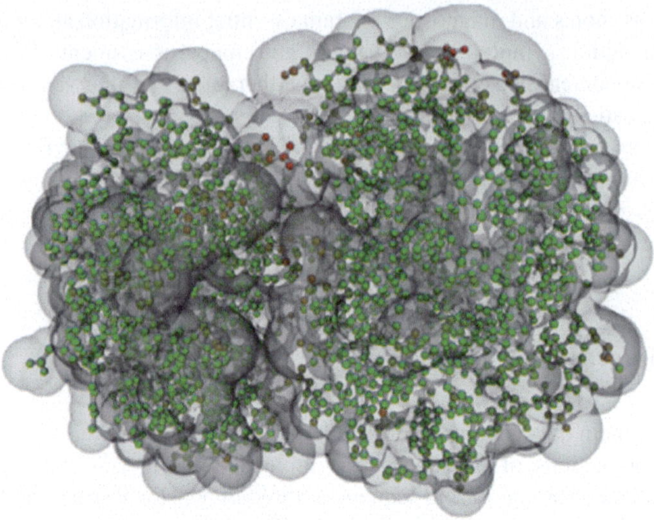

Fig. 8.6 Uncertainty-aware visualization of molecular data. Isosurfaces are used to indicate the uncertainty inherent in atomic positions (Maack et al., 2021)

in network data can arise from nodes or edges based on their potential existence and associated values.

Weiskopf (2022) provided a comprehensive overview of biological data and its related uncertainty visualization, as depicted in Fig. 8.7. The visualization employs different thicknesses and colors for corresponding proteins based on the uncertainty of their relation. Users can filter connections based on various parameters, enhancing the exploration of uncertainty in biological network data.

8.3.7 Abstraction of Clinical Data to Visual Analytics Data

As shown, the UAVA cycle starts with a dataset. In the Paper by Maack et al. (2023), data is divided into different types. In order to follow this scheme, we will order types of clinical data in the given types and summarize their sources of uncertainty.

Figure 8.8 shows the mapping of clinical data into the definition of high-level data type in the UAVA cycle. Here, we can observe that every category of clinical data can be mapped into a datatype.

Patient demographics can be mapped into high-dimensional data. Here, each dimension corresponds to one captured attribute. Patient monitoring can be represented by time-dependent data. Therefore, each measurement point in time can hold different attributes. Imaging data responds to grid data. Here, each pixel or voxel in the image is a grid point. Further, written reports can be mapped to text data easily.

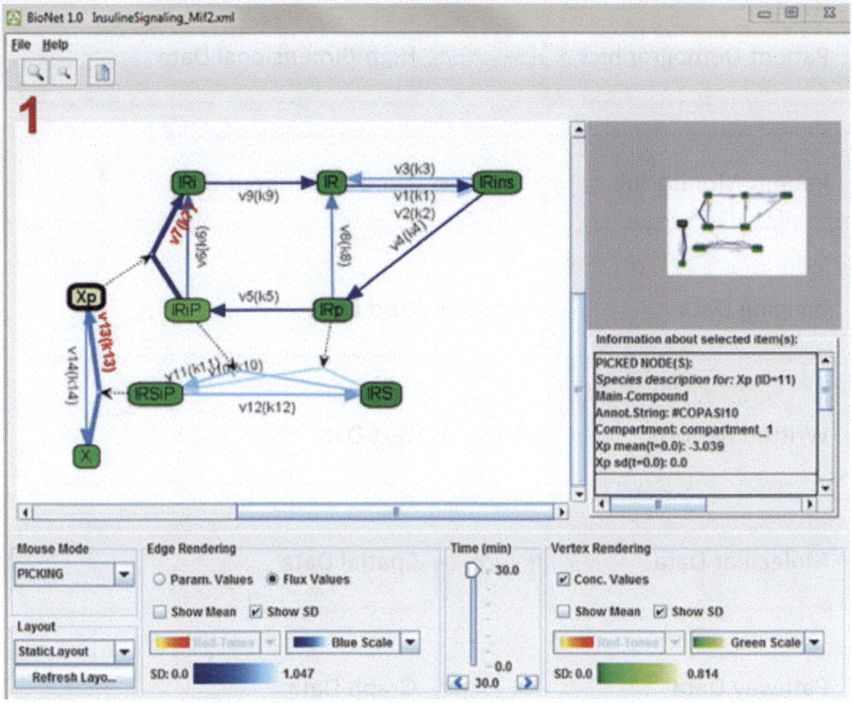

Fig. 8.7 UAVA for protein pathway analysis. Networks with uncertain edges are indicated with different thicknesses and colors (Weiskopf, 2022)

Molecular data provide an example of spatial data, whereas pathway data correspond to graph data.

8.4 Transferability to Predictive Sports

Section 8.4 shows that UAVA can be used for all data sources occurring in clinical data, and that it is a suitable tool to handle it. As a goal, this work aims to provide guidelines to use UAVA in predictive sports. In the following, we aim to summarize sources of data for predictive sports and aim for a similar categorization of abstract data in UAVA. Based on this, we will discuss how we can instantiate sources of uncertainty to predicte sports and give directions on how to use UAVA in this area.

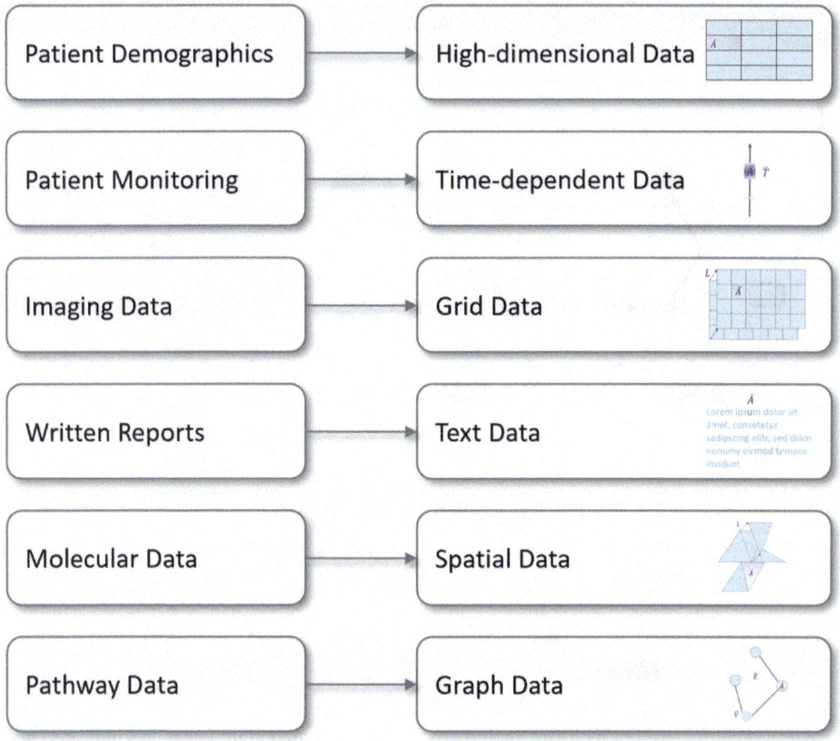

Fig. 8.8 Mapping of clinical data into the uncertainty-aware datatypes of the UAVA cycle. Each clinical data type can be assigned to an abstract data type

8.4.1 Data Sources for Predictive Sports Analysis

Predictive sports analysis, often referred to as sports analytics or sports data analysis, is the process of using statistical, mathematical, and computational techniques to analyze past and current sports data in order to make predictions and gain insights into various aspects of sports performance and outcomes (Bai & Bai, 2021). It involves collecting and analyzing a wide range of data related to sports, such as player statistics, team performance, game conditions, and more, to make informed predictions about future events in the sports world.

Player Performance Data compasses detailed statistics related to individual athletes, including metrics like points scored, assists, rebounds, shooting accuracy, and defensive contributions. This information is crucial for assessing a player's strengths, weaknesses, and overall impact on the team's success. Predictive models often leverage historical player performance data to anticipate future contributions and evaluate the potential outcomes of specific matchups.

Team performance data consists of aggregated statistics that reflect the collective performance of a sports team. Key metrics include win-loss records, average points scored and conceded, team chemistry, and strategic tendencies. Analyzing team-level data is fundamental for understanding overall team dynamics, strengths, and weaknesses, which are vital components in predicting game outcomes and tournament success.

Injury reports provide essential information about the health status of players, including current injuries, recovery timelines, and potential impact on performance. Predictive sports analysis takes into account the availability of key players, as injuries can significantly influence game strategies and outcomes. Integrating injury data allows analysts to adjust predictions based on the potential impact of absent or recovering players.

Weather data includes information on atmospheric conditions such as temperature, humidity, wind speed, and precipitation. In outdoor sports, weather can have a profound impact on game dynamics, affecting player performance and influencing strategic decisions. Incorporating weather data enables predictive models to consider environmental factors that may contribute to or hinder certain playing styles and strategies.

Game context data provides details about the circumstances surrounding a match, including whether the team is playing at home or away, the distance traveled, and the game schedule. Understanding the context helps analysts factor in variables like home-field advantage, fatigue from travel, and scheduling constraints, enhancing the accuracy of predictions by accounting for external influences on team performance.

Historical data forms the foundation for predictive sports analysis, encompassing past game results, player performances, and team trends. By identifying patterns and trends in historical data, analysts can build models that capture the dynamics of sports competitions over time. Historical data serves as a valuable resource for training predictive algorithms and understanding the evolving nature of sports.

Player tracking data involves real-time information on player movements, positioning, and physical exertion during a game. Technologies like GPS and motion sensors provide granular insights into an athlete's performance, including speed, acceleration, and spatial awareness. Integrating player tracking data enhances predictive models by considering the micro-level details of player behavior and decision-making.

Betting odds and market data from sportsbooks reflect the collective expectations and sentiments of the betting public. Analyzing betting odds helps analysts gauge the perceived probabilities of different outcomes and identify potential discrepancies between public perception and statistical models. This information can be valuable for understanding market dynamics and making informed predictions.

Social Media and News Feeds provide real-time updates on team dynamics, player sentiments, and public opinions. This qualitative data supplements quantitative metrics by offering insights into intangible factors such as team morale, external pressures, and public expectations. Integrating social media and news data enhances the contextual understanding of the sports environment.

8.4.2 Abstraction of Predictive Sports Data to Visual Analytics Data

To effectively apply UAVA to predictive sports, a comprehensive classification of predictive sports data is essential, mirroring the approach used for clinical data.

Figure 8.9 illustrates the mapping of predictive sports data onto the abstract data types of UAVA. A significant distinction from clinical data emerges, where predictive sports data can be amalgamated from diverse abstract data types.

Player performance data seamlessly fits into the category of high-dimensional data, a characteristic shared with team performance data and bidding odds data. Team performance data, however, may also be categorized as graph data when exploring relationships between different players alongside traditional high-dimensional attributes like the number of wins. Historical data aligns with time-dependent data, while injury reports exhibit versatility, classifiable as either time-dependent data, grid data (if imaging techniques are employed), or text data when considering written reports. Social media data presents itself as either grid data (if images are involved) or text data when dealing with textual content. Weather data and player tracking data find a natural classification as spatial data.

Despite the diversity in predictive sports data, it does not adhere to a singular category within UAVA. Nevertheless, the UAVA framework can be effectively applied. Building upon the work of Maack et al. (2023), who demonstrated the combination of UAVA data types in an arbitrary manner, it becomes evident that abstract data types can be viewed as attributes. For instance, time-dependent data can be enriched with spatial attributes at each time point, resulting in spatio-temporal data. Therefore, UAVA offers a flexible mechanism for the derivation of uncertainty events in predictive sports.

8.4.3 Derivation of Uncertainty Events in Predictive Sports

As detailed by Gillmann et al.(2023), a comprehensive list of uncertainty sources for various datatypes in VA has been established. However, this manuscript seeks to tailor this list specifically for predictive sports analytics. The objective is to empower domain scientists to articulate the specific types of uncertainty events present in their data.

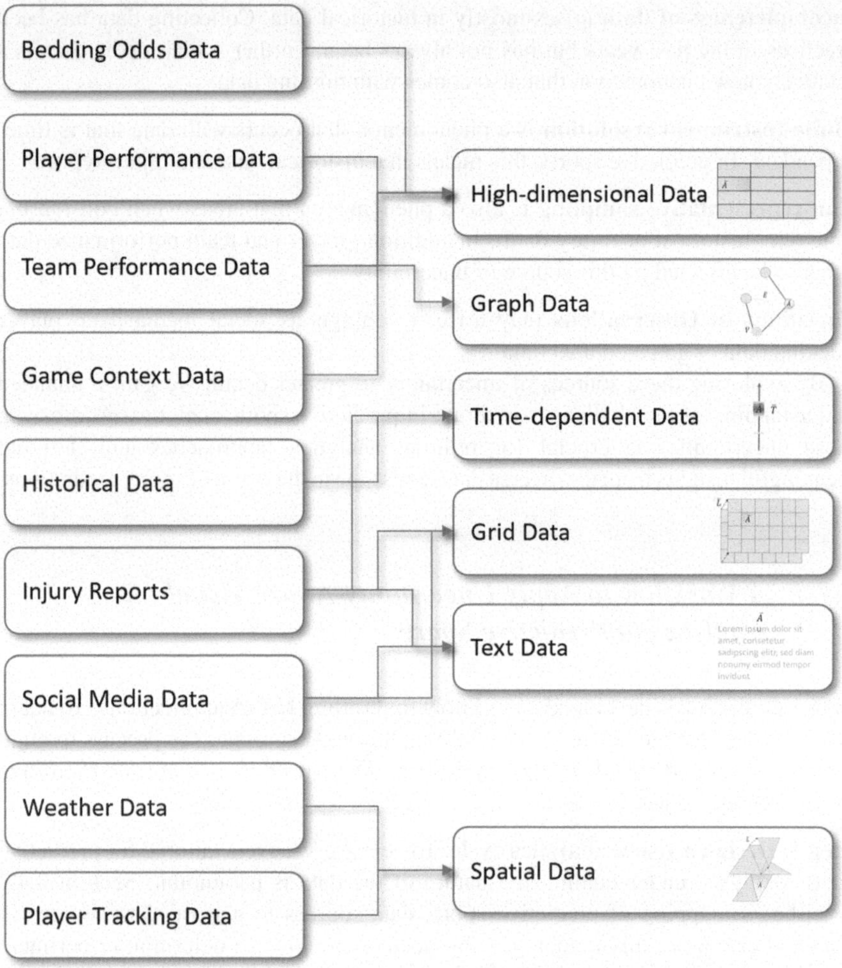

Fig. 8.9 Mapping of data sources in predictive sports to abstract data types of UAVA. In contrast to clinical data, predictive sports data sources can encompass multiple abstract data types of UAVA

Consequently, the sources of uncertainty within the dataset component can be refined. In other words, it becomes feasible to identify the inherent sources of uncertainty in the diverse data types characteristic of predictive sports.

To summarize, four primary sources of uncertainty exist in the dataset component: incompleteness of data, finite instrument resolution, non-representative sampling, and variations in observations. It is crucial to note that while all sources of uncertainty may potentially exist in any given case, they might not always be of paramount interest. The subsequent sections outline the data types where these uncertainties play a significant role.

Incompleteness of data arises mostly in historical data. Collecting data has been practices in the past years but has not always been. Further social media data is a relatively new phenomenon that also comes with missing data.

Finite Instrument resolution is a phenomenon that occurs with data that is time-dependent. In predictive sports, this means that historical data and injury reports.

Non-representative sampling is also a phenomenon that arisis when considering time (e.g. historical or injury data). In addition, player and team performance data can also be affected by this source of uncertainty.

Variations in Observations may arise in ambiguous social media data, player tracking data or game context data.

By exploring these sources of uncertainty in greater detail, we gain a nuanced understanding of the challenges inherent in predictive sports analytics. Addressing these uncertainties is crucial for refining analytical approaches and deriving meaningful insights from the diverse data landscape in the realm of sports predictions.

8.4.4 A Workflow to Apply Uncertainty-Aware Visual Analytics to Predictive Sports

Maack et al. (2023) developed a workflow for crafting UAVA applications. To adapt this workflow for predictive sports analysis, this section refines the process to align with the specific demands of the application. The workflow is delineated into five steps, each elucidated below.

Step 1: Design a visual analytics cycle. To devise a VA cycle tailored for predictive sports analysis, understanding the nature of the data is paramount. Section 8.4.2 furnishes a mapping of predictive sports data sources to general data sources in UAVA. Leveraging this mapping, subsequent steps involve determining pertinent analysis methods, including ML techniques and suitable visualization methods.

Step 2: Quantify system uncertainty of the given visual analytics cycle. Section 8.4.3 offers a derivation of uncertainty events specific to predictive sports analysis. The identification of crucial sources is imperative, with particular emphasis on discerning uncertainty in the hypothesis component. This uncertainty may vary depending on the chosen ML algorithm employed.

Step 3: Integrate and connect uncertainty-aware solutions. Based on the chosen hypothesis and visualization techniques from Step 1, seeking uncertainty-aware solutions for the selected algorithms becomes imperative. Work by Steinbach et al. (2022) provides insights into ML approaches adept at handling uncertainty events. Simultaneously, the work by Kamal et al. (2021) aids in identifying visualization approaches adept at managing uncertainty events.

Step 4: Separate the visual analytics cycle feedback loop into quantifiable and unquantifiable feedback. This crucial step involves splitting the feedback loop into quantifiable and unquantifiable feedback. If uncertainty-aware solutions are implemented in the hypothesis, they result in insights with a quantifiable feedback loop. To enhance uncertainty quantification, incorporating a feedback mechanism enabling users to provide subjective impressions of computed results is recommended.

Step 5: Generate provenance of uncertainty-aware components in the visual analytics cycle. To monitor the propagation and accumulation of uncertainty events throughout the runtime of a UAVA cycle, provenance becomes indispensable. Works such as Xu et al. (2020) offer an overview of potential techniques in this domain. Incorporating provenance ensures a comprehensive understanding of uncertainty events in the system.

8.5 Contribution

This paper offers a comprehensive overview of uncertainty-aware VA and its application to clinical data. Building upon this foundation, the manuscript endeavors to bridge insights from the clinical domain to the realm of predictive sports analysis.

Specifically, it presents an abstraction of predictive sports data into the framework of VA, a delineation of uncertainty events tailored for predictive sports analysis, and a refined workflow for constructing uncertainty-aware VA cycles within this domain.

In our future endeavors, we aspire to implement uncertainty-aware VA approaches across diverse use cases within predictive sports analysis. Additionally, we are committed to conducting a state-of-the-art analysis of uncertainty-aware VA methodologies in the context of predictive sports analysis.

References

Athawale, T. M., Johnson, K. A., Buston, C. R., & Johnson, C. R. (2019). A statistical framework for quantification and visualisation of positional uncertainty in deep brain stimulation electrodes. *Computer Methods in Biomechanics and Biomedical Engineering: Imaging & Visualization, 7*(4):438–449. PMID: 31186994.

Bai, Z., & Bai, X. (2021). Sports big data: Management, analysis, applications, and challenges. *Complexity, 2021*, 1–11.

Cheng, R., Emrich, T., Kriegel, H.-P., Mamoulis, N., Renz, M.,Trajcevski, G., & Züfle, A. (2014). Managing uncertainty in spatial and spatio-temporal data. In *2014 IEEE 30th International Conference on Data Engineering* (pp. 1302–1305). IEEE.

Conroy, M., Gillmann, C., Harvey, F., Mchedlidze, T., Fabrikant, S. I., Windhager, F., Scheuermann, G., Tangherlini, T. R., Warren, C. N., Weingart, S. B., et al. (2024). Uncertainty in humanities network visualization. *Frontiers in Communication, 8*, 1305137.

Engel, D. W., Jarman, K. D., Xu, Z., Zheng, B., Tartakovsky, A. M., Yang, X., Tipireddy, R., Lei, H., & Yin, J. (2015). *Uq methods for hpda and cybersecurity models, data, and use cases*. Technical report, Pacific Northwest National Lab.(PNNL), Richland, WA (United States).

Gillmann, C., Wischgoll, T., Hamann, B., & Ahrens, J. (2018). Modeling and visualization of uncertainty-aware geometry using multi-variate normal distributions. In *2018 IEEE Pacific Visualization Symposium (PacificVis)* (pp. 106–110). IEEE.

Gillmann, C., Saur, D., T., W., & G., S. (2021c). Uncertainty-aware visualization in medical imaging—a survey. In *EuroVis Conference—STAR Track.*

Gillmann, C., Saur, D., & Scheuermann, G. (2021b). How to deal with uncertainty in machine learning for medical imaging? In *2021 IEEE Workshop on TRust and EXpertise in Visual Analytics (TREX)* (pp. 52–58).

Gillmann, C., Maack, R. G. C., Raith, F., Pérez, J. F., & Scheuermann, G. (2023). A taxonomy of uncertainty events in visual analytics. *IEEE Computer Graphics and Applications.*

Gillmann, C., Peter, L., Schmidt, C., Saur, D., & Scheuermann, G. (2021a). Visualizing multimodal deep learning for lesion prediction. *IEEE Computer Graphics and Applications, 41*(5), 90–98.

Hansen, C. D., Chen, M., Johnson, C. R., Kaufman, A. E., & Hagen, H. (2014). *Scientific visualization: Uncertainty, multifield, biomedical, and scalable visualization.* Springer Publishing Company.

Hu, Z., Mahadevan, S., & Du, X. (2015). Uncertainty quantification in time-dependent reliability analysis. In *International Design Engineering Technical Conferences and Computers and Information in Engineering Conference* (Vol. 57083, pp. V02BT03A062). American Society of Mechanical Engineers.

Kamal, A., Dhakal, P., Javaid, A., Devabhaktuni, V., Kaur, D., Zaientz, J., & Marinier, R., III. (2021). Recent advances and challenges in uncertainty visualization: A survey. *Journal of Visualization, 24,* 1–30.

Kassiano, V., Gounaris, A., Papadopoulos, A. N., & Tsichlas, K. (2016). Mining uncertain graphs: An overview. In *International Workshop of Algorithmic Aspects of Cloud Computing* (pp. 87–116). Springer.

Keim, D. A., Mansmann, F., Schneidewind, J., Thomas, J. J., & Ziegler, H. (2008). Visual analytics: Scope and challenges. In *Visual data mining.*

Kerdjoudj, F. & Curé, O. (2015). Evaluating uncertainty in textual document. In *URSW at ISWC*, Bethlehem, United States.

Kretzschmar, V., Gillmann, C., Günther, F., Stommel, M., & Scheuermann, G. (2020). Statistically informed visualization framework for assisting interface optimization of hybrid component design. In *25th International Symposium on Vision, Modeling, and Visualization.*

Li, L., Ban, H., Wechsler, S., & Xu, B. (2017). *Spatial data uncertainty* (Vol. 1, pp. 313–340). Elsevier.

Lourdusamy, R. & Mattam, X. J. (2020). Clinical decision support systems and predictive analytics. In *Machine learning with health care perspective: Machine learning and healthcare* (pp. 317–355).

Maack, R. G. C., Raymer, M., Wischgoll, T., Hagen, H., and C., G. (2021). A framework for uncertainty-aware visual analytics of proteins.

Maack, R. G. C., Scheuermann, G., Hernandez, J., & Gillmann, C. (2023). Uncertainty-aware visual analytics: scope, opportunities, and challenges. *The Visual Computer, 39*(12), 6345–6366.

Maack, R. G. C., Scheuermann, G., Hernandez, J., & Gillmann, C. (2023). A workflow to systematically design uncertainty-aware visual analytics applications. *The Visual Computer.*

Nieradzik, L., Scheuermann, G., Saur, D., & Gillmann, C. (2021). *Effect of the output activation function on the probabilities and errors in medical image segmentation.* arXiv preprint arXiv: 2109.00903.

Potter, K., Rosen, P., & Johnson, C. R. (2011). From quantification to visualization: A taxonomy of uncertainty visualization approaches. In *IFIP Working Conference on Uncertainty Quantification* (pp. 226–249). Springer.

Preim, B., & Lawonn, K. (2020). A survey of visual analytics for public health. *Computer Graphics Forum, 39*(1), 543–580.

Raith, F., Scheuermann, G., & Gillmann, C. (2021). Uncertainty-aware detection and visualization of ocean eddies in ensemble flow fields a case study of the red sea. In *Proceedings of the Workshop on Visualisation in Environmental Sciences.*

Reiner, B. (2017). Quantitative analysis of uncertainty in medical reporting: Creating a standardized and objective methodology. *Journal of Digital Imaging, 31.*

Small, M. (2023). *The small man.* Accessed January 18, 2024.

Steinbach, P., Gernhardt, F., Tanveer, M., Schmerler, S., & Starke, S. (2022). *Machine learning state-of-the-art with uncertainties.*

Weiskopf, D. (2022). Uncertainty visualization: Concepts, methods, and applications in biological data visualization. *Frontiers in Bioinformatics, 2.*

Welle, F., Stoll, K., Gillmann, C., Henkelmann, J., Prasse, G., Kaiser, D. P., Kellner, E., Reisert, M., Schneider, H. R., Klingbeil, J., Stockert, A., Lobsien, D., Hofmann, K.T., Saur, D., & Wawrzyniak, M. (2023). Tissue outcome prediction in patients with proximal vessel occlusion and mechanical thrombectomy using logistic models. *Translational Stroke Research*, pp. 1–11

Xu, K., Ottley, A., Walchshofer, C., Streit, M., Chang, R., & Wenskovitch, J. (2020). Survey on the analysis of user interactions and visualization provenance. *Computer Graphics Forum, 39*(3), 757–783.

Yuan, J., Chen, C., Yang, W., Liu, M., Xia, J., & Liu, S. (2020). A survey of visual analytics techniques for machine learning. *Computational Visual Media, 7*, 3–36.

Part IV
Motion Capture and Feedback Systems

Chapter 9
Machine Learning in Biomechanics: Enhancing Human Movement Analysis

Bernd J. Stetter and Thorsten Stein

Abstract Biomechanical analysis of human movements is highly relevant for discovering strategies to prevent injury, treat disease, and enhance performance. In this context, high-dimensional datasets are typically collected using either laboratory-based biomechanical measurement systems or wearable sensors. In recent years, Machine Learning (ML) has become increasingly popular for exploiting the potential of high-dimensional biomechanical data. There are three major ML paradigms: supervised learning, unsupervised learning, and reinforcement learning, with the first two used primarily in biomechanics. In supervised learning, ML models are trained, for example, to classify knee injury status based on muscle activation patterns or to predict knee joint forces using wearable sensor data through regression algorithms. Unsupervised learning in biomechanical applications involves, for example, reducing high-dimensional kinematic data into compact low-dimensional representations or identifying characteristic groups of people, such as individuals with similar gait abnormalities. Reinforcement learning presents, for example, a promising approach to developing controllers for biomechanical models capable of generating physiologically feasible high-dimensional movements. ML-based analysis complements traditional biomechanical analysis well, as both have their own strengths and weaknesses. Overall, ML can support our understanding of human movement biomechanics and optimize movement patterns to prevent injuries and enhance human health and performance.

Keywords Gait Analysis · Biomechanical Modeling · Wearable Sensors · Kinematics · Kinetics · Machine Learning Algorithms · Data-Driven Approaches · Signal Processing · Daily Activities · Sport

B. J. Stetter (✉) · T. Stein
Institute of Sports and Sports Science, Karlsruhe Institute of Technology, Karlsruhe, Germany
e-mail: bernd.stetter@kit.edu

C. Dindorf et al. (eds.), *Artificial Intelligence in Sports, Movement, and Health*,
https://doi.org/10.1007/978-3-031-67256-9_9

9.1 Introduction

Movement is an important aspect of human life as it ensures physical mobility and thus interaction with the environment. Accordingly, human movement is an important topic for many scientific disciplines, including biomechanics. Biomechanics is a scientific discipline that deals, among other things, with the modeling, simulation and analysis of human movements to discover strategies to prevent injury, treat disease, and enhance performance (Seth et al., 2018). This requires an interdisciplinary research approach that profitably integrates knowledge from anatomy, physiology, physics, engineering, computer science and others. Today, biomechanics is a rapidly growing discipline that covers a wide variety of research questions and fields of application (e.g., Uchida and Delp (2021); https://isbweb.org/).

In biomechanics, human movements are usually studied under laboratory conditions with infrared camera systems, force plates and electromyography (EMG). The data collected using these systems, together with anthropometric data, form the input for biomechanical models that enable the calculation of additional variables that cannot simply be measured directly (e.g., joint angles, joint moments and joint forces). With this state-of-the-art approach it is possible to collect many high-dimensional datasets in a short period of time. This approach is very sophisticated and accurate, but also very expensive and limited to the laboratory (Dorschky et al., 2023). To enable a biomechanical analysis of human movements outside the laboratory, wearable sensors (e.g., IMUs) have been increasingly used in recent years (Díaz et al., 2020; Mundt, 2023). These sensors are worn close to the body, only slightly influence the wearer's movements, and offer the possibility to study human movements for extended periods of time in natural environments. These environments can be everyday day life or sports during training, rehabilitation and competition. Human movement analysis in these contexts is important for monitoring athletic performance, preventing injuries and managing disease progression (Preatoni et al., 2022). Wearable sensors are less expensive and enable an ecologically valid data collection. However, there are also some challenges when using wearable sensors, such as sensor drifts, noise, calibration errors, movement artifacts, data transmission errors and unmeasured signals (e.g., ground reaction forces), which must be considered (Dorschky et al., 2023; Hafer et al., 2023).

In principle, laboratory-based biomechanical measurement systems and wearable sensors can be used to collect many high-dimensional datasets. Depending on the research question (e.g., effect of gait training in knee osteoarthritis patients), the recorded or calculated biomechanical datasets (e.g., time series of knee joint moments during walking) are often reduced to a single discrete parameter (e.g., maximum knee adduction moment during the stance phase). Then statistical hypothesis testing is applied on such discrete parameters. With this well-founded approach, it cannot be completely ruled out that further important information is hidden in the high-dimensional datasets in the form of complex non-linear relationships that would be relevant in the context of the research question. In such situations, traditional simple statistical analyses reach their limits. In contrast, the field of Machine Learning (ML) focuses explicitly on the development of algorithms that can recognize patterns in high-dimensional datasets and make predictions.

The intersection of ML and biomechanics is precisely this topic that is the focus of this chapter. After a brief introduction to the topic of ML, the aim is to present selected applications in biomechanics according to the most important ML algorithms and thus give the reader an introductory overview of the topic. This chapter concludes with an outlook on future developments.

9.2 Fundamentals of Machine Learning

ML is a subfield of Artificial Intelligence (AI) that comprises among other things elements from statistics (e.g., Linear Regression and k-Means clustering), computer science (e.g., data structures and algorithms) as well as neuroscience (e.g., Neural Networks and learning). It involves the creation of algorithms that can automatically learn from data rather than through explicit programming and improve their performance over time based on some performance measure (Alpaydin, 2020).

ML includes three major learning paradigms, although hybrid forms exist (Alpaydin, 2020): (1) In supervised learning, algorithms are trained with input data which is associated with known output labels. Supervised learning includes classification (e.g., classification of gait pattern in patients with acute ACL injury; Sect. 9.3.1) and regression (e.g., prediction of knee joint forces based on wearable sensor data; Sect. 9.3.2), making it suitable for situations in which data with labeled features are available that define the meaning of the data. (2) Unsupervised learning involves discovering patterns in unlabeled data to understand the meaning of the data. Dimensionality reduction (e.g., reduction of high-dimensional kinematic data into a meaningful low-dimensional representation; Sect. 9.4.1) and clustering (e.g., grouping of patients with similar gait compensating strategies due to hip osteoarthritis; Sect. 9.4.2) represent unsupervised learning, enabling insights into data organization and relationships. (3) Finally, reinforcement learning employs a different approach, instead of training with sample data as in supervised learning, an agent interacts with an environment to learn optimal actions through trial and error. By receiving feedback in the form of rewards or penalties, successful actions are "reinforced" adapting the behavior to maximize cumulative reward (e.g., optimize prosthetic limb control based on feedback about movement success or failure; Sect. 9.5).

When a ML algorithm is trained with data, a ML model is created. For example, the training of a regression algorithm (i.e., learn regression coefficients) creates a predictive model. When the predictive model is fed with new, unseen data, the model can provide a prediction based on the data used to train the model. However, this process of developing a ML model is similar regardless of the type of ML algorithm motivated previously.

Figure 9.1 illustrates the primary steps involved in developing a ML model for biomechanical applications. It starts with data collection using various systems such as motion capture, wearable sensors, or EMG, to determine variables (e.g., joint angles, muscle activations) describing movement patterns on different levels. This is achieved through the application of signal processing and biomechanical modeling. Subsequently, when dealing with high-dimensional data, feature engineering is employed to derive a lower-dimensional representation. In the next step, an appropriate ML algorithm (e.g., Decision Tree for classification) must be selected based on the biomechanical task and the characteristics of the data. During the training process on a training set of the data, model parameters are adjusted to minimize error or maximize performance. When training a ML model, it's crucial to avoid both underfitting and overfitting. Underfitting arises when the model fails to adequately represent the training data, resulting in high training error, while overfitting occurs when the model excessively fits the training data (Dorschky et al., 2023). Finally, a test set of the data, also named as validation set, is utilized for validation to assess the performance of the trained model and ensure generalization to unseen data. Common validation approaches in biomechanical ML applications are the K-Fold Cross-Validation (KFCV) and the Leave-One-Subject-Out Cross-Validation (LOSOCV) (Dorschky et al., 2023; Halilaj et al., 2018). KFCV (e.g., 10FCV) divides the dataset into k subsets or "folds" (e.g., $k = 10$), training the algorithm k times with each fold as the test set once and the remaining data as the train set. LOSOCV allocates each subject's data solely to either training or test sets (i.e., the number of folds equals the number of subjects). Performance metrics are averaged across all iterations. Each approach has its strengths and limitations, and the choice depends on factors such as dataset size, computational resources, and the specific characteristics of the application scenario.

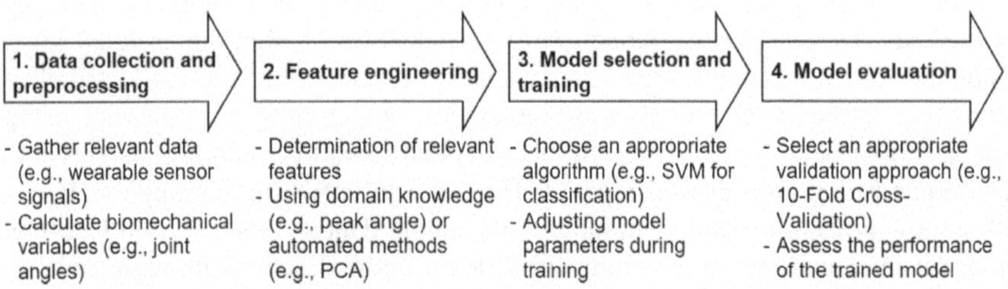

Fig. 9.1 The primary steps involved in developing a ML model, along with a brief description, occur before the model can be applied for biomechanical purposes. PCA: Principal Component Analysis; SVM: Support Vector Machine

9.3 Supervised Learning

Supervised learning is a ML paradigm where the algorithm is trained on a labeled dataset to learn the relationship between input features and corresponding output labels (Alpaydin, 2020). The term label, which is also known as response or dependent variable, refers to the output or outcome that an algorithm learns to predict (Halilaj et al., 2018). For example, in a ML model for diagnostics, it could represent disease status, while in a regression model, it signifies a biomechanical time series, such as the ground reaction force during a gait cycle. This entails using a dataset where both the input (e.g., joint kinematics) and the output (e.g., gait abnormalities) are known for model development. The goal is for the algorithm to learn a mapping function from the input to the desired output, enabling it to make predictions on new, unseen data. The labeled dataset would for example include instances of normal and abnormal gait, allowing the algorithm to discern patterns and make predictions about the gait characteristics of future individuals.

Supervised learning encompasses two primary subtypes: classification (Sect. 9.3.1), which involves predicting discrete categories, and regression (Sect. 9.3.2), which involves predicting continuous values.

9.3.1 Classification

9.3.1.1 Foundations and Biomechanical Applications

ML classification algorithms in biomechanics involve organizing high-dimensional data into meaningful groups or classes based on specific criteria, enabling analysis of human movement patterns. One example in biomechanics is the classification of muscle activation pattern, where classification models are trained to assess deficits in neuromuscular control after knee injury (Mohr et al., 2019). As described in Sect. 9.2, it begins with data collection and necessary calculations to obtain biomechanical variables of interest (e.g., joint angles, muscle activations).

Next, relevant features are extracted either through biomechanical domain knowledge or by utilizing dimensionality reduction on the raw or preprocessed data (see Sect. 9.4.1). The determined features serve as inputs for a classification algorithm. Common algorithms include Decision Trees, Support Vector Machines (SVM), and Artificial Neural Networks (ANN), which learn patterns and relationships in the data to accurately classify biomechanical data (Alpaydin, 2020; Halilaj et al., 2018). The algorithm selection can be a challenging part of developing good classification models due to the variety of possible algorithms (Alpaydin, 2020; Halilaj et al., 2018). Consequently, it may be worth testing different ones depending on the specific application, as not every algorithm will produce good results in every application (Richter et al., 2018).

After being trained on a dataset with known input and output, the classification model should undergo model evaluation for performance and generalization (see Sect. 9.2). The most commonly used performance metric for classification models is the accuracy, also named as classification rate, as the rate of correct classifications made by the model (Halilaj et al., 2018). Other metrics, such as the sensitivity (also true positive rate), specificity (also true negative rate), area under the receiver operating characteristic (ROC) curve, or the confusion matrix, can also be included to facilitate assessment and comparison with alternative models [see Alpaydin (2020); Halilaj et al. (2018) for more details].

Once the classification model is validated, it can be used to systematically classify participants or patients based on biomechanical data in various fields of application such as sports biomechanics and clinical biomechanics. Table 9.1 presents a selected overview of studies addressing classification scenarios in biomechanical applications.

Table 9.1 Exemplary studies utilize classification to investigate human movement biomechanics

Study	Purpose	Classification algorithm(s)	Finding
Christian et al. (2016)	Classification and assessment of gait pattern in patients with acute ACL injury	SVM	ACL injury and healthy individuals were classified with 100% accuracy, and the gait score of the injured group improved significantly after a therapeutic treatment
Richter et al. (2018)	Classification of movement strategies in change of direction tasks	RF, Corr2Mean, SVM, regression, ANN and others	Classification accuracy ranged from 82% (i.e., Corr2Mean) to 53% (i.e., discriminant analysis)
Mohr et al. (2019)	Classification of muscle activation pattern according to knee injury history	SVM	83% of the muscle activation patterns of the affected or unaffected leg were classified correctly, while females achieved 100% accuracy
Suda et al. (2020)	Classification of foot–ankle movement patterns among runners at varying experience levels	SVM	Foot–ankle kinematic and kinetic patterns showed classification accuracies of over 85% for less, moderately, and experienced runners

ACL anterior cruciate ligament; *RF* Random Forest; *SVM* Support Vector Machine; Corr2Mean: correlation to the cluster average; *ANN* Artificial Neural Network

9.3.1.2 Exemplary Study: "Support Vector Machine-Based Gait Pattern Classification"

Christian et al. (2016) conducted a study investigating the application of SVM in analyzing kinematic gait patterns of recently ACL-injured patients and assessing the impact of therapeutic intervention. By treating gait kinematics as high-dimensional data rather than discrete variables, a more comprehensive understanding of gait characteristics can be achieved, aiding in the objective assessment of gait and reducing subjective bias in observational gait analysis. The study involved recording 3D trajectories of 14 reflective markers of the lower body and thorax of seven male patients with acute unilateral anterior cruciate ligament (ACL) rupture and seven healthy males. Principal Component Analysis (PCA, Sect. 9.4.1) and Recursive Feature Elimination (i.e., algorithm to select a subset of features) were employed to extract features from 3D marker trajectories across the gait cycle, thus reducing dimensionality. In conjunction to this, a linear SVM was trained based on two Principal Components (PCs) to differentiate between the injured and healthy groups, with cross-validation performed to assess classification accuracy, yielding 100%.

The SVM model (Alpaydin, 2020) can be interpreted as a hyperplane, essentially a line in 2D in the specific case due to the two PCs, that separates the two groups in a manner that maximizes the margin, i.e. the distance between the hyperplane and the closest points from each group. This hyperplane is the decision boundary created by the SVM algorithm. The points closest to this hyperplane are the support vectors, which essentially determine the position and orientation of the hyperplane. By adjusting the position and orientation of this hyperplane, the SVM algorithm finds the optimal boundary that best divides the two groups.

Additionally, a classifier-oriented gait score was introduced by Christian et al. (2016) as a metric for gait quality. Therefore, the Euclidian distance along the normal vector of the hyperplane, indicating the direction of greatest separability, was calculated to rate the gait patterns. After manual therapeutic treatment, the injured group was re-evaluated using the SVM model. The results showed improved gait scores, indicating that the gait patterns of the injured group became closer to those of the healthy group. The improved gait score was consistent with the clinical rating of the patients.

The study demonstrates that a SVM model for classification effectively detects gait alterations caused by an ACL injury, with findings aligning with clinical assessments. Furthermore, the visualization capabilities facilitate the interpretation of key kinematic features, enhancing diagnostic integration.

9.3.2 *Regression*

9.3.2.1 Foundations and Biomechanical Applications

ML regression algorithms focus on predicting numerical values within a continuous range (i.e., output) based on input data (Alpaydin, 2020). This involves training an algorithm to learn the relationships in labeled datasets, enabling it to make future predictions about unseen data. These algorithms serve as an essential instrument for tackling the distinct challenges posed by biomechanical variables, which are often complicated to assess and interpret due to the complex interplay of biological and environmental factors. Through its systematic examination of complex relationships, regression provides a valuable framework for making predictions. For example, regression algorithms, when combined with wearable sensing, have recently been shown to achieve similar or even better performance for "in the wild" movement analysis compared to the use of traditional physics-based models (Dorschky et al., 2023).

The training of a regression algorithm starts with collected and often preprocessed data, such as the determination of biomechanical variables of interest by using biomechanical modeling (e.g., joint forces). Various regression algorithms such as Linear Regression, Polynomial Regression, SVM Regression, or ANN can be applied depending on the complexity of the relationships being studied (Alpaydin, 2020). Studies have indicated that the requisite algorithm complexity varies according to the complexity of the movement; basic algorithms such as linear or polynomial regression have demonstrated efficacy in predicting joint angles and joint moments of one-dimensional gym exercises, whereas more sophisticated algorithms have been necessitated for the prediction during gait (Mundt, 2023). Independent of the complexity of the algorithm, they learn from the labeled dataset (i.e., supervised learning) to establish relationships between input data (e.g., joint angles) and the output data (e.g., joint forces).

Following training, the regression model must undergo typical model evaluation to assess its performance and generalization (Sect. 9.2), which is crucial for determining the model's reliability and effectiveness. After validating the model and confirming its accuracy within the desired scope, it can be applied to the specific biomechanical task. Table 9.2 provides a selective overview of studies that utilized regression in biomechanical applications, with many focusing on predicting variables that are challenging to assess. Time series prediction using regression models plays a pivotal role in bridging the gap between laboratory-based research and real-world applications (Dorschky et al., 2023; Mundt, 2023). Both normal and pathological movement analysis across diverse domains, such as sports biomechanics and clinical biomechanics research, can benefit from joint angle, moment and force predictions.

Table 9.2 Exemplary studies utilize regression to investigate human movement biomechanics

Study	Purpose	Regression algorithm(s)	Finding
Argent et al. (2019)	Prediction of hip and knee angle time series using a wearable sensor during lower limb rehabilitation exercises	Linear Regression, Polynomial Regression, Decision Tree Regression, and RF	Depending on the exercise different models performed best with an average RMSE across all exercises of 4.81°
Stetter et al. (2019)	Prediction of knee joint force time series based on wearable sensor data in sports movements	ANN	The predicted vertical knee joint forces showed good agreement ($r \geq 0.81$ and rRMSE $\leq$ 20.3%) with reference values for most movements
Nicholson et al. (2022)	Prediction of pitching arm kinetics to mitigate shoulder stress	RF, SVM Regression, Gradient Boosting Machine, ANN, and Statistical Regression	The Gradient Boosting Machine exhibited the lowest RMSE of 0.013% BW*H for the elbow valgus torque and 1.7% BW for the shoulder distraction force
Moghadam et al. (2023)	Prediction of lower-limb joint kinematics, kinetics, and muscle force time series from wearable sensors	RF, SVM Regression, Multivariate Adaptive Regression Spline, and CNN	The RF and CNN outperformed the other algorithms: kinematics (RMSE: 3°–8°), kinetics (RMSE: 0.05–0.27 Nm/kg), and muscle forces (rRMSE: 18–36%)

RF Random Forest; *SVM* Support Vector Machine; *ANN* Artificial Neural Network; *CNN* Convolutional Neural Network; *r* correlation coefficient; *RMSE* root mean square error; *rRMSE* relative RMSE; *BW* body weight; *H* height

9.3.2.2 Exemplary Study: "Artificial Neural Network-Based Knee Joint Force Prediction"

We conducted a study using ANN to predict knee joint forces (KJF) during sport movements based on data obtained from two wearable sensors (Stetter et al., 2019). The motivation was to overcome limitations in mobile assessment of internal knee joint loading, which are crucial for providing adequate injury prevention strategies. Thirteen participants were instrumented with two wearable sensors (i.e., IMU) located on the right thigh and shank. Participants performed a variety of movements, including linear motions, changes of direction, and jumps, while IMU signals as well as full body kinematics and ground reaction forces were synchronously recorded. 3D KJF were determined using a full-body biomechanical model. An ANN was then trained on a dataset combining IMU signals as ANN inputs and 3D KJF as outputs for all movements, learning the association between the IMU signals and the time series of KJF.

The ANN model is illustrated in Fig. 9.2 and what happens during the training can be described as follows (Alpaydin, 2020): Weights, representing the strength of connections between neurons, and biases, which adjust the output along with the weighted sum of inputs, are initialized randomly. When the training starts, the input data are passed through the network, computing predictions. These predictions are compared with the actual outputs using a loss function to measure the disparity. Through backpropagation, gradients of the loss with respect to each weight and bias are computed, enabling adjustments to be made via an optimization algorithm. This iterative process, repeated for multiple rounds, called epochs, refines the algorithm's performance. To prevent overfitting, the algorithm's performance is periodically assessed on a validation set, halting training early if improvement plateaus. This training process was repeated 13 times to perform a LOSOCV (see Sect. 9.2) and assess the models predictive performance on new, unseen data.

The evaluation showed good agreement (correlation coefficients ≥ 0.81 and relative root mean square errors $\leq 20.3\%$) for the vertical KJF of the majority (11 out of 16) of the analyzed movements. Ten of the 16 movements showed comparable estimation accuracies (correlation coefficients ≥ 0.80 and relative root mean square errors $\leq 22.9\%$) for the anterior–posterior KJF. A pronounced drop in estimation accuracy for the medio-lateral KJF was observed (correlation coefficients ≤ 0.60 and relative root mean square errors $\geq 27.7\%$).

In summary, the study serves as an example of how ML regression combined with wearable sensors can be used to predict valuable biomechanical variables (i.e., KJF) for assessing joint loading. By addressing limitations in mobile KJF assessment, the study introduced new possibilities for in-field diagnosis potentially enhancing injury prevention strategies in the future.

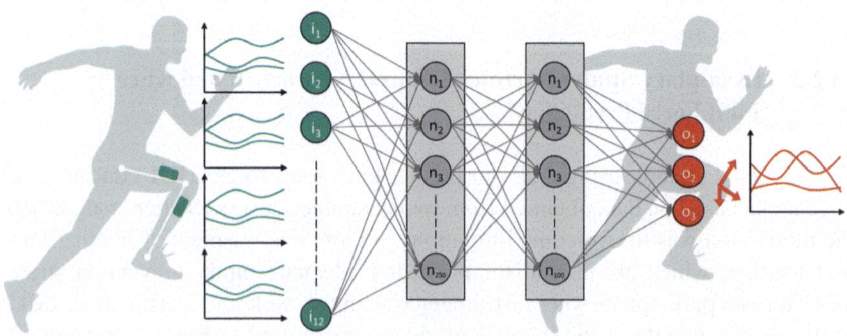

Fig. 9.2 Artificial Neural Network (ANN) using wearable sensors data as input (i1 to i12, illustrated in green) in order to predict three-dimensional knee joint forces as the biomechanical output (o1 to o3, illustrated in red) (mod. Stetter, 2021). The ANN shows two hidden layers (lightgrey boxes), one with 250 (n1 to n250) and one with 100 neurons (n1 to n100), which are connected to the input and output nodes. The circles represent the nodes of the ANN

9.4 Unsupervised Learning

Unsupervised learning is a ML paradigm where the algorithm analyzes unlabeled data to uncover inherent patterns or clusters without explicit guidance from predefined output labels (Alpaydin, 2020). In biomechanics, this can for example involve examining joint kinematics data without predefined categories or labels, with the aim of discovering meaningful relationships (e.g. coupled angular movements) or identifying characteristic groups (e.g., people with gait abnormalities) within high-dimensional data.

Unsupervised learning encompasses two primary subtypes: dimensionality reduction (Sect. 9.4.1), which aims to capture the essential features of the data, and clustering (Sect. 9.4.2), where data points are grouped based on similarities.

9.4.1 Dimensionality Reduction

9.4.1.1 Foundations and Biomechanical Applications

Dimensionality reduction involves algorithms aimed at reducing the number of features or variables in a dataset while preserving its essential information (Alpaydin, 2020). The process reflects the transformation of high-dimensional data into a lower-dimensional representation, making it more manageable for biomechanical analysis and ML model development (see Sect. 9.2). Over the past decades, two primary domains of biomechanical application of dimensionality reduction have been established:

(1) Reduction of high-dimensional biomechanical data into meaningful kinematic or muscle synergies following the idea of a modular control architecture to simplify control. This is motivated by the complexity of the musculoskeletal system, which is composed of approximately 700 muscles and 300 mechanical degrees of freedom (Bernstein, 1967). This highly redundant system enables us to achieve movement tasks in countless ways. A longstanding question in motor control and biomechanical research is how the central nervous system (CNS) resolves this redundancy. Furthermore, throughout our lives, we acquire numerous motor skills, such as walking or playing golf. This raises another key question in motor control and biomechanical research: how does the CNS represent this versatility? To provide answers to these fundamental scientific questions, dimensionality reduction algorithms come into play, as they offer a solution for extracting meaningful low-dimensional representations, often called synergies, from high-dimensional biomechanical data. Such synergies can exist either on a kinematic or muscular level (Daffertshofer et al., 2004; Tresch et al., 2006), and they typically represent compositional elements working together to produce results not obtainable by any of the elements alone (Fig. 4.1). For example, when conducting a PCA on high-dimensional kinematic data of

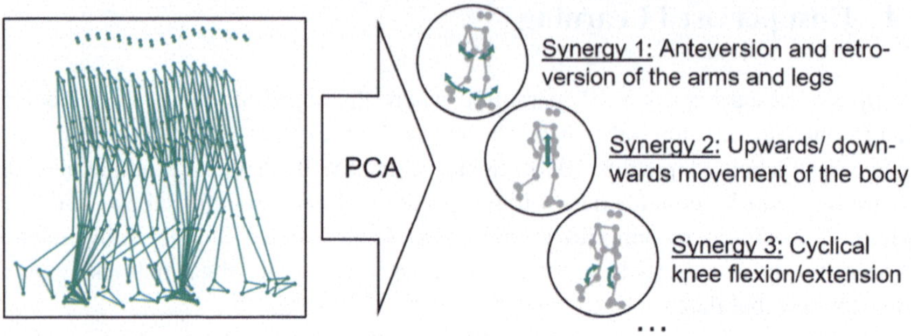

Fig. 9.3 Illustration for the application of dimensionality reduction, i.e. principal component analysis (PCA), to represent the high-dimensional walking movement by low-dimensional kinematic synergies. A short description of the aspects of the whole movement represented by each kinematic synergy is provided

straight-line walking, walking a 90° turn, and walking upstairs, the first five synergies explain more than 80% of the variance in a 54-dimensional space (18 markers × 3D coordinates) for each movement task (Stetter et al., 2020). Similar PCA-based approaches have been used to study postural control and to quantify technique in sports (Federolf, 2016). Alternative dimensionality reduction algorithms, such as nonnegative matrix factorization, have specifically been proven valuable in assessing the hypothesis that movements might be produced through the combination of a small number of muscle synergies (Tresch et al., 2006) (Fig. 9.3).

(2) Feature engineering or selection as a step in developing a ML model to improve performance for classification, regression or clustering. The foundation for that lies in the fact that the complexity of any ML algorithm (e.g., SVM) depends on the number of inputs. This determines both the runtime and required memory for computation, as well as the number of examples required to train such an algorithm (Alpaydin, 2020). Feature engineering involves selecting a subset of significant features from a dataset and discarding the rest, often achieved through dimensionality reduction algorithms. By eliminating redundant features, the complexity of ML models can be reduced and overfitting caused by highly correlated or noisy features can be mitigated (Mundt, 2023). Additionally, good feature engineering is an important step in developing a ML model from high-dimensional biomechanical data, as it can lead to high model performance even with simple algorithms, such as Logistic Regression (Halilaj et al., 2018). However, reducing data dimensionality while maintaining enough relevant information is a non-trivial challenge. For this purpose, features can be selected manually based on domain knowledge (e.g., peak knee angle during a cutting movement), or a data-driven approach is employed, such as calculating summary metrices of time series (e.g., average of the signal; Halilaj et al., 2018). Additionally, more open-source toolboxes [e.g., Tsfresh (Christ et al.,

2018), or Chameleon (Thilakeswaran et al., 2021)] including various dimensionality reduction algorithms have become available and are frequently used in ML applications in biomechanics (Mundt, 2023). For example, the study by Moghadam et al. (2023) (see Table 9.2) used the Tsfresh toolbox to extract features from EMG and IMU signals before training regression algorithms using the most important features. It's crucial to bear in mind that while automatic feature extraction techniques, such as the widely used PCA, can capture some of the data's significance, they may generate features that are difficult to interpret or lack relevance to a specific output (Halilaj et al., 2018). According to Halilaj et al. (2018), when combining features representing diverse biomechanical quantities (e.g., knee angles and moments), it's essential to rescale features, like z-score normalization, based on the intended ML algorithm for further analysis.

Table 9.3 provides a selected overview of studies utilizing dimensionality reduction algorithms. It focuses on the two primary domains of biomechanical application: meaningful reduction of high-dimensional biomechanical data and feature engineering.

9.4.1.2 Exemplary Study: "Dimensionality Reduction of Plantar Force Data for Assessing Effects of Different Running Shoes"

Trudeau et al. (2015) conducted a study investigating the application of a novel method, i.e. combining PCA and SVM, for assessing the effects of different footwear interventions on plantar loading. A PCA was used to extract different loading features, i.e. reducing the highly dimensional plantar loading patterns to its most important information, from the stance phase of running. Afterwards, a SVM model (see Sect. 9.3.1) was used to determine whether and how these loading features were different across three shoe conditions varying in weight, cushioning and sole construction. Plantar pressure data during the stance phase of ten running strides were recorded for each shoe condition from 42 active recreational runners using an insole consisting of 99 force cells (represented by a cell matrix of 105 elements, with six elements set to zero).

To begin the dimensionality reduction, a matrix with 126,000 rows (i.e., 42 participants $\times$ 3 shoes $\times$ 10 trials $\times$ 100 time points) and 105 columns (i.e., force cells) was created and standardized by subtraction of the mean force-vector of each shoe across trials and participants. A PCA was applied to this input matrix. This process can be described as follows (Alpaydin, 2020): First, the covariance matrix is calculated, summarizing the relationships between variables (i.e., force cells) by indicating how much they vary together. Next, PCA performs eigenvalue decomposition on the covariance matrix to find its eigenvectors and eigenvalues. Eigenvectors represent the directions of maximum variance in the data, while eigenvalues indicate the magnitude of variance along these directions. The eigenvectors are ranked by their corresponding eigenvalues, with the highest eigenvalue representing the first

Table 9.3 Exemplary studies utilize dimensionality reduction to investigate human movement biomechanics

Study	Purpose	Dimensionality reduction algorithm(s)	Finding
Daffertshofer et al. (2004)	Application of PCA for dimensionality reduction of high-dimensional kinematic and electromyography data	PCA	PCA reduced both kinematic and electromyography data into meaningful low-dimensional components
Tresch et al. (2006)	Comparison of different dimensionality reduction algorithms on electromyography data to extract muscle synergies	PCA, FA, ICA, and NMF	FA, ICA and NMF robustly identify muscle synergies and were similar in the solution they found
Phinyomark et al. (2012)	Dimensionality reduction as preprocessing step for hand motion classification	Different LDAs, and PCA	Extended LDA-based algorithms led to better classification results as without dimensionality reduction or using PCA
Christ et al. (2018)	Dimensionality reduction as preprocessing step for Machine Learning model development	63 time series characterization algorithms to extract meaningful features	A toolbox for feature selection from time series on basis of statistical hypothesis tests

PCA Principal Component Analysis; *FA* Factor Analysis; *ICA* Independent Component Analysis; *NMF* Nonnegative Matrix Factorization; *LDA* Linear Discriminant Analysis; *ML* Machine Learning

PC. Subsequent eigenvectors represent orthogonal directions of decreasing variance. Finally, PCA projects the original data onto the new orthogonal axes defined by the PCs. This transformation results in a lower-dimensional representation of the data, known as the PC scores, capturing the most important patterns of variation. In the study's application, the dimensionality was reduced to 35 PCs reflecting 99% of the data's variance and combined with three residual vectors for further analysis.

Following dimensionality reduction, pairwise linear SVM algorithms were applied to characterize systematic differences in force patterns between the shoe conditions by investigating the normal vector of the hyperplane (see Sect. 9.3.1). A LOSOCV was performed, and classification accuracies were higher than 94% for the three pairwise SVM models. Characteristic differences (e.g., greater force at the forefoot) between shoes were quantified and interpreted based on the PC scores, i.e. plantar loading features.

The study demonstrates that dimensionality reduction is a helpful step in ML model development to make high-dimensional data interpretable, as well as to successfully apply classification algorithms. From a practical perspective, this study serves as an example of how ML can assist in selecting appropriate footwear or guiding footwear interventions for specific populations such as neuropathic patients (Trudeau et al., 2015).

9.4.2 Clustering

9.4.2.1 Foundations and Biomechanical Applications

Clustering refers to ML algorithms that involve grouping similar data points together based on patterns or similarities within a dataset (Alpaydin, 2020). The objective of clustering is to discover inherent groupings in the data, where members within the same cluster share more similarities with each other than with those in other clusters. In the field of biomechanics, a common objective is to determine the optimal intervention tailored to individuals, such as selecting the ideal footwear or optimizing training protocols. While this task may sound almost trivial, it becomes quite challenging due to the fact that individuals respond to a given intervention in a person-dependent manner, resulting in the same intervention being beneficial for one person but not for another (Hoerzer et al., 2015). These individual responses have, for example, been observed across various interventions, including footwear, running surfaces, and orthotics (Hoerzer et al., 2015). Consequently, determine the most suitable intervention from a data analysis standpoint is far from straightforward. Exploratory data analysis, such as clustering movement patterns of individuals who react similarly to a specific intervention (e.g., a specific therapeutic treatment) or product (e.g., a running shoe), is a helpful concept to overcome this challenge.

The process starts with data preparation, including the determination of variables of interest using biomechanical modeling, for example joint kinematics. Subsequently, relevant features can be selected or extracted from the often high-dimensional dataset, which for example includes kinematic data from multiple joints and dimensions, with dimensionality reduction algorithms (see Sect. 9.4.1). Next, a clustering algorithm is chosen based on the dataset's characteristics and the specific biomechanical task. Typical algorithms are k-Means, Hierarchical Clustering, or Self-Organizing Maps. These algorithms partition the dataset into clusters of similar data points according to the underlying clustering approach (Xu & Tian, 2015). A common approach is centroid- or partition-based clustering (e.g., k-Means), which works on the closeness (e.g., Euclidean distance) of the data points to chosen central values. Connectivity-based clustering, such as Hierarchical Clustering, assigns data points to clusters based on their distance (e.g., Euclidean distance) to each other. Data points that are close to each are grouped into the same cluster. Further approaches exist, such as distribution-based clustering that uses statistical distributions (e.g., Gaussian distribution) to cluster the data (Xu & Tian, 2015). Self-Organizing Maps are an alternative clustering approach. They are ANN that project high-dimensional data on a low-dimensional grid of nodes, typically two-dimensional, enabling the identification of groups of similar data points (Kohonen, 2001). Once the clustering is complete, the quality of the clusters is evaluated using metrics such as silhouette

Table 9.4 Exemplary studies utilize clustering to investigate human movement biomechanics

Study	Purpose	Clustering algorithm(s)	Finding
van Drongelen et al. (2021)	Grouping of patients with similar gait compensating strategies due to unilateral hip OA	Hierarchical Clustering, and k-Means	Two clusters of patients with unilateral hip OA were identified, showing different deviations from healthy controls in spatio-temporal, kinematic, and kinetic parameters
Herzog et al. (2023)	Grouping of strategies during sit-to-stand and stand-to-sit movements in the context of rollator usage	Hierarchical Clustering, and k-Means	Three strategies for sit-to-stand (forward leaning, vertical rise, hybrid) and three strategies for stand-to-sit (backward lowering, vertical lowering, hybrid) were identified, each with two additional strategies observed in challenging balance conditions
Giles et al. (2023)	Grouping of different COD movement strategies in professional tennis	Hierarchical Clustering	Five clusters of different COD movement strategies were identified: cutters, gear changers, lateral changers, balanced changers, and passive changers
David and Barton (2024)	Objective assessment of individual movement strategies related to injury risk in athletes	Self-Organising Maps	Athletes with significantly different movement strategies when sidestepping were identified, with one strategy clearly associated with ACL injury risk factors

OA osteoarthritis; *COD* change of direction; *ACL* anterior cruciate ligament

score or within-cluster sum of squares (Halilaj et al., 2018). This evaluation helps assess how well and robust the clusters represent the underlying structure of the data. Finally, the clusters can be interpreted and visualized using techniques like scatter plots, or dendrograms to gain insights into the data's patterns. Clustering has been used in various biomechanical fields of application ranging from sports [e.g., grouping of individuals based on running kinematics (Hoerzer et al., 2015)] to clinical applications [e.g., grouping of distinct walking patterns in cerebral palsy (Roche et al., 2014)]. Table 9.4 presents a selected overview of studies that utilized clustering to investigate human movement biomechanics.

9.4.2.2 Exemplary Study: "Clustering to Identify Gait Compensating Strategies Due to Hip Osteoarthritis"

In a study by van Drongelen et al. (2021), clustering was utilized to group patients with unilateral hip osteoarthritis based on gait adaptations. These patients often show deficits in gait biomechanics even after total hip replacement surgery. A preoperative identification of patients at risk for persistent movement abnormalities after joint replacement is helpful for adapting or individualizing the rehabilitation program. Improved rehabilitation could for example prevent the development of degenerative joint disease in neighboring joints. The conducted analysis consisted of three consecutive steps: first, dimensionality reduction of gait kinematics; second, clustering the data of hip osteoarthritis patients ($n = 51$); and third, statistically comparing the gait biomechanics of the patients in the different clusters with healthy controls ($n = 46$).

PCA was used for dimensionality reduction, resulting in three PCs explaining 70% of the thorax, pelvis, hip, knee and foot kinematic gait cycle time series data. Hierarchical clustering based on the scores of the first three PCs was used for determining the appropriate number of clusters, and involved assessing the scree plots and silhouette coefficients. The scree plot illustrates the within-cluster sum of squares plotted against the number of clusters. As the number of clusters increases, the sum of squares decreases, but at a declining rate. The optimal number of clusters is indicated at the "elbow" of the curve, where the rate of decrease slows and the curve flattens. Silhouette coefficients measure the similarity of objects within clusters, when compared to points in other clusters, helping to select the number of clusters with the highest average silhouette score. These analyses helped identify the optimal number of two clusters. Using such tests is important to ensure that additional algorithms that determine cluster centers best represent the underlying structure of the data (Halilaj et al., 2018).

Subsequently, the k-Means algorithm with the defined number of two clusters was applied to identify the patients in the different subgroups. Thereby, the algorithm starts by randomly selecting centroids for each cluster, then assigns data points (i.e., patients) to the nearest centroid, updates centroids based on the mean of assigned data points, and iterates until convergence, meaning that the centroids no longer change significantly (Alpaydin, 2020). The goal is to minimize within-cluster variance, making data points within clusters similar and those in different clusters dissimilar.

The results of the study revealed that the clusters were characterized by differences in peak hip extension, with the cluster exhibiting less hip extension deviating significantly more from healthy controls. At least one year after total hip replacement, the gait pattern approached that of healthy individuals, but was not completely normalized, as both clusters still exhibited deviations from healthy controls. Overall, the study demonstrates that clustering is useful for identifying subgroups of hip OA patients exhibiting different types of gait adaptations. In the future, preoperative gait assessment and allocation to characteristic groups may help tailor rehabilitation programs for better postoperative outcomes.

9.5 Reinforcement Learning

Reinforcement learning is as ML paradigm based on the idea of an agent learning to take actions in an environment based on feedback in form of rewards and penalties to achieve specific goals (Alpaydin, 2020). In the context of biomechanics, reinforcement learning has traditionally played a minor role (Halilaj et al., 2018; Wu et al., 2021). However, with advancements in measurement technology, musculoskeletal modeling, and the emergence of technologies for ecological momentary assessment, such algorithms are becoming increasingly popular for addressing biomechanical research topics. For instance, reinforcement learning can optimize prosthetic limb control by enabling the algorithm to adapt its control strategy based on feedback about movement success or failure (Wen et al., 2020). Efforts to model control and biomechanics of movement have been ongoing in both the computer science and biomechanics communities (Halilaj et al., 2018; Seth et al., 2018). The simulation of physiologically accurate movement in diverse scenarios can support practitioners in tasks such as surgical planning and prototyping of assistive devices. However, existing methods are constrained by large and complex solution spaces of biomechanical models, restricting their applicability (Kidziński et al., 2018). Reinforcement learning presents a promising approach to develop model controllers capable of generating physiologically feasible movements in high-dimensional biomechanical systems (Kidziński et al., 2018). Additionally, reinforcement learning can offer alternatives to supervised ML or traditional analysis in biomechanics by estimating joint moments from electromyography or joint kinematics (Wu et al., 2021).

Overall, reinforcement learning in biomechanics holds new opportunities for optimizing movement patterns, personalized rehabilitation programs, and informing the development of adaptive assistive devices. Future research in this area holds the potential to significantly enhance human movement biomechanics and associated applications.

9.6 Summary and Outlook

The aim of this chapter was to provide an introductory overview of the application of ML in the context of human movement biomechanics. After a brief introduction to the topic in Sect. 9.2, examples of applications in biomechanics related to the three major ML paradigms of supervised learning (Sect. 9.3), unsupervised learning (Sect. 9.4), and reinforcement learning (Sect. 9.5) were presented. The focus was on ML algorithms related to the first two paradigms, which have primarily been used in biomechanics so far. In summary, ML complements traditional biomechanical analysis approaches by enhancing their analysis capabilities for high-dimensional data. In many applications of ML in biomechanics, the overall value is most likely dependent on both traditional biomechanical analysis steps and the quality of the ML model relevant to the specific biomechanical task. For example, the applied biomechanical measurement systems, signal processing procedures, and modeling techniques used to generate training data for a ML algorithm can significantly impact the outcome. In addition, interpreting the results of a ML model often requires incorporating biomechanical findings, which may have been derived using classic biomechanical approaches.

Looking ahead, the intersection of ML and biomechanics promises to enhance human movement analysis. ML algorithms enable researchers to extract nuanced patterns from high-dimensional biomechanical data, fundamentally altering our capabilities for analyzing human movement. One significant trend on the horizon is the deeper integration of advanced ML algorithms, such as Deep Learning. For example, Convolutional Neural Networks (CNN), ANN with many processing layers, are a type of Deep Learning algorithm (Alpaydin, 2020). In CNN, convolutional layers can automatically extract relevant features from the data. These layers prove effective for time series wearable sensor data due to the inherent correlation across both time and sensor axes (Dorschky et al., 2023). However, caution is warranted, as Deep Learning may only be appropriate when either a large dataset or a pretrained network is available (Halilaj et al., 2018).

The application of ML extends to real-time monitoring and feedback systems. By harnessing wearable sensors and biomechanical models, personalized feedback loops can be created to optimize movement patterns, prevent injuries, and enhance performance across various domains, including sports, rehabilitation, and ergonomics (Díaz et al., 2020; Dorschky et al., 2023). Interdisciplinary teams from diverse backgrounds and data sharing initiatives are expected to drive innovation in the field. As the prevalence of ML continues to grow, it's essential to establish good practices for conducting and reporting research at the intersection of biomechanics and ML, integrating important aspects such as rigorous model evaluation. This ensures that the conclusions drawn are valid and reproducible (Halilaj et al., 2018).

As ML becomes integrated into biomechanics, trust and confidence in the results are crucial for user acceptance. Explainable ML can help achieve this by making ML algorithms more transparent and traceable, specifically by developing white-box models instead of black-box models, for instance, through ML interpretability methods (Linardatos et al., 2021). Additionally, enhancing transparency would assist in practical solutions to meet legal requirements, such as the General Data Protection Regulation (GDPR) of the European Union, which mandates the traceability of ML models.

In conclusion, the outlook for ML in biomechanics is promising, with the potential to transform our understanding of human movement biomechanics and optimize movement patterns, prevent injuries, and enhance human health and performance. Through the responsible integration of advanced technology and collaborative efforts, we can unlock new insights that have far-reaching implications for human well-being.

References

Alpaydin, E. (2020). *Introduction to Machine Learning* (Vol. Fourth edition). The MIT Press.

Argent, R., Drummond, S., Remus, A., O'Reilly, M., & Caulfield, B. (2019). Evaluating the use of machine learning in the assessment of joint angle using a single inertial sensor. *Journal of Rehabilitation and Assistive Technologies, 6*, 2055668319868544. https://doi.org/10.1177/2055668319868544

Bernstein, N. (1967). *The co-ordination and regulation of movements.* Pergamon Press.

Christ, M., Braun, N., Neuffer, J., & Kempa-Liehr, A. W. (2018). Time series feature extraction on basis of scalable hypothesis tests (tsfresh—a python package). *Neurocomputing, 307*, 72–77. https://doi.org/10.1016/j.neucom.2018.03.067

Christian, J., Kröll, J., Strutzenberger, G., Alexander, N., Ofner, M., & Schwameder, H. (2016). Computer aided analysis of gait patterns in patients with acute anterior cruciate ligament injury. *Clinical Biomechanics, 33*, 55–60. https://doi.org/10.1016/j.clinbiomech.2016.02.008

Daffertshofer, A., Lamoth, C. J. C., Meijer, O. G., & Beek, P. J. (2004). PCA in studying coordination and variability: A tutorial. *Clinical Biomechanics, 19*(4), 415–428. https://doi.org/10.1016/j.clinbiomech.2004.01.005

David, S., & Barton, G. J. (2024). Characterization of movement patterns using unsupervised learning neural networks: Exploring a novel approach for monitoring athletes during sidestepping. *Journal of Sports Sciences.* https://doi.org/10.1080/02640414.2023.2300570

Díaz, S., Stephenson, J. B., & Labrador, M. A. (2020). Use of wearable sensor technology in gait, balance, and range of motion analysis. *Applied Sciences, 10*(1). https://doi.org/10.3390/app10010234

Dorschky, E., Camomilla, V., Davis, J., Federolf, P., Reenalda, J., & Koelewijn, A. D. (2023). Perspective on in the wild movement analysis using machine learning. *Human Movement Science, 87*, 103042. https://doi.org/10.1016/j.humov.2022.103042

Federolf, P. A. (2016). A novel approach to study human posture control: "Principal movements" obtained from a principal component analysis of kinematic marker data. *Journal of Biomechanics, 49*(3), 364–370. https://doi.org/10.1016/j.jbiomech.2015.12.030

Giles, B., Peeling, P., Kovalchik, S., & Reid, M. (2023). Differentiating movement styles in professional tennis: A machine learning and hierarchical clustering approach. *European Journal of Sport Science, 23*(1), 44–53. https://doi.org/10.1080/17461391.2021.2006800

Hafer, J. F., Vitali, R., Gurchiek, R., Curtze, C., Shull, P., & Cain, S. M. (2023). Challenges and advances in the use of wearable sensors for lower extremity biomechanics. *Journal of Biomechanics, 157*, 111714. https://doi.org/10.1016/j.jbiomech.2023.111714

Halilaj, E., Rajagopal, A., Fiterau, M., Hicks, J. L., Hastie, T. J., & Delp, S. L. (2018). Machine learning in human movement biomechanics: Best practices, common pitfalls, and new opportunities. *Journal of Biomechanics, 81*, 1–11. https://doi.org/10.1016/j.jbiomech.2018.09.009

Herzog, M., Krafft, F. C., Stetter, B. J., d'Avella, A., Sloot, L. H., & Stein, T. (2023). Rollator usage lets young individuals switch movement strategies in sit-to-stand and stand-to-sit tasks. *Scientific Reports, 13*(1). https://doi.org/10.1038/s41598-023-43401-6

Hoerzer, S., von Tscharner, V., Jacob, C., & Nigg, B. M. (2015). Defining functional groups based on running kinematics using self-organizing maps and support vector machines. *Journal of Biomechanics, 48*(10), 2072–2079. https://doi.org/10.1016/j.jbiomech.2015.03.017

Kidziński, Ł., Mohanty, S. P., Ong, C. F., Hicks, J. L., Carroll, S. F., Levine, S., Salathé, M., & Delp, S. L. (2018). Learning to run challenge: Synthesizing physiologically accurate motion using deep reinforcement learning. In *The NIPS '17 Competition: Building Intelligent Systems*, Cham.

Kohonen, T. (2001). *Self-organizing maps.* Springer.

Linardatos, P., Papastefanopoulos, V., & Kotsiantis, S. (2021). Explainable AI: A review of machine learning interpretability methods. *Entropy, 23*(1). https://doi.org/10.3390/e23010018

Moghadam, S. M., Yeung, T. D., & Choisne, J. (2023). A comparison of machine learning models' accuracy in predicting lower-limb joints' kinematics, kinetics, and muscle forces from wearable sensors. *Scientific Reports, 13*(1). https://doi.org/10.1038/s41598-023-31906-z

Mohr, M., von Tscharner, V., Emery, C. A., & Nigg, B. M. (2019). Classification of gait muscle activation patterns according to knee injury history using a support vector machine approach. *Human Movement Science, 66*, 335–346. https://doi.org/10.1016/j.humov.2019.05.006

Mundt, M. (2023). Bridging the lab-to-field gap using machine learning: a narrative review. *Sports Biomechanics*, 1–20. https://doi.org/10.1080/14763141.2023.2200749

Nicholson, K. F., Collins, G. S., Waterman, B. R., & Bullock, G. S. (2022). Machine learning and statistical prediction of pitching arm kinetics. *American Journal of Sports Medicine, 50*(1), 238–247. https://doi.org/10.1177/03635465211054506

Phinyomark, A., Hu, H., Phukpattaranont, P., & Limsakul, C. (2012). Application of linear discriminant analysis in dimensionality reduction for hand motion classification. *Measurement Science Review, 12*(3), 82–89. https://doi.org/10.2478/v10048-012-0015-8

Preatoni, E., Bergamini, E., Fantozzi, S., Giraud, L., Bustos, A. S. O., Vannozzi, G., & Camomilla, V. (2022). The use of wearable sensors for preventing, assessing, and informing recovery from sport-related musculoskeletal injuries: A systematic scoping review. *Sensors, 22*(9). https://doi.org/10.3390/s22093225

Richter, C., King, E., Falvey, E., & Franklyn-Miller, A. (2018). Supervised learning techniques and their ability to classify a change of direction task strategy using kinematic and kinetic features. *Journal of Biomechanics, 66*, 1–9. https://doi.org/10.1016/j.jbiomech.2017.10.025

Roche, N., Pradon, D., Cosson, J., Robertson, J., Marchiori, C., & Zory, R. (2014). Categorization of gait patterns in adults with cerebral palsy: A clustering approach. *Gait & Posture, 39*(1), 235–240. https://doi.org/10.1016/j.gaitpost.2013.07.110

Seth, A., Hicks, J. L., Uchida, T. K., Habib, A., Dembia, C. L., Dunne, J. J., Ong, C. F., DeMers, M. S., Rajagopal, A., Millard, M., Hamner, S. R., Arnold, E. M., Yong, J. R., Lakshmikanth, S. K., Sherman, M. A., Ku, J. P., & Delp, S. L. (2018). OpenSim: Simulating musculoskeletal dynamics and neuromuscular control to study human and animal movement. *Plos Computational Biology, 14*(7). https://doi.org/10.1371/journal.pcbi.1006223

Stetter, B. J., Ringhof, S., Krafft, F. C., Sell, S., & Stein, T. (2019). Estimation of knee joint forces in sport movements using wearable sensors and machine learning. *Sensors, 19*(17). https://doi.org/10.3390/s19173690

Stetter, B. J. (2021). *Wearable sensors and machine learning based human movement analysis—applications in sports and medicine*. Ph.D. thesis, Karlsruher Institut für Technologie (KIT). https://doi.org/10.5445/IR/1000131001

Stetter, B. J., Herzog, M., Mohler, F., Sell, S., & Stein, T. (2020). Modularity in motor control: Similarities in kinematic synergies across varying locomotion tasks. *Front Sports Act Living, 2*, 596063. https://doi.org/10.3389/fspor.2020.596063

Suda, E. Y., Watari, R., Matias, A. B., & Sacco, I. C. N. (2020). Recognition of foot-ankle movement patterns in long-distance runners with different experience levels using support vector machines. *Frontiers in Bioengineering and Biotechnology, 8*, 576. https://doi.org/10.3389/fbioe.2020.00576

Thilakeswaran, D., McManis, S., & Wang, X. R. (2021). Chameleon: A python workflow toolkit for feature selection. In *Data mining*. Singapore.

Tresch, M. C., Cheung, V. C. K., & d'Avella, A. (2006). Matrix factorization algorithms for the identification of muscle synergies: Evaluation on simulated and experimental data sets. *Journal of Neurophysiology, 95*(4), 2199–2212. https://doi.org/10.1152/jn.00222.2005

Trudeau, M. B., von Tscharner, V., Vienneau, J., Hoerzer, S., & Nigg, B. M. (2015). Assessing footwear effects from principal features of plantar loading during running. *Medicine and Science in Sports and Exercise, 47*(9), 1988–1996. https://doi.org/10.1249/MSS.0000000000000615

Uchida, T. K., & Delp, S. L. (2021). *Biomechanics of movement: The science of sports, robotics, and rehabilitation*. Mit Press.

van Drongelen, S., Stetter, B. J., Böhm, H., Stief, F., Stein, T., & Meurer, A. (2021). Identification of patients with similar gait compensating strategies due to unilateral hip osteoarthritis and the effect of total hip replacement: A secondary analysis. *Journal of Clinical Medicine, 10*(10). https://doi.org/10.3390/jcm10102167

Wen, Y., Si, J., Brandt, A., Gao, X., & Huang, H. (2020). Online reinforcement learning control for the personalization of a robotic knee prosthesis. *IEEE Transactions on Cybernetics, 50*(6), 2346–2356. https://doi.org/10.1109/Tcyb.2019.2890974

Wu, W., Saul, K. R., & Huang, H. (2021). Using reinforcement learning to estimate human joint moments from electromyography or joint kinematics: An alternative solution to musculoskeletal-based biomechanics. *Journal of Biomechanical Engineering-Transactions of the Asme, 143*(4). https://doi.org/10.1115/1.4049333

Xu, D., & Tian, Y. (2015). A comprehensive survey of clustering algorithms. *Annals of Data Science, 2*(2), 165–193. https://doi.org/10.1007/s40745-015-0040-1

Chapter 10
Artificial Intelligence-Based Motion Capture: Current Technologies, Applications and Challenges

Melanie Baldinger, Kevin Lippmann, and Veit Senner

Abstract Markerless motion capture has emerged as a significant technology in the research and application of motion capture systems. Unlike traditional marker-based approaches, markerless motion capture enables precise tracking and analysis of movements without the need for markers placed on the body. This offers a range of advantages, including improved user-friendliness, greater freedom of movement, and broader applicability in various environments, both within laboratories and outdoors. The aim of this chapter is to provide an overview of current markerless motion capture technologies, as well as their validity and applications in sports and health. We complement this literature review by providing two practical examples of our own research and summarize the main challenges that need to be tackled in future research.

Keywords Markerless Motion Capture · Pose Estimation · Depth Camera · Openpose · Kinect · Validation · Application

10.1 Markerless Motion Capture

Motion capture (MoCap) is used to study human movements in biomechanics, sports science, and clinical applications. MoCap helps analyze and optimize the performance of any kind of athletic movement, e.g. sprint start analysis or running analysis. Furthermore, motion analysis can be used to determine asymmetries and abnormalities in movements or for functional screening, balance, and agility testing. Rehabilitation or clinical applications include gait analysis, long-term monitoring of rehabilitation processes, or alteration in gait.

Current gold standard solutions use a marker-based approach where the subject is equipped with artificial markers on prominent anatomical landmarks. Movements

M. Baldinger (✉) · K. Lippmann · V. Senner
Sport Equipment and Sport Materials, TUM School of Engineering and Design, Technical University of Munich, Munich, Germany
e-mail: melanie.baldinger@tum.de

C. Dindorf et al. (eds.), *Artificial Intelligence in Sports, Movement, and Health*,
https://doi.org/10.1007/978-3-031-67256-9_10

are recorded using a set of video cameras in a calibrated movement space. Dedicated MoCap software tracks the markers and provides tools for kinematic analysis. This classical marker-based motion analysis is a highly specialized task that comes with constraints and challenges. It requires elaborate preparation of the measurement space as well as of the subject to be measured. A large number of high-precision and usually high-speed cameras that are calibrated and synchronized is necessary. Constant lighting conditions need to be ensured. In this way, the measurement is usually restricted to indoors and to a limited measurement volume. Therefore, the demands on the infrastructure result in a very costly procedure. Furthermore, the placement of the markers on subject's anatomical landmarks requires an expert to ensure the optimal placement. Light reflections, occlusions, and markers that are too close to each other can cause problems in tracking the markers, leading to inaccurate coordinates.

In recent years, markerless technologies have evolved in the field of MoCap. Considering the constraints and prerequisites of marker-based MoCap it becomes evident that markerless MoCap technologies could help overcome these challenges. They bear the potential to be used outside the laboratory, for everyday training environments, or during athletic competitions. Colyer et al. (2018) provide an overview of the evolution of motion analysis towards markerless systems that appear to be promising for motion analysis in daily training or competitions.

Three main technologies of markerless MoCap systems can be distinguished: wearable-based MoCap, typically consisting of **Inertial Measurement Units (IMUs)**, **Depth Cameras** that capture three-dimensional data using depth information, and so-called **Pose Estimation** algorithms that rely on computer vision. Figure 10.1 shows examples of these three technologies.

In the following section, all three technologies are briefly described. However, the focus of this chapter lies on methods using Artificial Intelligence, where we want to go further into detail.

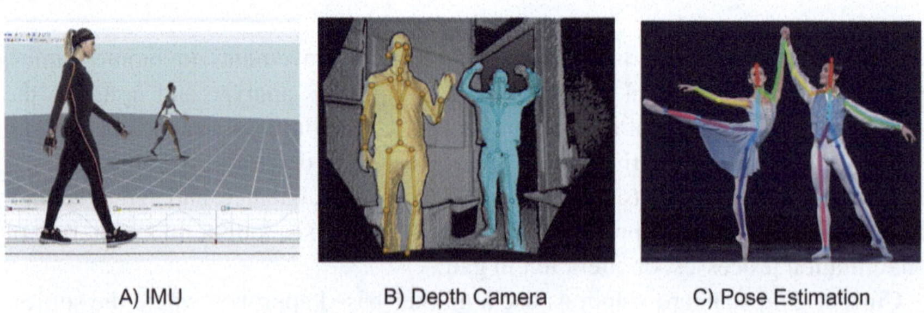

Fig. 10.1 Examples of markerless motion capture technologies: **a** Full body suit for IMU MoCap (Retrieved 07.02.2024 from https://www.movella.com/products/motion-capture/mvn-analyze). **b** 3D models of human subjects recorded and tracked using a Microsoft Kinect (Retrieved 07.02.2024 from https://docs.microsoft.com/de-de/azure/kinect-dk/body-sdk-setup). **c** Skeleton tracking of the OpenPose pose estimation algorithm (Cao et al., 2021)

10.1.1 IMU

IMUs contain a combination of accelerometers, gyroscopes, and magnetometers. Using the gyroscopes, the spatial orientation (position) of the body can be obtained in the form of three angular components (e.g., in Euler angles). Using the three acceleration components, the position-time curve can be calculated for all Cartesian spatial directions. Magnetometers are integrated to provide the orientation in the magnetic field of the earth (Poitras et al., 2019). A few specialized manufacturers, such as Xsens (XSens Technologies B.V.) or Rokoko (Rokoko Electronics), have developed wearable IMU full-body tracking systems for MoCap (see Fig. 10.1a).

Wearables or IMU sensors, in particular, offer, to some extent, advantages over marker-based MoCap systems. They are portable and do not require a lab environment, cameras or marker placements and in this way, enable the monitoring of athletes in real sports environments. Due to their small and lightweight design, they are unobtrusive for sports movements (Adesida et al., 2019). IMUs are potentially low cost and provided by numerous commercial suppliers. However, they also come with restrictions and challenges. Measurement accuracy of joint angles is highly dependent on the precise positioning of the sensors. Furthermore, ferromagnetic objects can disturb measurements, and a potential loss of signal during recording can occur when transferring the data wirelessly or due to interference with other devices (Adesida et al., 2019). Another issue to consider with IMUs is drift. Positional data is calculated via integration from acceleration data. Therefore, small deviations in the acceleration signal can result in considerable deviations in positional data, especially when integrating over a long period of time (Adesida et al., 2019).

10.1.2 Depth Camera

The second markerless MoCap technology we want to introduce is the depth camera or time-of-flight (TOF) camera. These cameras can capture three-dimensional models using depth information, which is based on the time-of-flight principle. A light impulse sent from the recording system is reflected by the object and sent back to the image sensor of the camera. Using the time that passes until the light is detected, the distance of the object to the camera can be inferred. In this way, the sensor captures the distances of each point in space from the camera instead of or in addition to the RGB data (Colyer et al., 2018). In this way, a three-dimensional image is created. One example of a TOF-camera is the *Microsoft Kinect*. A detailed description of the first and the second version of the Kinect is provided by Clark et al. (2019). In 2019 the latest version, the Azure Kinect, was introduced. Using the dedicated (human) body tracking algorithm (Shotton et al., 2013), a three-dimensional skeleton consisting of 32 joints can be extracted. From there on, kinematic parameters can be derived. Figure 10.1b shows an example of two 3D models tracked using the Kinect camera.

10.1.3 Pose Estimation

The third technology comes from the field of computer vision. Videos or images are digitally analyzed using image processing algorithms that rely on Artificial Intelligence. These so-called human pose estimation algorithms seek to predict position and orientation of body segments in images, thereby facilitating automated tracking and analysis of human kinetics and kinematics.

One of the big advantages of Pose Estimation is its ease of use. The algorithms only need video data or images as input for tracking and estimation of body poses. There is no need for specialized cameras or equipment, for example depth cameras, or instrumentation of the subject as in marker-based MoCap or IMU-based MoCap. This is a tremendous advantage in terms of financial and timely matters. Additionally, movements outside the lab can be recorded and analyzed. In this way, more diverse movements and sports can be studied. Moreover, even historical video data or videos from crashes can be studied. Hence, MoCap and motion analysis are available for a broader range of research questions, applications, and even for use in everyday life.

10.1.3.1 How Pose Estimation Works

Neural Networks and Deep Learning techniques are typically used for pose estimation. These models are trained on large datasets of images or videos containing annotated human poses, such as the Microsoft Common Objects in Context (COCO) Dataset (Lin et al., 2014) or the Max Planck Institute for Informatics (MPII) Human Pose Dataset (Andriluka et al., 2014).

Single-Person Pose Estimation detects the pose of a certain person in an image. The approaches can be distinguished between *regression-based methods* and *heatmap-based methods* depending on the key point detection (Dang et al., 2019; Zheng et al., 2023). The former method regresses key points directly by learning a mapping using a Deep Neural Network. In the heatmap-based approach, a heatmap with the key point existence probability is generated first. Key points are then predicted based on those heatmaps. A detailed overview of both methods is provided by Zheng et al. (2023).

In **Multi-Person Pose Estimation** body poses of more than one person can be tracked in the same image. Two main methodologies can be distinguished: *top-down* and *bottom-up*. In the top-down pipeline, the person is detected first. Key points of the body are estimated within the detected bounding box in the second step. In contrast, the bottom-up approach estimates all body joints first and groups them to form a pose of a person (Dang et al., 2019). Both pipelines are described in detail by Zheng et al. (2023).

Human body models are then usually represented as one of three types: skeleton model, planar model and volume model. The skeleton model is composed of a set of joints connected with each other. The planar model consists of different rectangles organically connected and the volume model is represented by geometric shapes (Ji et al., 2023).

The most commonly used Deep Learning methods applied for 2D pose estimation in the literature are: CNNs (Convolutional Neural Networks), GANs (Generative Adversarial Networks), GNNs (Graph Neural Networks), and RNNs (Recurrent Neural Networks) (Samkari et al., 2023).

A number of reviews investigated different 2D and 3D pose estimation algorithms evolving in recent years (Dang et al., 2019; Desmarais et al., 2021; El Kaid & Baïna, 2023; Ji et al., 2023; Munea et al., 2020; Samkari et al., 2023; Wang et al., 2021a, 2021b).

10.1.3.2 Examples of Pose Estimation Algorithms

OpenPose

One of the most prominent human pose estimation approaches is OpenPose (Cao et al., 2021). It is an open-source system that enables multi-person 2D pose estimation in images and videos or in real-time. This skeleton-based approach estimates 25 key points based on heatmaps and so-called Part Affinity Fields (PAFs). PAFs are sets of 2D vector fields that encode the position and orientation of body segments (Cao et al., 2021). Examples of movements tracked using OpenPose are shown in Fig. 10.2.

DeepPose

DeepPose is a single person pose estimation model and was one of the first human pose estimation approaches based on Deep Neural Networks (DNNs). Joint coordinates as key points are estimated by a cascade of DNN-based regressors (Toshev & Szegedy, 2014).

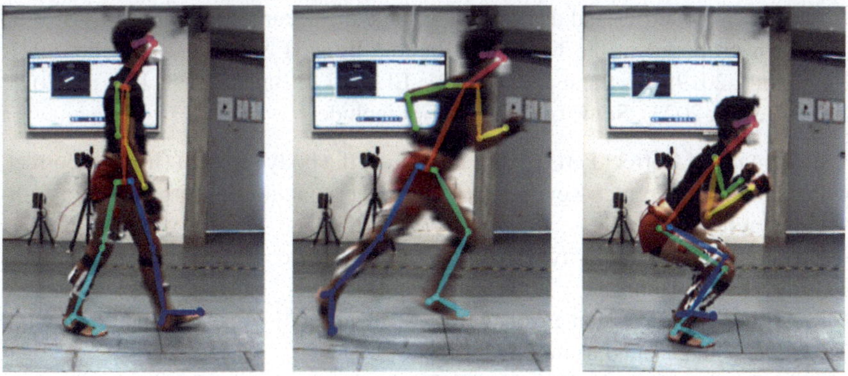

Fig. 10.2 Example of different movements tracked using the OpenPose algorithm

AlphaPose

Another example is AlphaPose. It is a regional multi-person pose estimation (RMPE) framework that is able to handle inaccurate human bounding boxes (Fang et al., 2017).

DensePose (Mask R-CNN)

DensePose represents a different approach in pose estimation. It aims to estimate the surface of the whole human body instead of joints as key points. The DensePose-COCO dataset is a manually annotated human body surface. Based on that, a DensePose-R-CNN (Region-based Convolutional Neural Network) is trained for pose estimation (Guler et al., 2018).

Theia3D

An example of commercial software for 3D human pose estimation based on Deep Learning techniques is Theia3D (Theia Markerless Inc., Kingston, ON, Canada). This software can be used together with standard commercial motion capture cameras and systems.

10.2 Validity of Markerless Motion Capture

10.2.1 Pose Estimation

10.2.1.1 Evaluation Against Datasets

Pose estimation algorithms can be validated against existing (annotated) datasets, such as the COCO Dataset (Lin et al., 2014) or the MPII Human Pose Dataset (Andriluka et al., 2014).

A number of metrics and datasets to evaluate the accuracy of markerless MoCap have been proposed in the literature (Badiola-Bengoa & Mendez-Zorrilla, 2021; Dang et al., 2019; Desmarais et al., 2021; El Kaid & Baïna, 2023; Ji et al., 2023; Samkari et al., 2023). Some of these metrics include:

- Percentage of Correct Parts (PCP): determine if a body segment (limb) is correct.
- Percentage of Correct Keypoints (PCK): determination of correctness of individual joints.
- Object Keypoint Similarity (OKS): measures how close the predicted keypoint is to the ground truth.
- Mean Per Joint Position Error (MPJPE): mean of Euclidean distance between estimated and ground truth coordinates.
- Mean Per Joint Velocity Error (MPJVE): the first derivative of the pose sequence.
- Mean Per Joint Angle Error (MPJAE): a measure of angle errors of joint segments.

Desmarais et al. (2021) and Zheng et al. (2023) report and discuss the accuracy of the best performing state-of-the-art markerless approaches against common datasets.

10.2.1.2 Evaluation Against Marker-Based MoCap

Another way to obtain markerless MoCap validity is to compare it with marker-based MoCap data. Accuracy is evaluated comparing kinematic variables of both methods. Colyer et al. (2018) give an overview of validation studies of different markerless technologies compared to marker-based systems.

Several studies exist that compare the performance of different pose estimation approaches. Needham et al. (2021) investigated three pose estimation algorithms based on Deep Learning: OpenPose, AlphaPose, DeepLabCut, with respect to the gold standard of marker-based motion capture. They compared 3D joint center locations of their participants during walking, running, and jumping. Results suggest that 3D joint center locations are not yet accurate enough. Still these technologies remain promising for out-of-the-lab environments. Mehdizadeh et al. (2021) examined the validity of gait variables using AlphaPose, OpenPose and Detectron. The evaluation against a 3D MoCap system revealed that temporal but not spatial gait measures correlate significantly with the marker-based system. Itokazu (2022) compared the reliability, validity, and accuracy of OpenPose and DeepLabCut against conventional marker-based MoCap software. Joint angles of the lower extremity were analyzed during standing up. Results confirmed high reliability and validity of both methods with an estimation error of fewer than 10° for hip and knee joints.

OpenPose Validation during Lunges, Counter Movement Jump and Rowing

We conducted a study comparing joint angles of OpenPose and a marker-based MoCap System (Vicon). 20 healthy subjects (8 female, 12 male; age: 25.1 ± 5.0 years; BMI: 23.11 ± 2.52 kg/m^2) took part and participated in a protocol of three different movements: a set of lunges, countermovement jump, and rowing on a rowing ergometer (see Fig. 10.3).

Movements were recorded using an RGB video camera (GoPro Hero10 Black) mounted on a tripod. Joint angles from the marker-based system were extracted directly from the Vicon Nexus Software (version 2.10.3) using the Plug-in Gait model with 31 markers. OpenPose key points were extracted, and joint angles were calculated using a custom Python script.

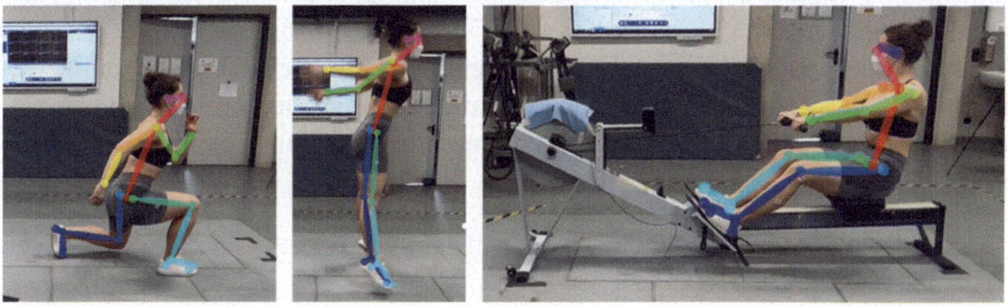

Fig. 10.3 Movements of the OpenPose validation study: lunges, counter movement jump and rowing on a rowing ergometer

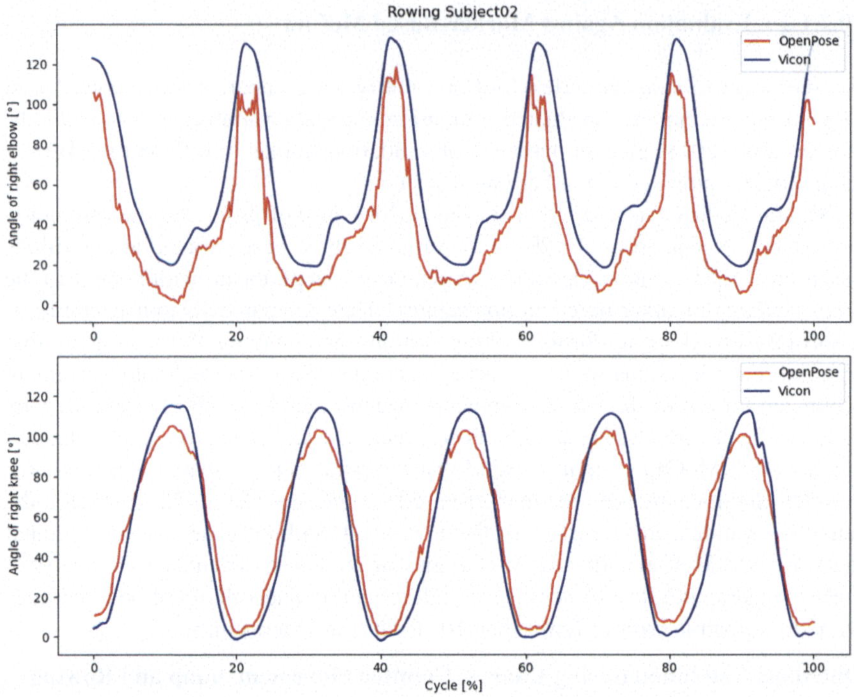

Fig. 10.4 Comparison of joint angles between OpenPose and the marker-based MoCap system (Vicon) for rowing for one subject

Exemplary results of the comparison between the marker-based MoCap system (Vicon) and OpenPose for the elbow and knee joint angle are shown in Fig. 10.4 for rowing and in Fig. 10.5 for lunges.

Moreover, OpenPose has been validated during gait analysis (D'Antonio et al., 2021; Ino et al., 2023; Stenum et al., 2021a, 2021b) bilateral squat (Ota et al., 2020), single-leg squat (Haberkamp et al., 2022), treadmill walking and running (Ota et al., 2021), and cycling (Bini et al., 2023). Nakano et al. (2020) investigated the accuracy of 3D motion capture using OpenPose during walking, countermovement jump, and ball throwing.

The validity and reliability of the commercial software Theia3D were examined in multiple studies. Gait kinematics (Kanko et al., 2021a), spatiotemporal gait parameters (Kanko et al., 2021c) and inter-session repeatability (Kanko et al., 2021b) show promising results.

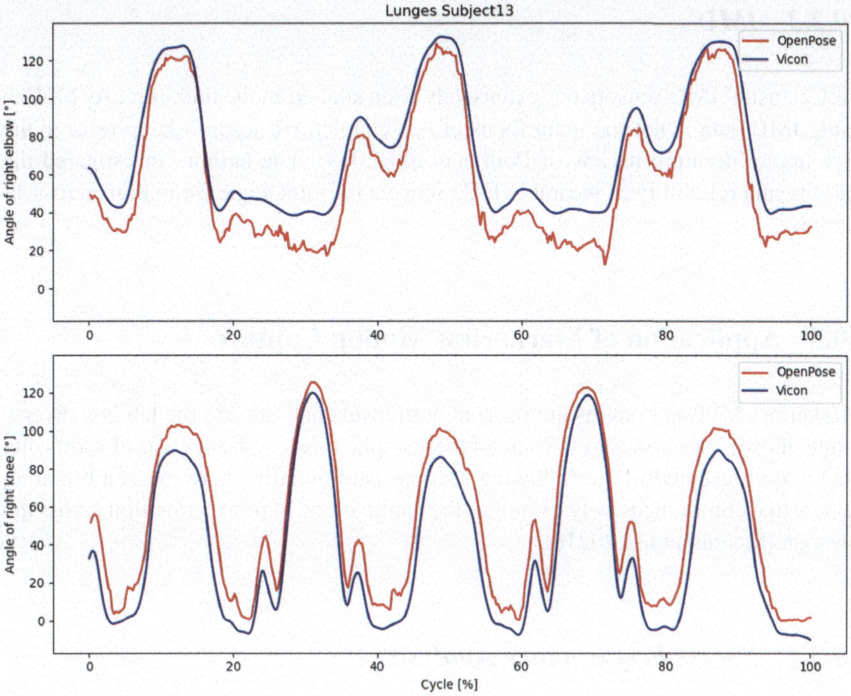

Fig. 10.5 Comparison of joint angles between OpenPose and the marker-based MoCap system (Vicon) for a set of lunges for one subject

10.2.2 Depth Camera

The validity of depth cameras, i.e., the Microsoft Kinect, is likewise evaluated in human movement studies against marker-based MoCap systems. A variety of validation studies exists in the literature. Springer and Yogev Seligmann (2016) provide an overview of studies evaluating the Kinect camera for gait analysis. Gray et al. (2017) validated the accuracy of Microsoft Kinect V2 during drop vertical jump. Ma et al. (2018) studied the measurement validity in upper-body movements using a rehabilitation game. Kinect's validity and reliability in upper body kinematics of stroke patients were furthermore investigated by Faity et al. (2022). Jo et al. (2022) examined the agreement of the Azure Kinect and a marker-based MoCap system during functional movements, such as squats, forward and lateral reach, and lunges. Thomas et al. (2022) validated the accuracy of the Azure Kinect during a sit-to-stand test. Bertram et al. (2023) evaluated the Azure Kinect as a clinical assessment tool testing static posture, postural transition, and locomotor function against a marker-based MoCap system.

10.2.3 IMU

MoCap using IMU sensors has extensively been studied in the literature. As MoCap using IMU data is not the main focus of this chapter, we would like to refer to the systematic literature review of Poitras et al. (2019). The authors investigated the validity and reliability of wearable IMU sensors for joint angle estimation across 42 studies.

10.3 Application of Markerless Motion Capture

Markerless MoCap systems are utilized both inside and outside the lab in a diverse range of use cases nowadays. Some of these applications in the context of sports and health are presented in the following section. Additionally, there exists a literature review that comprehensively examines the applications of pose estimation across the lifespan (Stenum et al., 2021a).

10.3.1 Sports Performance Analysis

In the field of sports and exercise science, there exist literature reviews addressing the applications of human pose estimation in general (Badiola-Bengoa & Mendez-Zorrilla, 2021) and OpenPose in particular (Baldinger & Senner, 2022). Use cases include bodyweight exercises, running, as well as team sports, such as soccer or volleyball, and even slower movements with more complexity, such for example, Taichi and Yoga. Pose estimation is used for detecting and predicting different parameters of specific sports, such as trajectories in table tennis, punching kinematics in boxing, or estimating jump height (Badiola-Bengoa & Mendez-Zorrilla, 2021; Baldinger & Senner, 2022).

A systematic review of the use of wearable technology in sports is provided by Adesida et al. (2019).

10.3.2 Training Assistance

Difini et al. (2021) summarize use cases of markerless motion capture as a training assistance tool. Sports include cheerleading, golf, skiing, and soccer, among others. Typical tasks are the analysis of the quality of movement to unburden the coach or instructor, give feedback on possible improvements in movements, or follow the expert's movement from a video or augmented reality.

10.3.3 Technique Evaluation (Bench Press)

In multiple exploratory studies, we examined the feasibility of the Azure Kinect in determining motion errors during bench press. As part of the validation, a number of studies were carried out on both powerlifters ("experts") and recreational athletes ("amateurs"). Both completed multiple sets of bench press motions. The expert additionally performed predefined error movements. Marker-based MoCap, the Azure Kinect, as well as IMUs mounted on the forehand and upper arm were used to capture the movements. The bench press motion and the Kinect's representation are shown in Fig. 10.6.

Kinematic parameters of the movements of the amateur and the expert were analyzed. Differences between the predefined error movements compared to the ideal movement were studied in detail. Based on that, an evaluation and comparison algorithm was implemented to provide automated feedback to the trainee.

A similar approach is presented by Wang et al. (2019). The authors propose an AI coach based on human pose estimation to provide personalized athletic training assistance for Freestyle Skiing. The framework consists of the following steps: detection and tracking of the athlete in the video, pose estimation, classification of "bad poses", and training suggestions.

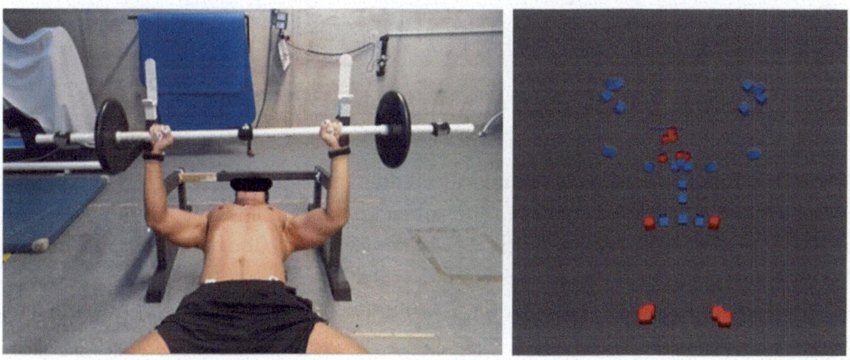

Fig. 10.6 Marker-based motion capture and body tracking using Azure Kinect during bench press

10.3.4 Clinical Applications

Knippenberg et al. (2017) give an overview of markerless MoCap systems used as part of a virtual reality (VR) training device in neurological rehabilitation. Application, target population, training content, and training efficacy are reported across eighteen selected studies. Results show that up to 2017, Kinect was used in the majority of studies. The target population of these training programs was mainly stroke patients, followed by persons with dementia, brain injury, cerebral palsy, Multiple sclerosis, and Parkinson's disease.

More recent reviews of clinical applications are provided by Hellsten et al. (2021), Wade et al. (2022), and Lam et al. (2023). Use cases include balance assessment to assess fall risk, and supervision and feedback on homebased exercises as part of therapy after surgery or stroke (Hellsten et al., 2021). Other tasks include automated clinical tests and continuous monitoring of patients in their homes (Wade et al., 2022). Furthermore, markerless MoCap has the potential to be used as an early screening tool for diseases by detecting and identifying symptoms (Lam et al., 2023). Kidziński et al. (2020), for example, developed a method to predict clinically relevant gait parameters from video data. The workflow uses the extracted keypoints from OpenPose and feeds them into a Neural Network to predict walking speed, cadence, knee flexion angle, and Gait Deviation Index. In this way, it enables outside-the-lab access to quantitative motion analysis for neurological and musculoskeletal disorders.

10.4 Current Challenges of Markerless Motion Capture

In our own experiments, we were mainly challenged by rare joint or body positions, such as in the bench press motion. The subject performing the bench press is lying on a bench instead of standing upright, which can impede the body pose estimation. Another issue we encountered was (self-) occlusions of body parts or occlusions of the sport equipment, for example, the rowing machine or the bar bell of the bench press.

This is consistent with the literature. Occlusion is often reported as a challenge in markerless MoCap (Desmarais et al., 2021; Jo et al., 2022; Zheng et al., 2023) and can be overcome by the use of multiple cameras (Difini et al., 2021). Furthermore, motion blur and fast movements hinder pose estimation (Wang et al., 2019). As many datasets are still captured indoors, generalization to in-the-wild scenarios is still challenging (Desmarais et al., 2021). Reduced accuracy due to loose-fitting clothes (Wade et al., 2022) or poor contrast between background and subject (Difini et al., 2021) are other issues to consider. Difini et al. (2021) summarize the limitations of pose estimation used as a training device for different types of sports and ideas to overcome those challenges, whereas shortcomings and research directions in clinical biomechanics are summarized by Wade et al. (2022).

Robustness of pose estimation can be further improved by more diverse datasets in terms of poses, movements, human shapes, and contexts (Desmarais et al., 2021; Wade et al., 2022).

References

Adesida, Y., Papi, E., & McGregor, A. H. (2019). Exploring the role of wearable technology in sport kinematics and kinetics: A systematic review. *Sensors (Basel, Switzerland), 19*(7). https://doi.org/10.3390/s19071597

Andriluka, M., Pishchulin, L., Gehler, P., & Schiele, B. (2014). 2D human pose estimation: New benchmark and state of the art analysis. In *CVPR 2014: 2014 IEEE Conference on Computer Vision and Pattern Recognition : proceedings : 23–28 June 2014, Columbus, Ohio* (pp. 3686–3693). IEEE Computer Society. https://doi.org/10.1109/CVPR.2014.471

Badiola-Bengoa, A., & Mendez-Zorrilla, A. (2021). A systematic review of the application of camera-based human pose estimation in the field of sport and physical exercise. *Sensors (Basel, Switzerland), 21*(18). https://doi.org/10.3390/s21185996

Baldinger, M., & Senner, V. (2022). Openpose and its current applications in sports and exercise science: A review. In D. Krumm, S. Schwanitz, & S. Odenwald (Eds.), *Spinfortec2022: Tagungsband zum 14. Symposium der Sektion Sportinformatik und Sporttechnologie der Deutschen Vereinigung für Sportwissenschaft (dvs), Chemnitz 29. - 30. September 2022* (pp. 14–17). Universitätsverlag Chemnitz. https://nbn-resolving.org/urn:nbn:de:bsz:ch1-qucosa2-807512

Bertram, J., Krüger, T., Röhling, H. M., Jelusic, A., Mansow-Model, S., Schniepp, R., Wuehr, M., & Otte, K. (2023). Accuracy and repeatability of the Microsoft Azure Kinect for clinical measurement of motor function. *PLoS ONE, 18*(1), e0279697. https://doi.org/10.1371/journal.pone.0279697

Bini, R. R., Serrancoli, G., Santiago, P. R. P., Pinto, A., & Moura, F. (2023). Criterion validity of neural networks to assess lower limb motion during cycling. *Journal of Sports Sciences, 41*(1), 36–44. https://doi.org/10.1080/02640414.2023.2194725

Cao, Z., Hidalgo, G., Simon, T., Wei, S.-E., & Sheikh, Y. (2021). Openpose: Realtime multi-person 2D pose estimation using part affinity fields. *IEEE Transactions on Pattern Analysis and Machine Intelligence, 43*(1), 172–186. https://doi.org/10.1109/TPAMI.2019.2929257

Clark, R. A., Mentiplay, B. F., Hough, E., & Pua, Y. H. (2019). Three-dimensional cameras and skeleton pose tracking for physical function assessment: A review of uses, validity, current developments and Kinect alternatives. *Gait & Posture, 68*, 193–200. https://doi.org/10.1016/j.gaitpost.2018.11.029

Colyer, S. L., Evans, M., Cosker, D. P., & Salo, A. I. T. (2018). A Review of the evolution of vision-based motion analysis and the integration of advanced computer vision methods towards developing a markerless system. *Sports Medicine—Open, 4*(1), 24. https://doi.org/10.1186/s40798-018-0139-y

Dang, Q., Yin, J., Wang, B., & Zheng, W. (2019). Deep learning based 2D human pose estimation: A survey. *Tsinghua Science and Technology, 24*(6), 663–676. https://doi.org/10.26599/TST.2018.9010100

D'Antonio, E., Taborri, J., Mileti, I., Rossi, S., & Patane, F. (2021). Validation of a 3D markerless system for gait analysis based on OpenPose and two RGB webcams. *IEEE Sensors Journal, 21*(15), 17064–17075. https://doi.org/10.1109/JSEN.2021.3081188

Desmarais, Y., Mottet, D., Slangen, P., & Montesinos, P. (2021). A review of 3D human pose estimation algorithms for markerless motion capture. *Computer Vision and Image Understanding, 212*, 103275. https://doi.org/10.1016/j.cviu.2021.103275

Difini, G. M., Martins, M. G., & Barbosa, J. L. V. (2021). Human pose estimation for training assistance. In A. C. M. Pereira & L. C. D. Da Rocha (Eds.), *Proceedings of the Brazilian*

Symposium on Multimedia and the Web (pp. 189–196). ACM. https://doi.org/10.1145/3470482.3479633

Faity, G., Mottet, D., & Froger, J. (2022). Validity and reliability of Kinect v2 for quantifying upper body kinematics during seated reaching. *Sensors (Basel, Switzerland), 22*(7). https://doi.org/10.3390/s22072735

Fang, H.-S., Xie, S., Tai, Y.-W., & Lu, C. (2017). Rmpe: Regional multi-person pose estimation. In *IEEE Xplore Digital Library, 2017 IEEE International Conference on Computer Vision: Iccv 2017 : Proceedings: October 22–29, 2017, Venice, Italy* (pp. 2353–2362). IEEE. https://doi.org/10.1109/ICCV.2017.256

Gray, A. D., Willis, B. W., Skubic, M., Huo, Z., Razu, S., Sherman, S. L., Guess, T. M., Jahandar, A., Gulbrandsen, T. R., Miller, S., & Siesener, N. J. (2017). Development and validation of a portable and inexpensive tool to measure the drop vertical jump using the Microsoft Kinect V2. *Sports Health, 9*(6), 537–544. https://doi.org/10.1177/1941738117726323

Guler, R. A., Neverova, N., & Kokkinos, I. (2018). DensePose: Dense human pose estimation in the wild. In *2018 IEEE/CVF Conference on Computer Vision and Pattern Recognition* (pp. 7297–7306). IEEE. https://doi.org/10.1109/CVPR.2018.00762

Haberkamp, L. D., Garcia, M. C., & Bazett-Jones, D. M. (2022). Validity of an artificial intelligence, human pose estimation model for measuring single-leg squat kinematics. *Journal of Biomechanics, 144*, 111333. https://doi.org/10.1016/j.jbiomech.2022.111333

Hellsten, T., Karlsson, J., Shamsuzzaman, M., & Pulkkis, G. (2021). The potential of computer vision-based marker-less human motion analysis for rehabilitation. *Rehabilitation Process and Outcome, 10*, 11795727211022330. https://doi.org/10.1177/11795727211022330

Ino, T., Samukawa, M., Ishida, T., Wada, N., Koshino, Y., Kasahara, S., & Tohyama, H. (2023). Validity of AI-based gait analysis for simultaneous measurement of bilateral lower limb kinematics using a single video camera. *Sensors (Basel, Switzerland), 23*(24). https://doi.org/10.3390/s23249799

Itokazu, M. (2022). Reliability and accuracy of 2D lower limb joint angles during a standing-up motion for markerless motion analysis software using deep learning. *Medicine in Novel Technology and Devices, 16*, 100188. https://doi.org/10.1016/j.medntd.2022.100188

Ji, H., Wang, L., Zhang, Y., Li, Z., & Wei, C. (2023). A review of human pose estimation methods in markerless motion capture. *Computer-Aided Design and Applications*, 392–423. https://doi.org/10.14733/cadaps.2024.392-423

Jo, S., Song, S., Kim, J., & Song, C. (2022). Agreement between azure Kinect and marker-based motion analysis during functional movements: A feasibility study. *Sensors (Basel, Switzerland), 22*(24). https://doi.org/10.3390/s22249819

El Kaid, A., & Baïna, K. (2023). A systematic review of recent deep learning approaches for 3D human pose estimation. *Journal of Imaging, 9*(12). https://doi.org/10.3390/jimaging9120275

Kanko, R. M., Laende, E. K., Davis, E. M., Selbie, W. S., & Deluzio, K. J. (2021a). Concurrent assessment of gait kinematics using marker-based and markerless motion capture. *Journal of Biomechanics, 127*, 110665. https://doi.org/10.1016/j.jbiomech.2021.110665

Kanko, R. M., Laende, E., Selbie, W. S., & Deluzio, K. J. (2021b). Inter-session repeatability of markerless motion capture gait kinematics. *Journal of Biomechanics, 121*, 110422. https://doi.org/10.1016/j.jbiomech.2021.110422

Kanko, R. M., Laende, E. K., Strutzenberger, G., Brown, M., Selbie, W. S., DePaul, V., Scott, S. H., & Deluzio, K. J. (2021c). Assessment of spatiotemporal gait parameters using a deep learning algorithm-based markerless motion capture system. *Journal of Biomechanics, 122*, 110414. https://doi.org/10.1016/j.jbiomech.2021.110414

Kidziński, Ł, Yang, B., Hicks, J. L., Rajagopal, A., Delp, S. L., & Schwartz, M. H. (2020). Deep neural networks enable quantitative movement analysis using single-camera videos. *Nature Communications, 11*(1), 4054. https://doi.org/10.1038/s41467-020-17807-z

Knippenberg, E., Verbrugghe, J., Lamers, I., Palmaers, S., Timmermans, A., & Spooren, A. (2017). Markerless motion capture systems as training device in neurological rehabilitation: A systematic review of their use, application, target population and efficacy. *Journal of Neuroengineering and Rehabilitation, 14*(1), 61. https://doi.org/10.1186/s12984-017-0270-x

Lam, W. W. T., Tang, Y. M., & Fong, K. N. K. (2023). A systematic review of the applications of markerless motion capture (MMC) technology for clinical measurement in rehabilitation. *Journal of Neuroengineering and Rehabilitation, 20*(1), 57. https://doi.org/10.1186/s12984-023-01186-9

Lin, T.-Y., Maire, M., Belongie, S., Hays, J., Perona, P., Ramanan, D., Dollár, P., & Zitnick, C. L. (2014). Microsoft COCO: Common objects in context. In D. Fleet, T. Pajdla, B. Schiele, & T. Tuytelaars (Eds.), *Lecture Notes in Computer Science: Vol. 8693. Computer vision—ECCV 2014: 13th European Conference, Zurich, Switzerland, September 6–12, 2014; proceedings* (Vol. 8693, pp. 740–755). Springer. https://doi.org/10.1007/978-3-319-10602-1_48

Ma, M., Proffitt, R., & Skubic, M. (2018). Validation of a Kinect V2 based rehabilitation game. *PLoS ONE, 13*(8), e0202338. https://doi.org/10.1371/journal.pone.0202338

Mehdizadeh, S., Nabavi, H., Sabo, A., Arora, T., Iaboni, A., & Taati, B. (2021). Concurrent validity of human pose tracking in video for measuring gait parameters in older adults: A preliminary analysis with multiple trackers, viewing angles, and walking directions. *Journal of Neuroengineering and Rehabilitation, 18*(1), 139. https://doi.org/10.1186/s12984-021-00933-0

Munea, T. L., Jembre, Y. Z., Weldegebriel, H. T., Chen, L., Huang, C., & Yang, C. (2020). The Progress of human pose estimation: A survey and taxonomy of models applied in 2D human pose estimation. *IEEE Access, 8*, 133330–133348. https://doi.org/10.1109/ACCESS.2020.3010248

Nakano, N., Sakura, T., Ueda, K., Omura, L., Kimura, A., Iino, Y., Fukashiro, S., & Yoshioka, S. (2020). Evaluation of 3D markerless motion capture accuracy using OpenPose with multiple video cameras. *Frontiers in Sports and Active Living, 2*(Article 50), 50. https://doi.org/10.3389/fspor.2020.00050

Needham, L., Evans, M., Cosker, D. P., Wade, L., McGuigan, P. M., Bilzon, J. L., & Colyer, S. L. (2021). The accuracy of several pose estimation methods for 3D joint centre localisation. *Scientific Reports, 11*(1), 20673. https://doi.org/10.1038/s41598-021-00212-x

Ota, M., Tateuchi, H., Hashiguchi, T., & Ichihashi, N. (2021). Verification of validity of gait analysis systems during treadmill walking and running using human pose tracking algorithm. *Gait & Posture, 85*, 290–297. https://doi.org/10.1016/j.gaitpost.2021.02.006

Ota, M., Tateuchi, H., Hashiguchi, T., Kato, T., Ogino, Y., Yamagata, M., & Ichihashi, N. (2020). Verification of reliability and validity of motion analysis systems during bilateral squat using human pose tracking algorithm. *Gait & Posture, 80*, 62–67. https://doi.org/10.1016/j.gaitpost.2020.05.027

Poitras, I., Dupuis, F., Bielmann, M., Campeau-Lecours, A., Mercier, C., Bouyer, L. J., & Roy, J.-S. (2019). Validity and reliability of wearable sensors for joint angle estimation: A systematic review. *Sensors (Basel, Switzerland), 19*(7). https://doi.org/10.3390/s19071555

Samkari, E., Arif, M., Alghamdi, M., & Al Ghamdi, M. A. (2023). Human pose estimation using deep learning: A systematic literature review. *Machine Learning and Knowledge Extraction, 5*(4), 1612–1659. https://doi.org/10.3390/make5040081

Shotton, J., Sharp, T., Kipman, A., Fitzgibbon, A., Finocchio, M., Blake, A., Cook, M., & Moore, R. (2013). Real-time human pose recognition in parts from single depth images. *Communications of the ACM, 56*(1), 116–124. https://doi.org/10.1145/2398356.2398381

Springer, S., & Yogev Seligmann, G. (2016). Validity of the Kinect for gait assessment: A focused review. *Sensors (basel, Switzerland), 16*(2), 194. https://doi.org/10.3390/s16020194

Stenum, J., Cherry-Allen, K. M., Pyles, C. O., Reetzke, R. D., Vignos, M. F., & Roemmich, R. T. (2021). Applications of pose estimation in human health and performance across the lifespan. *Sensors (Basel, Switzerland), 21*(21). https://doi.org/10.3390/s21217315

Stenum, J., Rossi, C., & Roemmich, R. T. (2021b). Two-dimensional video-based analysis of human gait using pose estimation. *PLoS Computational Biology, 17*(4), e1008935. https://doi.org/10.1371/journal.pcbi.1008935

Thomas, J., Hall, J. B., Bliss, R., & Guess, T. M. (2022). Comparison of Azure Kinect and optical retroreflective motion capture for kinematic and spatiotemporal evaluation of the sit-to-stand test. *Gait & Posture, 94*, 153–159. https://doi.org/10.1016/j.gaitpost.2022.03.011

Toshev, A., & Szegedy, C. (2014). DeepPose: Human pose estimation via deep neural networks. In *CVPR 2014: 2014 IEEE Conference on Computer Vision and Pattern Recognition : proceedings : 23–28 June 2014, Columbus, Ohio* (pp. 1653–1660). IEEE Computer Society. https://doi.org/10.1109/CVPR.2014.214

Wade, L., Needham, L., McGuigan, P., & Bilzon, J. (2022). Applications and limitations of current markerless motion capture methods for clinical gait biomechanics. *PeerJ, 10*, e12995. https://doi.org/10.7717/peerj.12995

Wang, J., Qiu, K., Peng, H., Fu, J., & Zhu, J. (2019). Ai coach: Deep human pose estimation and analysis for personalized athletic training assistance. In L. Amsaleg (Ed.), *ACM Digital Library, Proceedings of the 27th ACM International Conference on Multimedia* (pp. 374–382). Association for Computing Machinery. https://doi.org/10.1145/3343031.3350910

Wang, C., Zhang, F., & Ge, S. S. (2021a). A comprehensive survey on 2D multi-person pose estimation methods. *Engineering Applications of Artificial Intelligence, 102*, 104260. https://doi.org/10.1016/j.engappai.2021.104260

Wang, J., Tan, S., Zhen, X., Xu, S., Zheng, F., He, Z., & Shao, L. (2021). Deep 3D human pose estimation: A review. *Computer Vision and Image Understanding, 210*, 103225. https://doi.org/10.1016/j.cviu.2021.103225

Zheng, C., Wu, W., Chen, C., Yang, T., Zhu, S., Shen, J., Kehtarnavaz, N., & Shah, M. (2023). Deep Learning-based human pose estimation: A survey. *ACM Computing Surveys, 56*(1), 1–37. https://doi.org/10.1145/3603618

Part V
Practical Examples of Machine Learning and Predictive Analytics

Chapter 11
Machine Learning in Tennis

Fernando Vives, Javier Lázaro, José Francisco Guzmán, Miguel Crespo, and Rafael Martínez-Gallego

Abstract The analysis of sporting performance, particularly in tennis, has been studied for several decades. The use of new technologies and tracking systems, such as Hawk-Eye, has advanced research in this field. A review of scientific articles shows the recent evolution of Machine Learning (ML) techniques and their potential impact on tennis. Finally, a practical example of a predictive model is presented to demonstrate the process and results of this study.

Keywords Performance Analysis · Sport Analytics · Coaching · Tracking Technology · Tactical

11.1 Introduction

The study of sports performance has been the subject of numerous investigations, utilizing biomechanics and notational analysis during both competition and training sessions. This has become an invaluable tool for coaches in their technical-tactical planning, for players to achieve greater performance, and for researchers to gain a better understanding of sporting performance (Hughes & Bartlett, 2008; O'Donoghue, 2014).

In tennis, as in other sports, there has been significant evolution in obtaining and interpreting records. These records can be used to optimise the training process or prepare more effectively and specifically for competition (Morgulev et al., 2018). Currently, a wide range of devices, such as high-speed cameras, GPS, tracking, and

F. Vives (✉) · J. Lázaro · J. F. Guzmán · M. Crespo · R. Martínez-Gallego
Department of Sport and Physical Education, University of Valencia, Valencia, Spain
e-mail: fervial@alumni.uv.es

J. Lázaro
Independent researcher, Valencia, Spain

M. Crespo
Development Department, International Tennis Federation, London, UK

C. Dindorf et al. (eds.), *Artificial Intelligence in Sports, Movement, and Health*,
https://doi.org/10.1007/978-3-031-67256-9_11

tagging systems, are used for data collection (Barris & Button, 2008; Jindo et al., 2022).

Hawk-Eye (HE) technology was first used on 21 April 2001 during a cricket match between Pakistan and England at Lord's Cricket Ground. The technology uses high-speed cameras, computers, and electronic screens to track the ball's trajectory. It was later introduced to professional tennis tournaments, with the Hopman Cup in Perth being the first to use it in 2006 (Shigh Bal & Dureja, 2012). This system employs ten cameras positioned around the court to track the three-dimensional position of the ball during each point using an algorithm. The estimated average error is 3.6 mm (Baodong, 2014; Mecheri et al., 2016).

The introduction of Hawk-Eye technology in tennis has allowed access to a wide range of data that has been the subject of study in various research projects. One of the most analysed aspects has been the serve, given its fundamental role in initiating the point and the advantage it can provide to the player. Studies such as Kolbinger and Lames (2013) examined the distribution of the serve in right-handed male hard court players. Other studies, such as Rioult et al. (2015) and Mecheri et al. (2016), evaluated serve efficiency and factors such as speed, direction and court surface. In addition, Kovalchik and Albert (2017) developed a model to analyse pre-serve routines, while Whiteside and Reid (2017) identified the characteristics of first serves to achieve an ace. More recently, the serve has been studied in the doubles discipline (Martínez-Gallego et al., 2021a, 2021b; Vives et al., 2022). Theoretical models have also been proposed to improve serve and return efficiency in elite tennis, such as Vives et al. (2023) and Fitzpatrick et al. (2023).

In addition to the serve, playing strategies and physical characteristics of players have been explored. Studies such as Loffing et al. (2010) analysed the presumed tactical advantages of left-handed players, while Reid et al. (2016) examined gender differences in hitting and movement dynamics in Grand Slam. Differences between junior and professional players have also been studied for better training planning, as demonstrated by Kovalchik and Reid (2018). Cui et al. (2019) explored performance indicators based on anthropometric characteristics and self-assessments in different groups of players. Finally, Meurs et al. (2021) investigated the Positional Advantage Index as a tool to identify a player's on-court advantage over his opponent.

11.2 Machine Learning in Tennis

11.2.1 Machine Learning in Sport

As discussed in the previous section, the introduction of Hawk-Eye technology in tennis has enabled access to a vast amount of data, which has been utilized to develop various research projects.

Similarly, other sports also generate a plethora of data that can be analyzed or used to predict future events. In the field of sports, Machine Learning (ML) algorithms aim

Table 11.1 Use of ML algorithms in team sports (Beal et al., 2019; Horvat & Job, 2020)

	SVM	Random forest/ Decision tree	Linear/Logistic regression	Neural networks	Other
Football	✔	✔	✔	✔	✔
Basketball	✔	✔	✔	✔	✔
American football	✔	✔	✔	✔	
Cricket	✔	✔	✔		

to assist in evaluating player or team performance, preventing injuries, identifying talent, and aiding decision-making by players and coaches (Horvat & Job, 2020).

Table 11.1 below displays the primary ML methods used in various team sports, including football, basketball, American football, and cricket.

11.2.2 Machine Learning Techniques for Tennis

The use of ML in tennis is a recent development, primarily due to advancements in technology for data collection through tagging and tracking systems. This is a brief overview of the evolution of ML in tennis, from the earliest studies to the present day.

The prediction of results is a major field of study in the world of tennis. Innovative approaches have been implemented to address specific considerations, such as the type of playing surface, the variability of players' skills, and the use of historical data from professional tournaments. Various algorithms, such as Logistic Regression (LR), Random Forest (RF), Decision Tree (DT), Artificial Neural Networks (ANNs), Naive Bayes (NB) and Support Vector Machine (SVM), have been used to predict outcomes. However, their effectiveness varies, highlighting the importance of considering multiple factors and data quality (Cornman et al., 2017; Learning, 2017; Peters, 2017).

Different ML techniques have been used by various authors to obtain effective predictive models in tennis. One of the pioneering studies in this field is that of Boulier and Stekler (1999), who evaluated the effectiveness of classification in basketball and tennis as predictors of results using base rate forecasts and Brier scores. In a similar context, Kovalchik (2016) investigated 11 predictive models to predict the results of more than 2000 men's professional tennis matches. Hostačný (2018) analysed the accuracy of LR models, RF, DT and ANNs using data from individual men's matches. In comparative studies, Ghosh et al. (2019) and Sekar (2019) evaluated the performance of different classification algorithms, concluding that the decision tree outperformed other algorithms.

In addition, novel approaches have been proposed, such as Lerner et al. (2019), who used live match data and recurrent neural networks to calculate win probabilities, and Bayram et al. (2021), who used network analysis to derive a surface-specific, time-varying score for professional tennis players. More recent research in 2022, such as that of Yue et al. (2022) and Solanki et al. (2022), has continued to explore statistical methods and ML models to improve score prediction in tennis, while Bunker et al. (2023) compared Elo and Weighted Elo scoring methods, highlighting the accuracy of the alternating DT and LR model in the experimental framework Sports Result Prediction Cross Industry Standard Process for Data Mining (CRISP-DM).

The serve is considered the most decisive stroke in modern tennis, one of the first major analyses of the serve was conducted by Mecheri et al. in 2016, with a sample of 262,596 serves they determined that the serve has a significant effect on the outcome of the point. Service direction has also been addressed in other studies such as that of Wei et al. (2015), by a specific player in a given context, or that of Zhu and Naikar (2022) who found an accuracy on first serves of 49% for men and 44% for women. Attempts have also been made to determine the main features to achieve an ace in both singles (Whiteside & Reid, 2017) and doubles (Vives et al., 2023). Finally, Gao and Kowalczyk (2021) identified the serve as a crucial predictor of match outcome.

Besides the service, other game situations have been studied, thus Wei et al. (2016) used spatio-temporal tracking data to make predictions of the direction of the next shot during a match in real time. Along the same lines, Shimizu et al. (2019) proposed a method for predicting the direction of the next shot using Long Short-Term Memory (LSTM) networks, based on sequential information about the player's posture and position on the court. In contrast, Makino et al. (2020) analyzed in detail the rallies of professional players with the aim of developing a predictive model of point outcome. Lastly, Zhou and Liu (2024) found that the player's position and the court area of the stroke determined the selection of groundstroke stances.

Several authors have conducted different studies to classify different stroke types and patterns. Kovalchik and Reid (2018) developed a classification of stroke types used by professional players during a match based on various criteria, such as speed, direction, spin and intention of the stroke. The rest was also analysed in depth in 2022 by Kovalchik and Albert, identifying six unique impact styles of returned serves in professional tennis. The latest study by Martínez-Gallego et al. (2021b) determined specific patterns of volley positions in both men and women. Such information may prove valuable for player-specific preparation and the creation of effective strategies for competition.

Tennis is a dynamic and highly competitive sport, several studies have tried to analyse and understand other aspects of the game. For example, Cui et al. (2019) analysed the performance of male Grand Slam tennis players using a point-by-point approach to identify key success factors. Other study of Giles et al. (2020) developed an approach for the automatic detection and classification of change of direction movements in professional players. Giles et al., (2021, 2023) continued this same line of research with two further studies to differentiate the movement styles of professional players. Future sport performance has also been examined in different studies through the morphological characteristics of athletes. Such as Panjan et al., (2010) with Slovenian junior tennis players, Deshpande and Klotzman (2022) with top 100 ranked professional female players, or Siener et al. (2021) who analysed different ML techniques used as a tool to predict future success.

Finally, other areas have also been addressed in different recent studies. Filipcic et al. (2014) analysed the criteria for identifying and ranking players, providing relevant information on the characteristics that distinguish the best male tennis players. On the other hand, Rosker and Majcen Rosker (2021) examined how visual adaptive ability influences performance in tennis and Hao and Hu (2023) investigated how technological applications can contribute to the development and improvement of tennis performance. The application of sensors has also started to be used in work such as that of Perri et al. (2022) or Wu et al. (2023), looking for improved real-time assessment during training sessions.

A table-summary (Table 11.2) has been created to display the primary tennis-specific contributions in the area of Sport Sciences. The focus has been on sports performance analysis of both male and female players. These contributions have practical implications in the preparation of training sessions and technical-tactical decision making during matches. The table includes information on the authors, data collection and processing, the study field area, and the ML techniques used in the process.

11.3 Application of a Novel Method

To enhance reader comprehension of the various techniques employed in an ML model, we will present a case study of a previous investigation on the first serves in men's professional doubles tennis as an example.

11.3.1 Object of the Study

The study aimed to identify differences between first services ending in 1 (Type 1), 2 (Type 2), 3 (Type 3), and 4 or more shots (Type 4) in terms of their incidence at the point. Analysis revealed significant differences only between Type 1 and Type 4 effectiveness. We therefore identified the most relevant characteristics in the first type of services (Type 1) and trained the model to determine the variables and their values that best predicted service effectiveness.

11.3.2 Methodology

A pipeline that included all XAI (Explainable Artificial Intelligence) processes from Data Processing to training the predictive model (Deep Neural Network) was built to calculate the most important variable (Feature Importance), select values that maximize probabilities (Probabilistic and Statistical Inference), and test the results on a synthetic dataset.

Table 11.2 Main tennis-specific papers of ML published in the area of sports sciences

Author(s)	Data set	Data collection	ML
Wei et al. (2015)	4.758 first serves 2.292 secod serves Men's singles (2012–2014)	Hawk-Eye	Logistic Regression Decision Tree
Kovalchik (2016)	2.395 matches Men's singles (2014)	ATP website	Regression-based (4) Point-based (3) Paired comparison (2) Bookmaker consensus
Whiteside and Reid (2017)	25.680 first serves Men's singles (2012–2015)	Hawk-Eye	Decision Tree K-Means Clustering
Kovalchik and Reid (2018)	Men's singles: 270.023 shots Women's singles 178.136 shots (2015–2017)	Hawk-Eye	Multi-stage Clustering
Cui et al. (2019)	29.675 points Men's singles (2011–2016)	Australian Open, Roland Garros, Wimbledon and US Open website Doppler radar (IBM)	Classification Tree (CHAID)
Makino et al. (2020)	Men's professional singles from 1970	Match charting project (MCP)	L1-regularized Logistic Regression
Giles et al. (2021)	157.841 change of direction 513 matches (2016–2018)	Hawk-Eye	Hierarchical Clustering
Kovalchik and Albert (2022)	142.803 returns serve Men's singles (2018–2020)	Tracking data	Latent Style Allocation Model Finite Mixture Models
Vives et al. (2023)	14.146 serves 97 doubles matches Davis Cup (2010–2019)	Hawk-Eye	Feature Importance Deep Neural Network
Zhou and Liu (2024)	36 players Men's singles (2019– 2021)	Kinovea	Bayesan Network

The process is shown in Fig. 11.1.

Exploratory Data Analysis and Data Processing

The study analysed a total of 14.146 first serves in Davis Cup men's doubles matches played from 2010 to 2019. It involved 160 players in 123 teams from 34 different countries, with an average age of 30.03 ± 4.73 years.

The dataset consisted of the variables presented in Table 11.3.

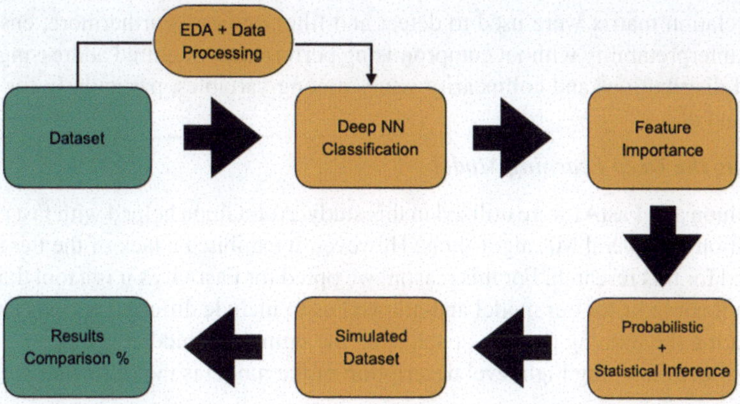

Fig. 11.1 Pipeline workflow architecture

Table 11.3 The derived variables included

Target variables	Input features
Court side:	SPEED: Mean speed of the serve
DEUCE/AD	POSITION: Position of the server when hitting the serve
Efectiveness:	TIME: Time between ball impact and ball bounce
TYPE 1: The point finishes with 1 shot	SPEED LOSS: Loss of speed of the ball after its bounce
TYPE 2: The point finishes with 2 shots	IMPACT Z: Height of the ball at impact
TYPE 3: The point finishes with 3 shots	NET CLEARANCE: Height of the ball when passing over the net
TYPE 4: The point finishes with 4 shots	SERVE ANGLE: The angle formed between the bounce of the ball and the centre of the service box from the position of the server
	VERTICAL PROJECTION ANGLE: The angle formed by the bounce of the ball, the point of impact, and the trajectory of the ball from the ground
	dL: Distance from ball bounce to the sideline of the service box

Following the Exploratory Data Analysis, which included correlation matrices, boxplots, histograms, and Kernel Density Estimation plots (KDE), the data was prepared for the application of ML classification algorithms. Non-informative variables, with a variance equal to or close to 0, were identified. To address class imbalance, weak target samples were oversampled. Feature selection was performed using a combination of tennis knowledge criteria, correlation analysis, and feature selection algorithms like Permutation feature importance and SHAP importance (Rajbahadur et al., 2021). Statistical methods like histogram analysis, boxplot analysis or analysis of correlation matrix were used to detect and filter outliers. Furthermore, ensuring model interpretability without compromising performance required addressing non-normal distributions and collinearity issues among variables, particularly for serve angle and dL.

Training the Deep Learning Model

AutoGluon and FastAI were utilized in this study. AutoGluon helped with fast experimentation on several ML algorithms. However, it exhibited a lack of the flexibility required for this research. For this reason, we opted for FastAI, as it is a tool that was a more flexible fit for our model and allowed us to include different options such as automating the training process or selecting the number of hidden layers.

The Deep Learning high level description of the model is the following:

1. Backbone Network:
   A model with 5 layers of feature size [256, 128, 128, 128, 64]. The basic layer block (named LinBnDrop) is formed by the next transformations:
   - Linear Layer (torch.nn.linear)
   - Reactified Linear Unit—ReLU (torch.nn.relu)
   - Batch Normalization—BatchNorm1d (torch.nn. BatchNorm1d)
2. Loss Function:
   Focal Loss Flat (Lin et al., 2017). The focal loss works specially well with imbalanced data as it adapts its weights to focus learning on hard misclassified examples.
3. Optimization Algorithm:
   Adam (Kingma & Ba, 2015).

Feature Importance Algorithms

The SHAP (SHapley Additive exPlanations) and Feature Permutation Importance techniques, which indicate the relative importance of each variable, were used to identify the most important variables of the first serves. However, only the results obtained with the first method (SHAP) were finally published.

SHAP Summary Plots are visual tools used to determine how each feature contributes to the predictions of a model. To do this, the algorithm proceeds to calculate the SHAP values, then they are sorted by their relative importance in the prediction and finally, the results are displayed graphically (Lundberg & Lee, 2017).

Probabilistic and Statistical Analysis

In order to optimize the effectiveness of the serve and understand how the selected characteristics affect the target variables, an innovative semi-automated algorithm based on classical statistical methods was designed.

The Kernel Density Estimation (KDE) algorithm was applied to model a smoothed distribution of the data for each class, using statistical estimators such as the mean, Maximum Likelihood Estimation (MLE) and the percentiles 5 and 95 for the relevant characteristics.

Finally, optimal values were identified by selecting regions on the graph that exhibited a higher density of points corresponding to the desired outcome (type 1 effectiveness) and a lower density for the undesired outcome (type 4 effectiveness). The integration of these statistical estimators was essential to understand the underlying probability distribution and guide the value selection process.

Synthetic Data-Set Generation

In the final step a synthetic dataset using the selected values was generated, and the prediction was simulated. The values outside the desired selected threshold were substituted by random values inside the new calculated limits for the most important variables. Finally, predictions on the whole dataset were performed using the Deep Learning Model previously trained. Then the final rate of type 1 and type 4 was calculated. By doing this, the approach was validated. Note that this step is using the model trained beforehand. We consider the predictions using this model reliable because the evaluation metric of the model (averaged f1-score) reached 93%.

11.3.3 Results

Our proposed pipeline obtained an F1-score of 95% for the type 1 and 94% for the type 4. Likewise, the overall classification accuracy on the evaluation test set was 94%, precision and recall values of the model also exhibited high levels, close to 90%. Hence, this model has demonstrated its reliability in delineating the attributes of first serves that culminate in an ace and the first serves enduring for 4 or more shots.

The next step was to identify the most relevant variables of the model for each type of effectiveness (Type 1 and Type 4). SHAP was used to determine the most important variable, which turned out to be serve angle and dL, in addition to the speed, for both the Deuce and Advantage sides. SHAP is a technique that provides values indicating the average impact of each variable on the model's outputs. These results highlight the significance of serve angle and dL, besides of the speed, in predicting the effectiveness of the first serve in men's double tennis.

The final step involved generating a dataset where the original values were replaced with the recommended values for the most important variable obtained in the previous step. The results with the recommended values, as shown in Table 11.4, demonstrated a significant improvement for both the variable dL (between 0 and 28 cm) and the serve angle (between 5.7° and 8.7°), regardless of the serving side. In contrast, the speed variable showed minimal variation once it reached 187 km/h.

Table 11.4 Results of the predictions using the trained model

Variable	Side	Values (min–max)	Effectiveness before (%)	Effectiveness after (%)
dL (m)	Deuce	0–0.28	33.05	83.40
	AD		30.64	81.26
	Both		33.49	88.48
Serve angle (deg)	Deuce	5.7–8.7	33.70	88.68
	AD		29.77	88.21
	Both		33.25	89.04
Speed (km/h)	Deuce	187–220	35.17	45.75
	AD		34.36	44.13
	Both		30.38	39.91

11.3.4 Discussion

The serve has become the most decisive shot in modern tennis, allowing servers to gain an advantage over their opponents. This study identifies key variables for achieving an ace in men's professional doubles tennis. The serve angle and the distance from the ball bounce to the sideline were found to be crucial in producing an ace, along with the speed variable. The model enhances the effectiveness of first serves to almost 90% when the serve angle values are between 5.7° and 8.7°. Similarly, recommended values below 29 cm for the distance from the ball bounce to the sideline would push the model's effectiveness beyond 85%. These findings are consistent with previous research in men's singles tennis, where it was observed that when the service angle was equal to or greater than 5.88° and the bounce distance from the line was less than 15.27 cm, the probability of hitting a direct serve reached almost 80% (Whiteside & Reid, 2017).

However, speed does not exhibit the same pattern once it exceeds 187 km/h. Unlike in individual tennis, where previous studies have identified speed as the determining factor for a direct serve (Rioult et al., 2015; Brown, 2021), our findings suggest a more nuanced relationship in doubles tennis.

11.3.5 Conclusion

Based on the results of this study, it can be observed that, while the speed of the serve is relevant, extremely high speeds do not guarantee greater success in direct serves. Instead, factors such as the angle of the serve and the accuracy of the bounce near the sidelines have a significant impact on the likelihood of hitting an ace.

These results could prove highly valuable for coaches and players when planning training sessions focused on serving and making technical-tactical decisions during competition, optimizing the performance of the first serve in high-performance matches.

References

Baodong, Y. (2014). Hawkeye technology using tennis match. *Computer Modelling New Technologies, 18*(12C), 400–402.

Barris, S., & Button, C. (2008). A review of vision-based motion analysis in sport. *Sports Medicine, 38*, 1025–1043.

Bayram, F., Garbarino, D. & Barla, A. (2021). Predicting tennis match outcomes with network analysis and machine learning. In *SOFSEM 2021: Theory and practice of computer science: 47th international conference on current trends in theory and practice of computer science, SOFSEM 2021, Bolzano-Bozen, Italy, January 25–29, 2021, Proceedings 47* (pp. 505–518). Springer.

Beal, R., Norman, T. J., & Ramchurn, S. D. (2019). Artificial intelligence for team sports: A survey. *The Knowledge Engineering Review, 34*, e28.

Boulier, B. L., & Stekler, H. O. (1999). Are sports seedings good predictors? An evaluation. *International Journal of Forecasting, 15*(1), 83–91.

Brown, E. G. (2021). A faster serve has more impact on success for female elite tennis players than males. *International Journal of Performance Analysis in Sport, 21*(4), 600–610.

Bunker, R., Yeung, C., Susnjak, T., Espie, C., & Fujii, K. (2023). A comparative evaluation of Elo ratings-and machine learning-based methods for tennis match result prediction. *Proceedings of the Institution of Mechanical Engineers, Part P: Journal of Sports Engineering and Technology, 12*, 17543371231212236.

Cornman, A., Spellman, G., & Wright, D. (2017). *Machine learning for professional tennis match prediction and betting*. Working Paper, Stanford University.

Cui, Y., Liu, H., Liu, H., & Gómez, M. Á. (2019). Data-driven analysis of point-by-point performance for male tennis player in Grand Slams. *Motricidade, 15*(1), 49–61.

Deshpande, S., & Klotzman, V. (2022). How can machine learning determine whether a women's tennis player will make it to top 100? *Journal of Student Research, 11*(2), 2847.

Filipcic, A., Panjan, A., & Sarabon, N. (2014). Classification of top male tennis players. *International Journal of Computer Science in Sport, 13*(1), 36–42.

Fitzpatrick, A., Stone, J. A., Choppin, S., & Kelley, J. (2023). Analysing Hawk-Eye ball-tracking data to explore successful serving and returning strategies at Wimbledon. *International Journal of Performance Analysis in Sport, 21*, 5487. https://doi.org/10.1080/24748668.2023.2291238

Gao, Z., & Kowalczyk, A. (2021). Random forest model identifies serve strength as a key predictor of tennis match outcome. *Journal of Sports Analytics, 7*(4), 255–262.

Ghosh, S., Sadhu, S., Biswas, S., Sarkar, D., & Sarkar, P. P. (2019). A comparison between different classifiers for tennis match result prediction. *Malaysian Journal of Computer Science, 32*(2), 97–111.

Giles, B., Kovalchik, S., & Reid, M. (2020). A machine learning approach for automatic detection and classification of changes of direction from player tracking data in professional tennis. *Journal of Sports Sciences, 38*(1), 106–113. https://doi.org/10.1080/02640414.2019.1684132

Giles, B., Peeling, P., Kovalchik, S., & Reid, M. (2021). Differentiating movement styles in professional tennis: A machine learning and hierarchical clustering approach. *European Journal of Sport Science, 23*(1), 44–53. https://doi.org/10.1080/17461391.2021.2006800

Giles, B., Peeling, P., Kovalchik, S., & Reid, M. (2023). Differentiating movement styles in professional tennis: A machine learning and hierarchical clustering approach. *European Journal of Sport Science, 23*(1), 44–53. https://doi.org/10.1080/17461391.2021.2006800

Hao, J., & Hu, H. (2023). Beyond the coach: Exploring the efficacy of a machine learning application for improving tennis players' performance. In *CS and IT Conference Proceedings* (Vol. 13, No. 9). CS & IT Conference Proceedings.

Horvat, T., & Job, J. (2020). The use of machine learning in sport outcome prediction: A review. *Wiley Interdisciplinary Reviews: Data Mining and Knowledge Discovery, 10*(5), e1380.

Hostačný, J. (2018). Non-linear classification as a tool for predicting tennis matches.

Hughes, M., & Bartlett, R. (2008). What is performance analysis? In M. Hughes & I. M. Franks (Eds.), *The essentials of performance analysis: An introduction* (pp. 8–20). Routledge.

Jindo, T., Mitsuhashi, D., & Kubota, T. (2022). Accuracy of subjective stats of key performance indicators in tennis. *International Journal of Racket Sports Science, 4*(2), 40–55.

Kingma, D. P., & Ba, J. (2015). Adam: a method for stochastic optimization. In *Conference Paper at ICLR 2015*. arXiv preprint arXiv:1412.6980.

Kolbinger, O., & Lames, M. (2013). Ball trajectories in tennis-Lateral and vertical placement of right handed men's singles serves. *International Journal of Performance Analysis in Sport, 13*(3), 750–758.

Kovalchik, S. A., & Albert, J. (2022). A statistical model of serve return impact patterns in professional tennis. arXiv preprint arXiv:2202.00583

Kovalchik, S. (2016). Searching for the GOAT of tennis win prediction. *Journal of Quantitative Analysis in Sports, 12*(3), 127–138.

Kovalchik, S., & Albert, J. (2017). A multilevel Bayesian approach for modeling the time-to-serve in professional tennis. *Journal of Quantitative Analysis in Sports, 13*(2), 49–62. https://doi.org/10.1515/jqas-2016-0091

Kovalchik, S., & Reid, M. (2018). A shot taxonomy in the era of tracking data in professional tennis. *Journal of Sports Sciences, 36*(18), 2096–2104. https://doi.org/10.1080/02640414.2018.1438094

Learning, M. (2017). Final project report: Real time tennis match prediction using machine learning.

Lerner, S., Badri, D., & Monogue, K. (2019). DeepTennis: Mid-match tennis predictions CS230-fall.

Lin, T. Y., Goyal, P., Girshick, R., He, K., & Dollár, P. (2017). Focal loss for dense object detection. In *Proceedings of the IEEE international conference on computer vision* (pp. 2980–2988).

Loffing, F., Hagemann, N., & Strauss, B. (2010). Automated processes in tennis: Do left-handed players benefit from the tactical preferences of their opponents? *Journal of Sports Sciences, 28*(4), 435–443. https://doi.org/10.1080/02640410903536459

Lundberg, S. M., & Lee, S. I. (2017). A unified approach to interpreting model predictions. *Advances in Neural Information Processing Systems, 30*, 546.

Makino, M., Odaka, T., Kuroiwa, J., Suwa, I., & Shirai, H. (2020). Feature selection to win the point of atp tennis players using rally information. *International Journal of Computer Science in Sport, 19*(1), 37–50.

Martínez-Gallego, R., Crespo, M., & Jiménez, J. (2021a). Analysis of the differences in serve effectiveness between Billie Jean King Cup (former Fed Cup) and Davis Cup doubles tennis matches. *International Journal of Sports Science and Coaching, 16*(3), 777–783.

Martínez-Gallego, R., Ramón-Llin, J., & Crespo, M. (2021b). A cluster analysis approach to profile men and women's volley positions in professional tennis matches (doubles). *Sustainability, 13*(11), 6370.

Mecheri, S., Rioult, F., Mantel, B., Kauffmann, F., & Benguigui, N. (2016). The serve impact in tennis: First large-scale study of big Hawk-Eye data. *Statistical Analysis and Data Mining: THe ASA Data Science Journal, 9*, 310–325. https://doi.org/10.1002/sam.11316

Meurs, E. V., Buszard, T., Kovalchik, S., Farrow, D., & Reid, M. (2021). Interpersonal coordination in tennis: assessing the positional advantage index with Australian Open Hawkeye data. *International Journal of Performance Analysis in Sport, 21*(1), 22–32. https://doi.org/10.1080/24748668.2020.1843213

Morgulev, E., Azar, O. H., & Lidor, R. (2018). Sports analytics and the big-data era. *International Journal of Data Science and Analytics, 5*, 213–222.

O'Donoghue, P. (2014). *An introduction to performance analysis of sport*. Routledge.

Panjan, A., Šarabon, N., & Filipčič, A. (2010). Prediction of the successfulness of tennis players with machine learning methods. *Kinesiology, 42*(1), 98–106.

Perri, T., Reid, M., Murphy, A., Howle, K., & Duffield, R. (2022). Prototype machine learning algorithms from wearable technology to detect tennis stroke and movement actions. *Sensors, 22*, 8868. https://doi.org/10.3390/s22228868

Peters, J. (2017). *Predicting the outcomes of professional tennis matches*. University of Edinburg.

Rajbahadur, G. K., Wang, S., Oliva, G. A., Kamei, Y., & Hassan, A. E. (2021). The impact of feature importance methods on the interpretation of defect classifiers. *IEEE Transactions on Software Engineering, 48*(7), 2245–2261.

Reid, M., Morgan, S., & Whiteside, D. (2016). Matchplay characteristics of Grand Slam tennis: implications for training and conditioning. *Journal of Sports Sciences, 34*(19), 1791–1798. https://doi.org/10.1080/02640414.2016.1139161

Rioult, F. Mecheri, S., Mantel, B., Kauffmann,F. & Benguigui, N. (2015). What can Hawk-Eye data reveal about serve performance in tennis? In MLSA15: Machine learning and data mining for sports analytics workshop (ECML/PKDD 2015) (pp. 36–45). Porto.

Rosker, J., & Majcen Rosker, Z. (2021). Skill level in tennis serve return is related to adaptability in visual search behavior. *Frontiers in Psychology, 12*, 689378.

Sekar, A. (2019). *Predicting the winner of a tennis match using machine learning techniques*. Masters thesis, Dublin, National College of Ireland.

Shimizu, T., Hachiuma, R., Saito, H., Yoshikawa, T., & Lee, C. (2019, October). Prediction of future shot direction using pose and position of tennis player. In *Proceedings Proceedings of the 2nd International Workshop on Multimedia Content Analysis in Sports* (pp. 59–66).

Siener, M., Faber, I., & Hohmann, A. (2021). Prognostic validity of statistical prediction methods used for talent identification in youth tennis players based on motor abilities. *Applied Sciences, 11*, 7051. https://doi.org/10.3390/app11157051

Singh Bal, B., & Dureja, G. (2012). Hawk-Eye: A logical innovative technology use in sports for effective decision making. *Sport Science Review, 21*(1–2), 107–119.

Solanki, S., Jakir, V., Jatav, A., & Sharma, D. (2022). Prediction of tennis match using machine learning. *International Journal of Progressive Research in Engineering Management and Science (IJPREMS), 2*(6), 59–7.

Vives, F., Crespo, M., Guzmán, J. F., & Martínez-Gallego, R. (2022). Effective serving strategies in men's doubles Davis cup matches: An analysis using tracking technology. *International Journal of Performance Analysis in Sport, 22*(4), 638–648.

Vives, F., Lázaro, J., Guzmán, J. F., Martínez-Gallego, R., & Crespo, M. (2023). Optimizing sporting actions effectiveness: A machine learning approach to uncover key variables in the men's professional doubles tennis serve. *Applied Sciences, 13*(24), 13213.

Wei, X., Lucey, P., Morgan, S., Carr, P., Reid, M., & Sridharan, S. (2015, August). Predicting serves in tennis using style priors. In Proceedings of the 21th ACM SIGKDD International Conference on Knowledge Discovery and Data Mining (pp. 2207–2215).

Wei, X., Lucey, P., Morgan, S., & Sridharan, S. (2016). Forecasting the next shot location in tennis using fine-grained spatiotemporal tracking data. *IEEE Transactions on Knowledge and Data Engineering, 28*(11), 2988–2997.

Whiteside, D., & Reid, M. (2017). Spatial characteristics of professional tennis serves with implications for serving aces: A machine learning approach. *Journal of Sports Sciences, 35*(7), 648–654. https://doi.org/10.1080/02640414.2016.1183805

Wu, M., Wang, R., Hu, Y., et al. (2023). Invisible experience to real-time assessment in elite tennis athlete training: Sport-specific movement classification based on wearable MEMS sensor data. *Proceedings of the Institution of Mechanical Engineers, Part p: Journal of Sports Engineering and Technology, 237*(4), 271–282. https://doi.org/10.1177/17543371211050312

Yue, J. C., Chou, E. P., Hsieh, M.-H., & Hsiao, L.-C. (2022). A study of forecasting tennis matches via the Glicko model. *PLoS ONE, 17*(4), e0266838. https://doi.org/10.1371/journal.pone.0266838

Zhou, J. Q., & Liu, Y. (2024). Probability prediction of groundstroke stances among male professional tennis players using a tree-augmented Bayesian network. *International Journal of Performance Analysis in Sport, 14*, 1–13. https://doi.org/10.1080/24748668.2024.2314646

Zhu, Y., & Naikar, R. (2022). Predicting tennis serve directions with machine learning. In international workshop on machine learning and data mining for sports analytics (pp. 89–100). Springer.

Chapter 12
Using Convolutional Neural Network to Predict Sports

Arisoa S. Randrianasolo

Abstract Convolutional Neural Networks, powerful Machine Learning tools for image classifications, can also be employed to perform sports outcome predictions. To use a Convolutional Neural Network for sports predictions, we arranged the statistics of the two opposing teams or players into a grid representation. We have exploited this two-dimensional input arrangement to expand the training set for our Convolutional Neural Network. The expansion consisted of shifting each grid that represented a game by one and two columns to the right. This shifting idea made it possible to employ Convolutional Neural Networks in predicting sports events without relying on extensive historical data. We used the Men Euro 2020 and Women US Open 2021 as test cases to illustrate this approach. The most performant models from our exploration registered a 70.2% accuracy in predicting the Women US Open 2021 and a 69.8% accuracy in predicting the Men Euro 2020. These accuracies are considered as improvements. The ensemble techniques we previously used on these datasets had an accuracy of 64.9% on the Women US Open 2021 and 67% on the Men Euro 2020.

Keywords Sports Predictions · Convolutional Neural Networks · Machine Learning

12.1 Introduction

Predicting the outcome of a sporting event is an activity that is popular among fans, players, coaches, team managers, and team owners. Fans want to know ahead of time the probability of their favorite team winning a particular game. They may be interested in such forecasts just for the fun of the game or for betting purposes. The users of popular sports betting sites like bet365, betway, and many more, will fall under this case. Coaches on the other hand want to know their chances of winning to

A. S. Randrianasolo (✉)
School of Information, Technology and Computing, Abilene Christian University, 1600 Campus Ct, Abilene, TX 79601, USA
e-mail: sar04b@acu.edu

C. Dindorf et al. (eds.), *Artificial Intelligence in Sports, Movement, and Health*,
https://doi.org/10.1007/978-3-031-67256-9_12

select the best tactics to use against the opponents. Whether the reason is fun, money, marketing, or strategy, sporting event stakeholders are always interested in predicting the outcome of competitive games. Along with the evolution and improvement of technology, more data is generated about games, tournaments, and competitions. The abundance of data has led many researchers to look into the possibility of using Machine Learning algorithms to predict the outcome of head-to-head games. A small collection of the research done in this area is summarized in the related section below. The application of Machine Learning to predict sporting events, for the most part, is reserved for events where plenty of historical data is available to train the algorithms. To list a few examples, the research conducted by Hsu (2021) that used candlestick charts and a Convolutional Neural Network used more than 18 thousand games. The research conducted by Candila and Palazzo (2020) that used Artificial Neural Networks to predict the outcome of tennis games used more than 26 thousand of games. The research conducted by Alfredo and Isa (2019) that used various tree-based Machine Learning algorithms used more than 3 thousand games. What do we do then if we want to predict an event that lacks extensive historical data? This is where we believe that the usage of Convolutional Neural Networks can come in handy. Convolutional Neural Networks accept the input as a 2-dimensional grid. We can exploit this grid representation to shift the input by one or more columns to create new inputs and therefore expand the training data.

12.2 Related Work

In the last few years, Machine Learning algorithms have slowly become the preferred tool for researchers working on sports predictions. Pretorius and Parry (2016) and Parry employed a Random Forest to forecast the 2015 Rugby World Cup. Wilkens (2021) created an ensemble technique to predict the 2010–2019 tennis games. Alfredo and Isa (2019) tested C5.0, Random Forest, and Extreme Gradient Boosting on the games from the 2007–2017 season of the English Premier League (EPL). Beal et al. (2021) used a Random Forest to predict the games from the 2016 to 2019 season of the EPL. Saiedy et al. (2020) used a Support Vector Machine and a Random Forest to predict the EPL games from the 2018–2019 season.

Neural networks and their variants have also been used in sports predictions. Rahman (2020) utilized Long Short-Term Memory units to construct a Deep Neural Network to predict the 2018 FIFA World Cup. A deep network containing 2 hidden layers of 10 and 2 units respectively was trained on a dataset that contained international football game results from 1872 to 2018. This approach had an accuracy of 63.3% in predicting the group stage of the 2018 FIFA World Cup. Cheng et al. (2003) used backpropagation networks and a learning vector quantization to predict the outcomes of football games from the Italian Serie A. Three different backpropagation networks were created for each team in the league. The first network captured the situation where the team was playing a weaker team. The second network captured the situation where the team was playing another team of equal strength. The third network captured the situation where the team was playing a stronger team. Given input data about a game, the difference between the two teams' scores and net goals was calculated, then the learning vector quantization would select which backpropagation network should be used. Data from the days 6 to 17 of the 2001–2002 Serie A season were used to train this approach. The approach had an accuracy of 52.29% in predicting the games for the days 18–34.

Convolutional Neural Networks have also been used in different ways in sports predictions. Shen et al. (2024) utilized a Convolutional Neural Network to extract football players' abilities from game recordings. The Convolutional Neural Network was trained on 10 randomly selected 10-min videos from the European Women's Champions League in 2021–2022. The network's accuracy in classifying football actions and goal angles from the 2021–2022 dataset exceeded the 95% mark.

Lin et al. (2018) used a Convolutional Neural Network to predict the outcome of games from the National Basketball Association (NBA). The data used to train the network consisted of games from October 2014 to April 2017 for a total of 4147 games. Each game was represented by a 16 × 16 grid that contained the performance comparison between the 16 players from each team. The network had two convolutional layers. The first convolutional layer had 8 × 8 units followed by a pooling layer of size 3 × 3. The second convolutional layer had 2 × 2 units followed by a polling layer of size 2 × 2. The fully connected neural network part of this network had 3 hidden layers. The optimization used was the Adam optimizer. By using a tenfold cross-validation, this approach had an accuracy of 79% in predicting the games from the dataset.

Hsu (2021) trained a Convolutional Neural Network on a dataset that contained 18,944 American football games. The network used as an input a 10 × 10 candlestick chart image with 4 channels. The network had two convolutional layers that used a 3 × 3 local receptive field. The first layer had 8 channels and the second layer had 16 channels. Two max-pooling layers with a 2 × 2 window and two drop-out layers with 0.5 probability were also used. One drop-out layer was placed after the last max-pooling and the other was placed before the output layer in the fully connected neural network. The fully connected neural network had one layer of 128 units followed by another layer that had 2 units. The network used a rectified linear activation function in the units. The Convolutional Neural Network outputted the winning probabilities. This output was combined with the past head-to-head results between the two teams and was injected into a Logistic Regression to produce the final predictions. This approach had an accuracy of 69.29% in predicting the test set from the American National Football League games.

12.3 Short Introduction to Convolutional Neural Network

This section will briefly explain the various sections of a Convolutional Neural Network. This section is aimed to provide a general overview. Readers who need more details are encouraged to refer to Fukushima (1980) and Lecun et al. (1998).

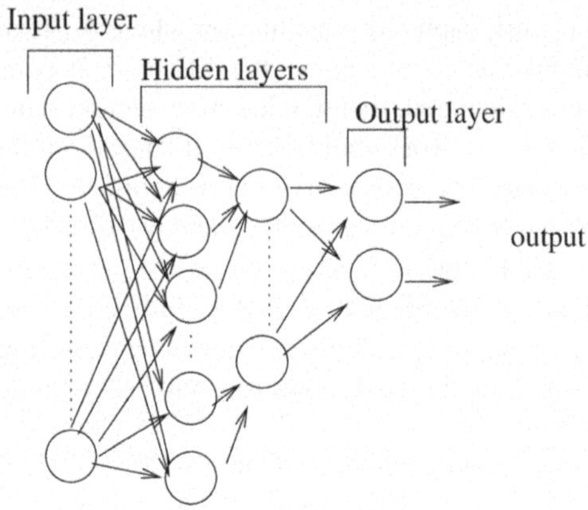

Fig. 12.1 Topology of a Neutral Network with two hidden layers

12.3.1 Neural Network

A neural network is a Machine Learning technique that was inspired by the way the brain works. The network consists of one or more layers. Each layer represents a column of units. Each unit simulates the functionality of the neuron in the brain. Each unit receives multiple inputs, calculates a weighted sum of the inputs, plugs the weighted sum into an activation function, and finally fires out an output signal. Theoretically, a neural network can represent any function by using more layers and more units. Usually, a neural network is fully connected; this means each unit in a layer is sending a signal to all units in the next layer. A neural network contains an input layer, one or more hidden layers, and an output layer. The network learns by backpropagating the errors from the expected output and the produced output back to units in each layer. A simple topology of a neural network can be seen in Fig. 12.1.

12.3.2 Convolutional Neural Network

A Convolutional Neural Network is a variant of a neural network. A Convolutional Neural Network is characterized by the presence of one or more convolutional layers placed before the fully connected neural network. The input to the network is a grid, a 2-dimensional pixel image, and not a 1-dimensional like the regular neural network. The convolutional layers are not fully connected. A smaller group of units, of size 3 $\times$ 3 for example, is connected to another unit in the next layer. This smaller window can be slid by one column to the right or one row down to make sure that all units from the previous layer are connected to some units in the next layer. To further simplify the output of the convolutional layer, a pooling layer is usually used. A unit in the pooling layer takes a group of convolutional units, 2 $\times$ 2 for example, and outputs a value like the maximum of the 2 $\times$ 2 area, or the average, or the L2. The usage of the convolutional layer and the pooling layer is based on the principle that

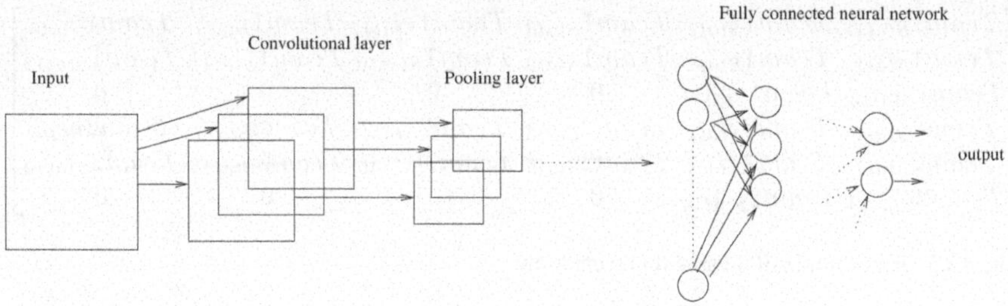

Fig. 12.2 Simplified topology of a Convolutional Neural Network

the existence of the pattern is what is important and not the location of the pattern. The last convolutional layer or pooling layer, depending on the structure, is flattened into a 1-dimensional column of units and is connected to a fully connected neural network. Convolutional Neural Networks also have the particularity of not having just one grid of units in the convolutional or pooling layer. Multiple grids of units can exist in the layers. The number of grids in each layer is called the layer's channel. Figure 12.2 describes an example of a Convolutional Neural Network.

Convolutional Neural Networks are commonly used for image classification. In image classification, pixels' values are extracted from the pictures. The pixels are sent to the convolutional layers so that the network can perform feature extractions. The extracted features are finally sent to a fully connected neural network to perform the actual classification. Various researchers have applied Convolutional Neural Networks to image classification tasks. To list a few examples, Wang et al. (2021) used a Convolutional Neural Network to classify flowers. Hao et al. (2023) used a Convolutional Neural Network to classify images of Alzheimer's disease from a set of magnetic resonance images. Tan and Teoh Teik (2023) used a Convolutional Neural Network to classify Pneumonia images from X-rays.

12.4 The Approach

Let us start by explaining how to represent each game that will be used to train the Convolutional Neural Network. Each game is represented by a $n \times n$ grid. The top half, $n/2 \times n$, of the grid contains the statistics for the first team, and the bottom half, $n/2 \times n$, contains the statistics for the second team. Rows in the $n/2 \times n$ can be padded with 0 s if the statistics from each team cannot fill the $n/2 \times n$ grid assigned to them. Figure 12.3 illustrates an example of a game representation. The grid shall be, on purpose, made a bit larger to allow shifting to happen in order to expand the training data.

As already mentioned in the introduction, the training set is expanded by shifting each game representation. Each game representation can be shifted by one, two, or three positions to the right to create a new representation. As each representation

$$\begin{bmatrix} Team1_{Stat1} & Team1_{Stat2} & Team1_{Stat3} & Team1_{Stat4} & Team1_{Stat5} & Team1_{Stat6} \\ Team1_{Stat7} & Team1_{Stat8} & Team1_{Stat9} & Team1_{Stat10} & Team1_{Stat11} & Team1_{Stat12} \\ Team1_{Stat13} & Team1_{Stat14} & 0 & 0 & 0 & 0 \\ Team2_{Stat1} & Team2_{Stat2} & Team2_{Stat3} & Team2_{Stat4} & Team2_{Stat5} & Team2_{Stat6} \\ Team2_{Stat7} & Team2_{Stat8} & Team2_{Stat9} & Team2_{Stat10} & Team2_{Stat11} & Team2_{Stat12} \\ Team2_{Stat13} & Team2_{Stat14} & 0 & 0 & 0 & 0 \end{bmatrix}$$

Fig. 12.3 An example of a game representation

$$\begin{bmatrix} 0 & Team1_{Stat1} & Team1_{Stat2} & Team1_{Stat3} & Team1_{Stat4} & Team1_{Stat5} \\ Team1_{Stat6} & Team1_{Stat7} & Team1_{Stat8} & Team1_{Stat9} & Team1_{Stat10} & Team1_{Stat11} \\ Team1_{Stat12} & Team1_{Stat13} & Team1_{Stat13} & 0 & 0 & 0 \\ 0 & Team2_{Stat1} & Team2_{Stat2} & Team2_{Stat3} & Team2_{Stat4} & Team2_{Stat5} \\ Team2_{Stat6} & Team2_{Stat7} & Team2_{Stat8} & Team2_{Stat9} & Team2_{Stat10} & Team2_{Stat11} \\ Team2_{Stat12} & Team2_{Stat13} & Team2_{Stat14} & 0 & 0 & 0 \end{bmatrix}$$

Fig. 12.4 An example of a game representation shifted by one position

is shifted, we have to make sure that we do not lose any of the statistics from each team. A wrap-around approach can be taken if not enough room is available to do more shifting. The picture below, Fig. 12.4, illustrates this case.

This idea of shifting the data in the grid representation to expand the training set is a common practice in using Convolutional Neural Networks to perform image classification. In the image classification cases, pixel values are moved one or more columns to the right. We are adapting this very same technique to a grid that contains the team's statistics and not pixel values. In addition, we add a restriction that any shift we perform shall not make us lose any of the statistics from the grid.

In addition to the shifting, the training dataset is also balanced by listing each game twice. In the second listing, the order of the teams is changed and the outcome is set to the opposite of the outcome in the first listing.

12.5 Case Studies

We picked two cases to illustrate the application of this approach. In both cases, we created a Convolutional Neural Network that comprised a 6×6 input grid, followed by a convolutional layer that had 6 channels of 4×4 units, followed by a max-pooling layer that contained 6 channels of 2×2 units. The fully connected neural network end had $6 \times 2 \times 2 = 24$ input units. The structure of the fully connected network was different for each of the case studies we considered.

The two Convolutional Neural Networks we created used a stochastic gradient descent optimization function with the following setting: learning rate $= 0.00001$, momentum $= 0.9$, and batch size $= 1$. A rectified linear unit function was used as an activation in the convolutional layer, the first hidden layer of the fully connected neural network, and the second hidden layer of the fully connected neural network. A linear activation function was used in the two units on the output layer. The game-winner was determined by applying a one-hot encoding on the outputs from these two units.

12.5.1 The Case of Tennis

We collected statistics of women tennis players from wtatennis.com for the year 2020. We used these statistics to create game representations for the Women US Open in 2021. After performing the correlation analysis in Fig. 12.5, we used a total of 10 predictors: player's rank, number of matches, and the percentages for the following: first serve, first serve points, breakpoints, service games won, first return points, second return points, return games won, and break points converted. Most of these predictors were percentages and were in the range of 0–100.

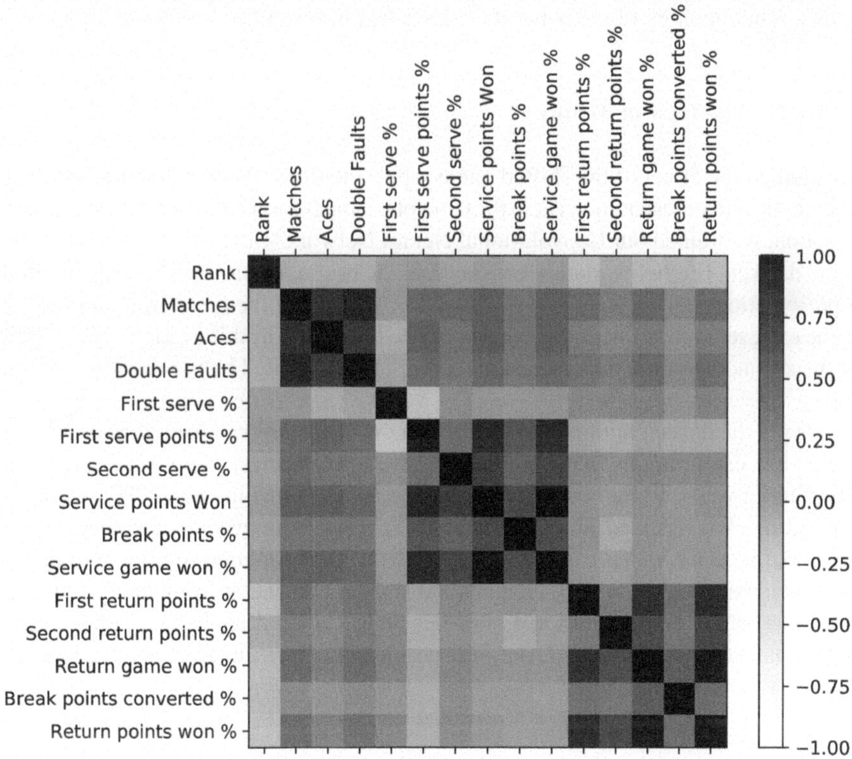

Fig. 12.5 Correlation analysis of Women US Open 2021 predictors

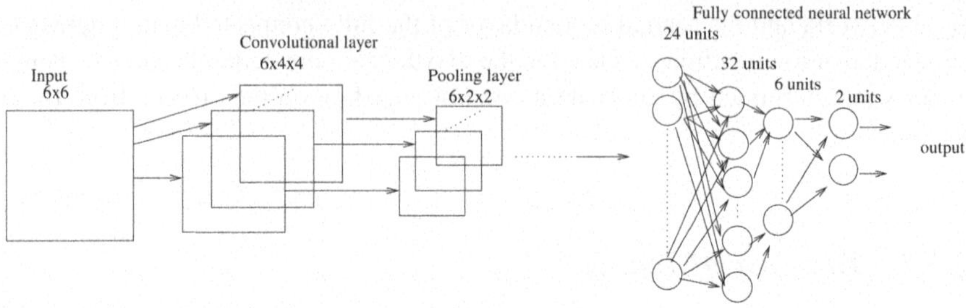

Fig. 12.6 Topology of the Convolutional Neural Network for the Women US Open 2021

The Convolutional Neural Network was trained on the game representations from the first round of the Women US Open 2021. As stated in the approach section, we added to the training set the shifted representations. For this case, we shifted each representation by one and two positions to the right. We started with 60 unbalanced games. When the balancing was performed, the training set had 120 games. The shift by one position resulted in 240 games. The shift by two positions resulted in 360 games. The topology of the network is described in Fig. 12.6.

12.5.1.1 The Case of Tennis

We studied the effect of the shifted game representations. We wondered whether or not the shifted representations help the Convolutional Neural Network. To answer this question, we trained our Convolutional Neural Network with three variations of the same dataset. The first variation consisted of the original dataset without the shifted representations added. The second variation consisted of the first variation plus the game representations shifted by one position to the right. The third variation consisted of the second variation plus the game representations shifted by two positions to the right.

We ran the dataset multiple times through the Convolutional Neural Network. At the end of each run, also known as epoch, we tested the accuracy of the network. The dataset was split into two sets. 80% were used for training and 20% were used for testing. We repeated this experiment 100 times. The average accuracy of the network for each epoch is captured in Fig. 12.7. We also captured additional statistics such as maximum, minimum, median, and standard deviation from the 100 runs in the experiment. These additional statistics were captured at the last epochs. The Additional statistics for shift 2, our best-performing representation, are available in Fig. 12.8.

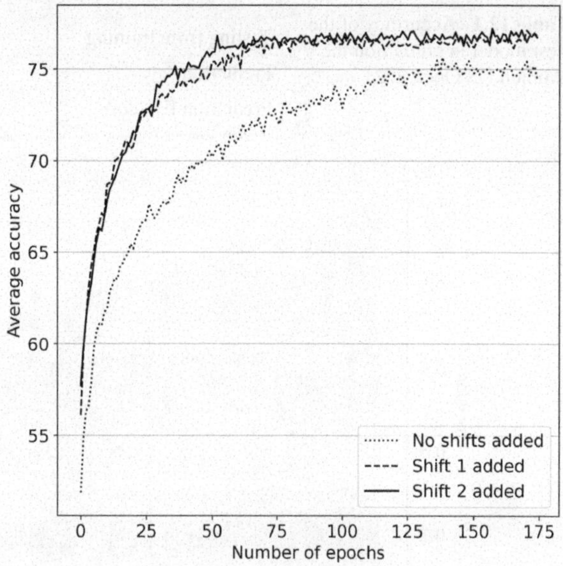

Fig. 12.7 Effect of the shifted game representations on the Women US Open 2021 dataset

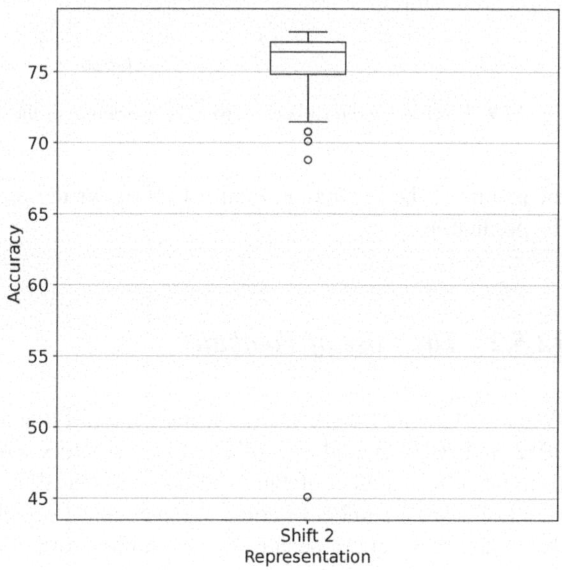

Fig. 12.8 Box plot of the additional statistic captured at the last epochs for shift 2 on the Women US Open 2021 dataset

12.5.1.2 Prediction

The Convolutional Neural Network model produced from the training was used to predict the second, third, and fourth rounds, quarterfinals, semifinals, and the final of the Women US Open 2021. In total, we predicted 57 games. Table 12.1 captures

Table 12.1 Accurracy of the best model in prediction the Women US Open 2021

Testing from training	77.1%
Prediction	70.2%
Prediction F1-score	0.7118

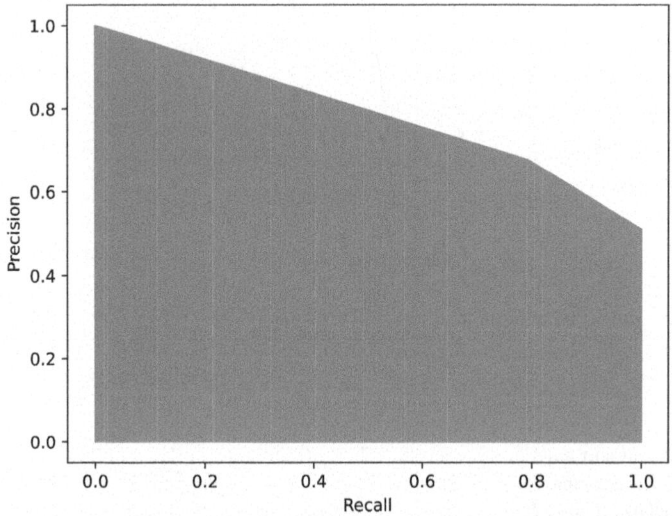

Fig. 12.9 Precision and recall curve from the prediction of the Women US Open 2021

the results of the prediction. Figure 12.9 shows the precision and recall curve from the prediction.

12.5.2 The Case of Football

We gathered data from uefa.com from the qualifying stages of the Men Euro 2008, 2012, and 2016. In total, we collected 17 predictors and they are: goals scored, goals from penalties, number of games, shots on target, shots off target, shots blocked, the count of assists, number of corners, the count of offsides, goals saved, goals taken, the count of own goals, penalties saved, number of fouls committed, numbered fouls endured, the amount of yellow cards collected, and the amount of red cards collected. The correlation analysis for these predictors is captured in Fig. 12.10.

These predictors served to craft the 6×6 grid game representations for the head-to-head matches from the Euro tournaments in 2008, 2012, and 2016. The Convolutional Neural Network was trained on these game representations. There were 88 unbalanced games. After the balancing, this number doubled to 176. The shift by one position resulted in 352 games and the shift by two positions resulted in 528 games. Figure 12.11 describes the topology of the network.

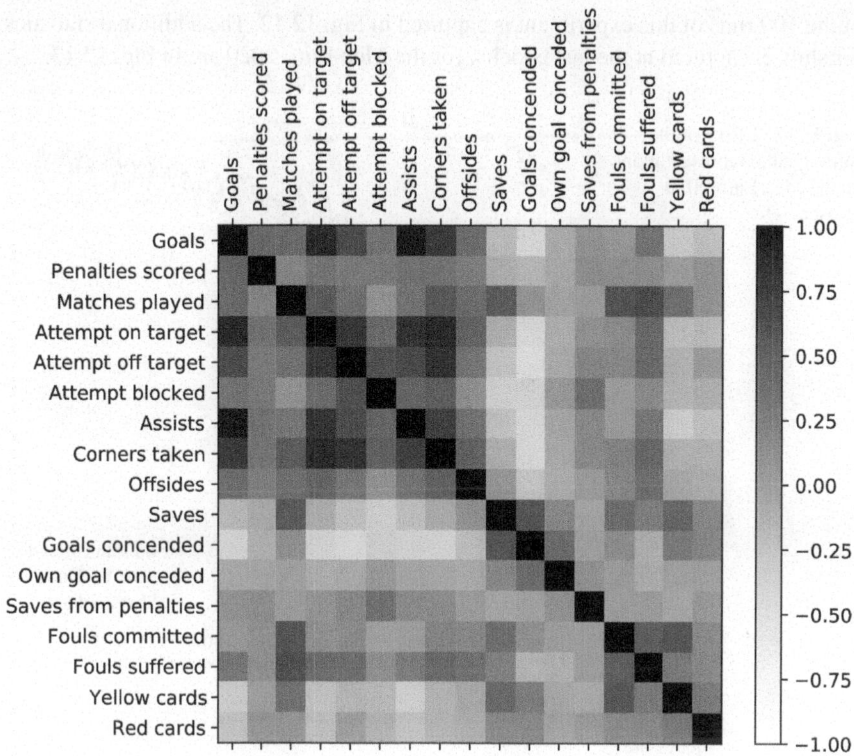

Fig. 12.10 Correlation analysis of the Men Euro 2008, 2012, and 2016 predictors

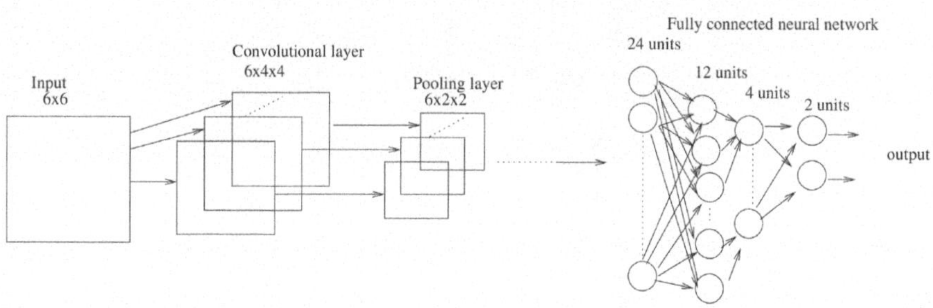

Fig. 12.11 Topology of the Convolutional Neural Network for the Men Euro 2020

12.5.2.1 Effect of the Shifts

We ran a similar study as what we did in the case of tennis, in the previous section, for the case of football. The goal was to discover whether or not the shifted representations helped the convolutional network reach a better accuracy or not. The average of the 100 runs of this experiment is captured in Fig. 12.12. The additional statistics for shift 2, captured at the last epochs, for the Men Euro 2020 are in Fig. 12.13.

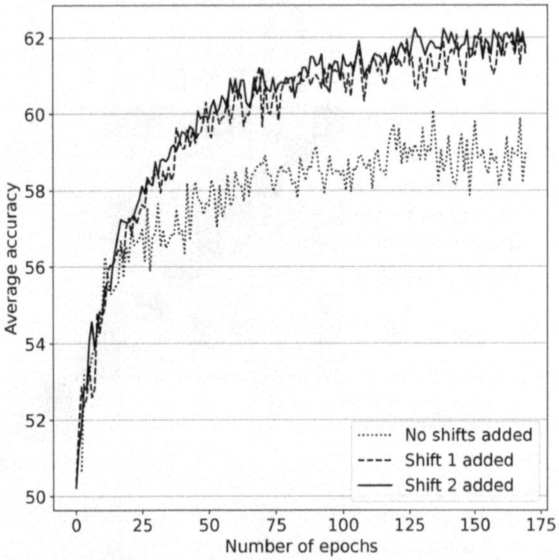

Fig. 12.12 Effect of the shifted game representations on the Men Euro 2020 dataset

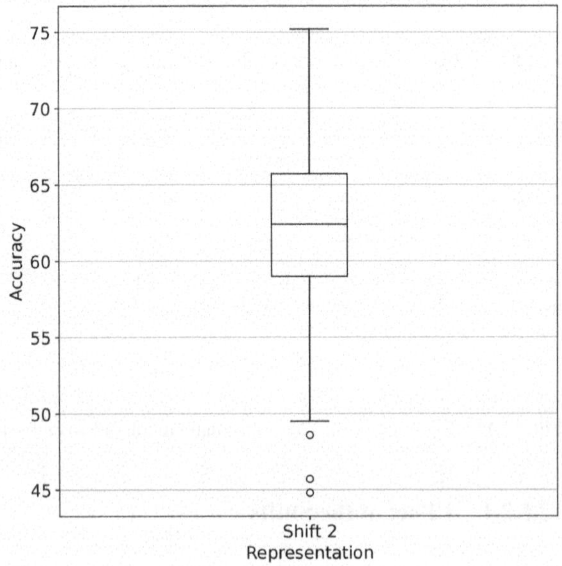

Fig. 12.13 Box plot of the additional statistic captured at the last epochs for shift 2 Men Euro 2020 dataset

Table 12.2 Accuracy of the best model in predicting the Men Euro 2020

Testing from training	75.2%
Prediction	69.8%
Prediction F1-score	0.7234

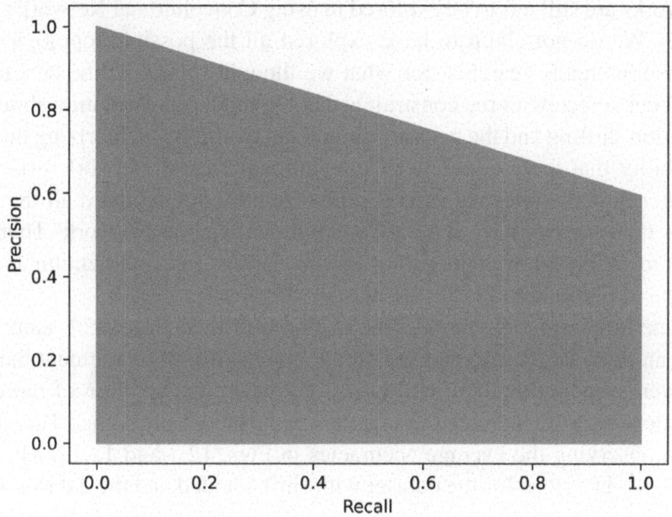

Fig. 12.14 Precision and recall curve from the prediction of the Men Euro 2020

12.5.2.2 Prediction

After training on the game representations from the Men Euro 2008, 2016, and 2012, the model produced was used to predict the Men Euro 2020. The data from the qualifying stage of the Euro 2020 was used to create the game representations for the main tournament. None of the game representations from the Men Euro 2020 were used in the training. In total, we predicted 43 games. Table 12.2 captures the results of the prediction. Figure 12.14 shows the precision and recall curve from the prediction.

12.6 Discussion

Convolutional Neural Networks can be useful tools in sports predictions. The 2-dimensional grid demanded by Convolutional Neural Networks provides opportunities to augment the dataset by shifting the input. We have shown from the case studies, previously described, that the accuracies of the Convolutional Neural Networks that we used got better when shifted representations were added to the dataset. The most performant models, Tables 12.1 and 12.2, from our exploration registered a 70.2%

accuracy in predicting the Women US Open 2021 and a 69.8% accuracy in predicting the Men Euro 2020. These accuracies are an improvement. The ensemble techniques we previously used on these datasets had an accuracy of 64.9%, in Randrianasolo and Pyeatt (2023), on the Women US Open 2021 and 67%, in Randrianasolo (2023), on the Men Euro 2020.

More works are still left to be explored in using Convolutional Networks in sports predictions. We do not claim to have explored all the possible topologies for the network. We manually searched for what we thought should be the best topology. We guided our search with the constraints that the input representation should allow representation shifting and the network should not overfit by memorizing the dataset. The possibility that there is another Convolutional Neural Network structure that can do better than the ones we used is high. We have not explored all the possible parameters that one can have with a Convolutional Neural Network. There is still more work to do in exploring the values for the learning rate, momentum, batch size, and the type of optimizer.

The game representation can also be explored further. Instead of using a 6×6 grid, one can use a larger grid that will allow more shiftings to augment the dataset. We, however, suspect that there will be a point where the addition of more shifted representations may not increase the accuracy of the model any higher. This suspicion came from observing the average accuracies in Figs. 12.7 and 12.12. The average accuracies are very close for the dataset with shift 1 added and the dataset with shift 2 added.

12.7 Conclusion

The ability to predict the outcomes of games is an important advantage in competitive sports. Such ability can help in coaching teams and players and can help in improving financial gains as well. In this paper, we summarized our attempt to predict the outcomes of sports games using a Convolutional Neural Network. Our approach expanded the training set by shifting each grid that represented a game by one and two columns to the right. With this approach, we slightly improved our accuracy in predicting the Men Euro 2020 and Women US Open 2021.

As stated in the discussion, we have not explored all the possible configurations and parameters involved with a Convolutional Neural Network. We are convinced that Convolutional Neural Networks have a lot of potential that can still be explored within the arena of sports predictions.

References

Alfredo, Y. F., & Isa, S. M. (2019). Football match prediction with tree based model classification. *International Journal of Intelligent Systems and Applications, 11*, 20–28.

Beal, R., Middleton, S. E., Norman, T. J., & Ramchurn, S. D. (2021). Combining machine learning and human experts to predict match outcomes in football: A baseline model. *Proceedings of the AAAI Conference on Artificial Intelligence, 35*(17), 15447–15451. https://doi.org/10.1609/aaai.v35i17.17815

Candila, V., & Palazzo, L. (2020). Neural networks and betting strategies for tennis. *Risks, 8*(3), 11542.

Cheng, T., Cui, D., Fan, Z., Zhou, J., Lu, S. (2003) A new model to forecast the results of matches based on hybrid neural networks in the soccer rating system. In *Proceedings fifth international conference on computational intelligence and multimedia applications.* ICCIMA 2003 (pp. 308–313).

Fukushima, K. (1980). Neocognitron: A self-organizing neural network model for a mechanism of pattern recognition unaffected by shift in position. *Biological Cybernetics, 36*, 193–202.

Hao, Y., Pengzhou, C., Moyuan, F., & Toe, T. T. (2023). Alzheimer's disease image classification based on efficient convolutional neural network. In *Proceedings of the 2022 7th international conference on biomedical imaging, signal processing. ICBSP '22* (pp. 6–11). Association for Computing Machinery, New York. https://doi.org/10.1145/3578892.3578894

Hsu, Y.-C. (2021). Using convolutional neural network and candlestick representation to predict sports match outcomes. *Applied Sciences, 11*(14), 46594. https://doi.org/10.3390/app11146594

Lecun, Y., Bottou, L., Bengio, Y., & Haffner, P. (1998). Gradient-based learning applied to document recognition. *Proceedings of the IEEE, 86*(11), 2278–2324. https://doi.org/10.1109/5.726791

Lin, S.-H., Chen, M.-Y., & Chiang, H.-S. (2018) Forecasting results of sport events through deep learning. In *Proceedings of the 2018 international conference on machine learning and cybernetics (ICMLC), vol. 2* (pp. 501–506). https://doi.org/10.1109/ICMLC.2018.8526954

Pretorius, A., & Parry, D. A. (2016). Human decision making and artificial intelligence: A comparison in the domain of sports prediction. In *Proceedings of the annual conference of the South African institute of computer scientists and information technologists. SAICSIT '16*. Association for Computing Machinery, New York. https://doi.org/10.1145/2987491.2987493

Rahman, M. A. (2020). A deep learning framework for football match prediction. *SN Applied Sciences, 2*(165), 1821. https://doi.org/10.1007/s42452-019-1821-5

Randrianasolo, A. S., & Pyeatt, L. D. (2023). Using genetic algorithm to create an ensemble machine learning models to predict tennis. In *Proceedings of the future technologies conference. FTC 2022*, vol. 1 (pp. 681–695). Springer, Cham.

Randrianasolo, A. S. (2023). Predicting euro games using an ensemble technique involving genetic algorithms and machine learning. In *Proceedings of the IEEE 13th annual computing and communication workshop and conference. CCWC 2023* (pp. 0470–0475).

Saiedy, S., Qachmas, M., & Amanullah, F. (2020). Predicting epl football matches results using machine learning algorithms. *International Journal of Engineering Applied Sciences and Technology, 5*, 83–91.

Shen, L., Tan, Z., Li, Z., Li, Q., & Jiang, G. (2024). Tactics analysis and evaluation of women football team based on convolutional neural network. *Scientific Reports, 14*, 255.

Tan, Y., & Teoh Teik, T. (2023). Pneumonia image classification method based on improved convolutional neural network. In *Proceedings of the 2022 5th international conference on sensors, signal and image processing. SSIP '22* (pp. 6–12). Association for Computing Machinery, New York, NY. https://doi.org/10.1145/3577148.3577150

Wang, Z., Wang, K., Wang, X., & Pan, S. (2021) A convolutional neural network ensemble for flower image classification. In *Proceedings of the 2020 9th international conference on computing and pattern recognition. ICCPR '20* (pp. 225–230). Association for Computing Machinery, New York, NY. https://doi.org/10.1145/3436369.3437427

Wilkens, S. (2021). Sports prediction and betting models in the machine learning age: The case of tennis. *Journal of Sports Analytics, 7*, 1–19.

Chapter 13
Learning to Run Marathons: On the Applications of Machine Learning to Recreational Marathon Running

Barry Smyth, Ciara Feely, Jakim Berndsen, Brian Caulfield, and Aonghus Lawlor

Abstract The widespread adoption of mobile devices and wearable sensors has created an explosion of exercise-related data. In this chapter we consider how these data can be used to support individuals as they train and compete, focusing in particular on recreational marathon runners. We discuss why the marathon is an interesting data science application domain, and we present several case studies to demonstrate how ideas from machine learning and recommender systems can be used to help marathon runners.

Keywords Marathon Running · Machine Learning · Performance Prediction · Injury Prediction · Pacing Recommendation

13.1 Introduction

As we have come to better appreciate the important role that exercise has to play in our increasingly sedentary lives (Lieberman, 2015), more and more people, from all walks of life, are turning to various forms of endurance exercise to improve their cardiovascular fitness, mental health and general well-being (Sharma et al., 2006; Vina et al., 2012). Running is one of the most popular forms of exercise due to its low barrier to entry and well-documented physiological and mental health benefits (Cantwell, 1985; Grunseit et al., 2018; Pedisic et al., 2020; Shipway & Holloway, 2010; Szabo & Àbrahám, 2013). Among runners the marathon is widely considered to be one of the ultimate endurance challenges. Every year big-city marathons attract tens of thousands of runners to tackle these challenging 26.2 mile (42.2 km) events. This level of interest, combined with the widespread adoption of mobile devices and wearable sensors, and all the data produced as a result, makes marathon running

B. Smyth (✉) · C. Feely · J. Berndsen · B. Caulfield · A. Lawlor
Insight Research Centre for Data Analytics, University College Dublin, Dublin, Ireland
e-mail: barry.smyth@ucd.ie

C. Dindorf et al. (eds.), *Artificial Intelligence in Sports, Movement, and Health*,
https://doi.org/10.1007/978-3-031-67256-9_13

an exciting application domain from a Machine Learning perspective (Brady et al., 2005; Dunne et al., 2005; Kiernan et al., 2018; Willy, 2018).

In this chapter, we outline a growing body of research on this topic and present several case studies on the use of Machine Learning for recreational runners as they train for, and compete in, marathon events. The purpose of this chapter is not to introduce new research—expanded versions of the case studies presented have been published elsewhere (Berndsen et al., 2019a; Feely et al., 2021, 2022, 2023)—but rather to provide an integrated vision of a body of research targeted at recreational marathon runners. In doing so we highlight several important research opportunities worthy of explanation.

13.2 Related Work

Activity data has the potential to tell us not just about how we have been exercising, but also how we should be exercising (Smyth et al., 2022). This is especially true for recreational marathon runners because of the many challenges they face. These challenges present several opportunities for technological intervention as summarised in Fig. 13.1; the interested reader is referred to Smyth et al. (2022) for further examples and additional discussion.

13.2.1 Supporting the Physical Aspects of Marathon Training

Not surprisingly, current research on the application of Machine Learning for the marathon has focused on ways to support the physical aspects of training, from the estimation of important fitness metrics to the provision of more targeted and personalized training advice, to predicting race performance.

13.2.1.1 Estimating Physiological Fitness Indicators

Sports scientists use a variety of metrics to estimate the fitness levels of individuals, such as the well-known VO_2max score (Noakes, 2003; Daniels, 2013; Billat et al., 1994). VO_2max measures the maximum rate of oxygen consumption during exercise and serves as a key indicator of physiological fitness. With the advent of smartwatches and wearable sensors, it is now possible to estimate VO_2max directly from training data using variables such as training load, intensity, heart rate response etc. (Akay et al., 2011, 2013; Abut et al., 2016; De Brabandere et al., 2018; Webb et al., 2014), but without the need for expensive laboratory tests. Similar approaches can be applied to predict other key fitness-related metrics too (Billat et al., 2003; Faude et al., 2009; Poole et al., 2008). These problems can be framed as supervised learning tasks, and the resulting models have the potential to improve training programs by providing

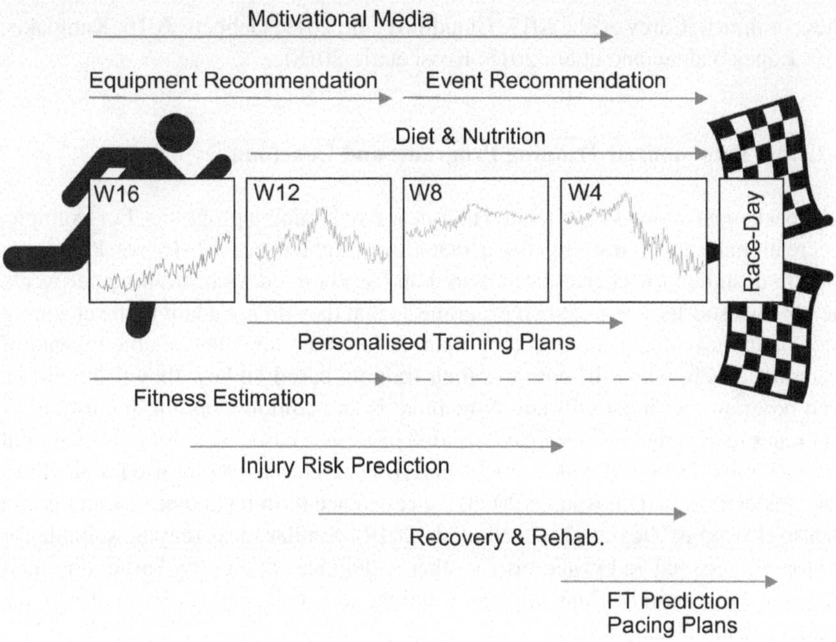

Fig. 13.1 The opportunities for technological interventions in marathon running, during training, on race-day and beyond. Several opportunities relate to supporting the runner with the physiological aspects of training and recovery, but other opportunities exist too, to help runners stay motivated and interested during the long months of training; see also (Smyth et al., 2022)

more targeted, personalized advice, and tailored recommendations to athletes, based on their evolving fitness levels and realistic performance goals.

13.2.1.2 Recovery and Injury Risk

How a runner recovers is a critical part of marathon training (Noakes, 2000). The right recovery strategy can help to maximise fitness gains and minimise injury risk, but exactly what this strategy should be is not always clear, especially for recreational runners. Therefore, an important opportunity exists to estimate recovery needs, based on an athlete's current fitness levels and recent training effort, and to recommend appropriate recovery actions; see (Barros et al., 2017; Bowen et al., 2019; Lazarus et al., 2017; Malisoux et al., 2015; Thornton et al., 2017). Although modern fitness devices often include some recovery estimation features, there is considerable room for improvement (Pulkkinen & Saarikoski, 2010) by generating more insightful and actionable recovery recommendations (Glaros et al., 2003). It may soon be possible to use activity data to identify novel patterns of behaviour linking training, recovery, and injury. This may lead to novel early warning systems for athletes, alerting them to changes in their performance efficiency, which may be a precursor to the onset of illness or injury (Carey et al., 2017; Claudino et al., 2019; Gabbett, 2016; Kampakis, 2016; López-Valenciano et al., 2018; Rossi et al., 2018).

13.2.1.3 Personalized Training Programs and Coaching

In the past, most athletes have tended to follow fixed training programs. For example, a recreational runner training for a marathon might use a 12–16 week training program designed to achieve a 4-h marathon based on 4 days of training per week. The obvious shortcoming of such programs is that they do not adapt to the changing needs of an individual runner as they train. A fortunate few may be able to avail of a personal coach, who will optimise their training based on how they respond to a given program, but most will not. Now there is an additional option: the use of AI techniques to generate *personalized training programs* based on a runner's goals and training habits. Indeed, the idea of a *virtual AI coach* has been proposed in the literature (Fister et al., 2015; Rauter, 2018) for resistance training and mountain biking; see also (Loepp & Ziegler, 2018; Ni et al., 2019). Similar ideas may be suitable for developing personalized programs for other endurance athletes, by harnessing real-time data about an individual's fitness, training, and goals; e.g. (Feely et al., 2020a, b; Tragos et al., 2023).

13.2.1.4 Performance Prediction and Race Planning

As race day approaches, runners will begin to carefully consider their goal time and their race strategy. In the marathon, participants must plan how to pace their race to maximise their performance across the full marathon distance. In doing so, they will need to consider their current fitness level, the topology of the course, weather conditions on the day, and their fueling strategy. Starting too fast can cause late race slowdowns, but starting too cautiously can be equally detrimental (Smyth, 2018) and if a runner gets their pacing or fueling strategy wrong, then they can even hit the dreaded wall (Buman et al., 2008; Ely et al., 2008; Smyth, 2018). Planning pacing correctly requires an accurate estimate of a runner's likely finish time. A runner can use this to determine a suitable average pace, which can be adjusted for different stages of the race to accommodate the start section, hills, etc. The existing literature uses linear models to predict future race times from previous race times (Bartolucci & Murphy, 2015; Keogh et al., 2019; Schmid et al., 2012) but translating a goal time into a specific pacing plan is less well explored, although some preliminary work has been conducted (Smyth & Cunningham, 2017b, 2018a, b).

13.2.2 Supporting the Secondary Aspects of Marathon Training

In addition to the physical aspects of marathon training, Fig. 13.1 highlights several secondary interventions, from keeping runners motivated to recommending suitable races and suggesting appropriate equipment. Many of these are familiar recommendation tasks (suggesting products, people, places, etc.), but the connection with marathon running adds an interesting new dimension.

13.2.2.1 Recommending Races and Events

In the recommender systems literature there are several examples of event recommendation (Macedo et al., 2015; Minkov et al., 2010; Qiao et al., 2014) and it is likely that similar techniques could be easily adapted for marathon runners. Many of these approaches rely on social network information to identify events that friends plan to attend. With the rise of social networks for sports (e.g., Strava) it should be possible to use similar ideas to identify upcoming races or other events that may suit a target runner. Moreover, by incorporating information about a runner's current training progress and goals, it may be possible to recommend specific races that will challenge the runner in the right way and at the right time. This may improve their training outcome as well as adding a new training component to help with motivation.

13.2.2.2 Recommending Training Routes and Training Partners

In the past, recommender systems have also been used for route planning (McGinty & Smyth, 2001; Chakraborty, 2012), often in tourism applications (Borràs et al., 2014; Gavalas et al., 2014; Ricci, 2002; Werthner & Ricci, 2004). Once again, similar ideas can be used to suggest interesting and challenging training routes to runners, especially when a runner travels to a new location; indeed, combining aspects of tourism with activities like running or cycling is increasingly popular. Moreover, since running can be a social activity, it may also be useful to recommend training partners, perhaps based on availability and ability, or even based on their interests, so that the conversation can flow during long runs; see, for example, (Goyal et al., 2018; Kurade, 2014; O'Donovan et al., 2008, 2009; Tang et al., 2013).

13.2.2.3 Recommending Equipment and Content

Even though running places a relatively low equipment burden on a runner, matching the right equipment with the right runner is important (Ryan et al., 2011). Recommender systems have a long history in product recommendation and by profiling a runner based on their sex, age, gait characteristics, training, running routes, home weather, etc., it should be possible to make personalized gear recommendations; see, for example, (Frejlichowski et al., 2016; Hwangbo et al., 2018; Marks, 2017; Wakita et al., 2015; Zrenner et al., 2018). Similarly, recommending relevant content (articles, podcasts etc.) based on a runner's current training and interests (Álvarez et al., 2019, 2020; Chen et al., 2020; Vall et al., 2019) may also help to motivate runners (Pilloni et al., 2017) and distract them from their toughest long runs (Han & Xu, 2016). For example, recommending a podcast about the importance of interval training may be a useful way to motivate a runner about their next (interval) training session, while suggesting an article to read about fueling their long runs might help them succeed with their next long run.

13.3 The Strava Dataset

This work is based on research conducted using an anonymized dataset of training activities (2014–2017) made available under a data-sharing agreement between Strava Inc. and the authors' institution. Each logged activity, for some runner, r, includes distance, timing and elevation data, sampled at various frequencies depending on the tracking device [smartphone, smartwatch, Global Position Systems (GPS) sensor, etc.] used. Thus, each runner is associated with a set of training activities $A(r) = \{A_1, \ldots A_n\}$ with each $A_i = (d_i, D_i, T_i, E_i, C_i, HR_i)$, where d_i is the activity date and D_i, T_i, E_i correspond to distance (m), time (sec), elevation (m) time-series data. $\mathrm{C_i}$ and $\mathrm{HR_i}$ correspond to cadence and heartrate data when present. Due to variations in sampling frequencies and signal errors, we resampled these raw data at 100 m intervals to produce a new set of time-series representing the meantime, elevation, cadence, and heartrate for each 100 m intervals of an activity. We also calculated the average pace (mins/km) for each 100 m interval from the distance and time data.

We extracted marathon races by identifying runners with marathon-length activities in the same location at a similar time on a specific date, to focus primarily on organised marathon events. The resulting dataset is summarised in Table 13.1. In the case studies that follow, we used various subsets of this marathon dataset depending on the requirement of the study and the complexity of the analysis required.

13.4 Case Study 1: Predicting Marathon Performance

A very common question from marathon runners concerns the link between their training efforts and their expected marathon performance (Doherty et al., 2019). Most runners follow a training plan to prepare them for a finish time range (e.g. 4–4:30 h), but many are interested in more precise finish time estimates or revised estimates as training progresses. We describe a case study, based on (Feely et al., 2022), to explore the relationship between different aspects of marathon training

Table 13.1 The Strava dataset of marathon runners used in this work shows summary runner details (sex, age) and key training and performance metrics (marathon finish time, training sessions per week and total distance per week) for each dataset year

Year	Sex	Runners	Age	Race-time (mins)	Sessions/ week	Distance/week
2014	F	6340	41.2 ± 60.4	261.1 ± 50.6	3.4 ± 1.5	35.6 ± 17.9
	M	36,636	41.7 ± 34.7	240.4 ± 50.9	3.5 ± 1.6	38.5 ± 21.0
2015	F	14,725	39.9 ± 33.0	263.6 ± 51.8	3.6 ± 1.6	37.0 ± 21.1
	M	73,194	41.2 ± 30.5	241.1 ± 52.8	3.6 ± 1.7	39.5 ± 21.2
2016	F	27,396	29.1 ± 29.4	266.2 ± 51.7	3.6 ± 1.6	36.8 ± 18.0
	M	119,946	40.7 ± 29.4	243.0 ± 53.6	3.6 ± 1.7	39.6 ± 21.6
2017	F	43,207	38.2 ± 24.0	267.8 ± 51.2	3.7 ± 1.6	36.9 ± 18.39
	M	167,078	39.8 ± 21.8	244.8 ± 54.1	3.6 ± 1.7	39.8 ± 21.4

In the case of age, racetime, sessions and distance per week, the data is presented as mean with standard deviation values

and race performance. We use Case-Based Reasoning (CBR) for this, which is a popular Machine Learning approach in which new problems are solved by retrieving and adapting the solutions to similar problems (*cases*) that have occurred in the past (de Mántaras et al., 2005; Bridge et al., 2005). Each case corresponds to a feature-based summary of a runner's training history (the *case description*) and an actual marathon time (case solution) and we predict the performance of a new runner, using the marathon times of cases with *similar* training histories.

13.4.1 Feature Representation

$C(r, w)$ is a case for runner *r*, *w* weeks before their race; see Eq. 13.1. MT is the marathon time achieved and F (r, w) consists of the features used to represent the training for week *w* (weekly) and the training weeks up to week *w* (*cumulative*); see Table 13.2. We also extract the previous (fastest) marathon finish time (PMT) for runners, because the work of (Smyth & Cunningham, 2017a, b) has shown that past race times can be very effective when it comes to predicting future times.

$$C(r, w) = (F(r, w), MT, PMT) \tag{13.1}$$

Table 13.2 A summary of the training activities feature-set

Feature	Unit	When	Description
Total distance	km	Weekly	Total weekly distance
Max (total distance)	km	Cumulative	Max weekly distance
Mean (total distance)	km	Cumulative	Avg. weekly distance
Long run	km	Weekly	Max activity distance (in week)
Max (long run)	km	Cumulative	Max long run distance
Mean (long run)	km	Cumulative	Mean long run distance
Training days	Unit	Weekly	Num active days
Max (training days)	Unit	Cumulative	Max weekly activities
Mean (training days)	Unit	Cumulative	Mean weekly activities
Mean pace	(mins/km)	Weekly	Mean pace (in week)
Min (mean pace)	(mins/km)	Cumulative	Fastest weekly pace
Mean (mean pace)	(mins/km)	Cumulative	mean weekly pace
Fastest 10 km	(mins/km)	Weekly	Fastest 10 km pace (in week)
Min (fastest 10 km)	(mins/km)	Cumulative	Min fastest 10 km pace
Mean (fastest 10 km)	(mins/km)	Cumulative	Mean fastest 10 km pace

13.4.2 Case-Based Prediction Models

We use the following approaches to predict the finish time for a target runner r_t in week w, by selecting the k most similar cases, using a standard Euclidean distance metric, and calculating the average of their finish times (Feely et al., 2022).

13.4.2.1 Previous Marathon Time (PMT) Model

This model uses only the past marathon time (PMT) and the sex of the runner to identify a set of similar cases. It is included as a benchmark, based on the work of (Smyth & Cunningham, 2017a, b, 2018a, b), against which to evaluate the influence of training history data.

13.4.2.2 Training Activity Model (TA)

This model uses a stepwise, forward, sequential feature selection process to identify the subset of training features to use each week, as the basis for case similarity. This means a case for week w can include a different set of features depending on which features were found to be most useful in predicting marathon times at that point in training. For reasons of space we do not include any further details on the feature selection process here, but the interested reader is referred to Feely et al. (2022) where it is discussed in detail.

13.4.2.3 Combined (C) and Ensemble (E) Models

We also include two ways to combine these models: (i) in C the past race times and training features are combined into a single representation; (ii) in E the race time and training features remain separate but the predictions from each are averaged.

13.4.3 Evaluation

To evaluate these prediction models we generate marathon time predictions for Strava runners, at various points in their training, and compare the predicted times to the actual marathon times that these runners went on to achieve.

13.4.3.1 Dataset

The dataset used includes just over 160,000 16-week training histories from 85,000 unique runners, comprising more than 8 million training activities.

13.4.3.2 Method

A standard tenfold cross-validation approach is used to evaluate the marathon time predictions for the various techniques, using the mean absolute percentage error as a performance metric; e.g. an error of 10% means that the predicted marathon time differs from the actual marathon time by 10%.

13.4.3.3 Performance vs. Training Week

Figure 13.2 shows the predicted performance for males (a) and females (b). The predictions from the PMT model (and the actual previous marathon time) remain static with training week, as they do not depend on training. Interestingly, using the actual previous marathon time of rt outperforms the use of past marathon times from similar runners (*kNN*). Using information about r_t's recent training improves predictions for males and females as training progresses; the more we know about a runner's training, and the closer we get to race day, the more accurate the predictions. Combining past race times and training information improves predictions further and using a single combined representation (C) outperforms the ensemble approach (E).

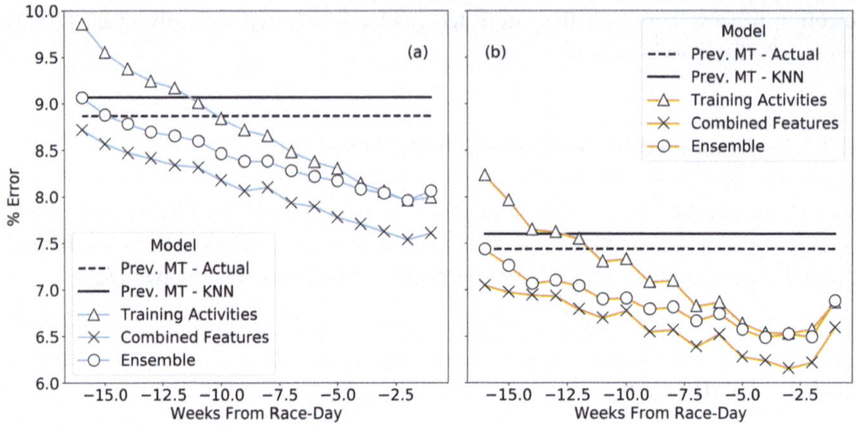

Fig. 13.2 Percentage error for different weeks in training for each of the previous race-time, training activities, and combined models for males (**a**) and females (**b**)

13.4.3.4 Performance Versus Ability

To evaluate the influence of runner ability on prediction accuracy, Fig. 13.3 shows the prediction accuracy of model *C* at different points in training based on runner ability. Faster runners (<3:30 marathoners) and slower runners (>4:30 marathoners) are associated with less accurate predictions than the recreational runners who complete the marathon in the 3.5–4.5 h range. Arguably, these are likely to be runners who are most focused on achieving improvements in their finish times, especially those targeting the iconic sub-4-h marathon. The results also show slightly better predictions closer to race day when we control for runner ability. Of course, additional factors may be at play here. For example, injuries during training can certainly impact performance and how a runner paces their race can also determine their finish time. Both of these issues will be discussed in the case studies that follow.

13.4.4 Discussion

This case study is important for several reasons. First, many marathon programs design sessions based on a runner's eventual race pace; for example, a particular session might be specified as 30 min at marathon pace or a long run at 40 s per km slower than marathon pace. Thus, runners need to know their marathon time/pace so that they can correctly tune their training. Second, providing a runner with regular marathon time predictions can help them to understand how their training is progressing. Improving finish time predictions can build a runner's confidence, while a lack of improvement may signal a need for some change in training (Feely et al., 2023). Finally, as race day approaches, a runner needs to know their likely

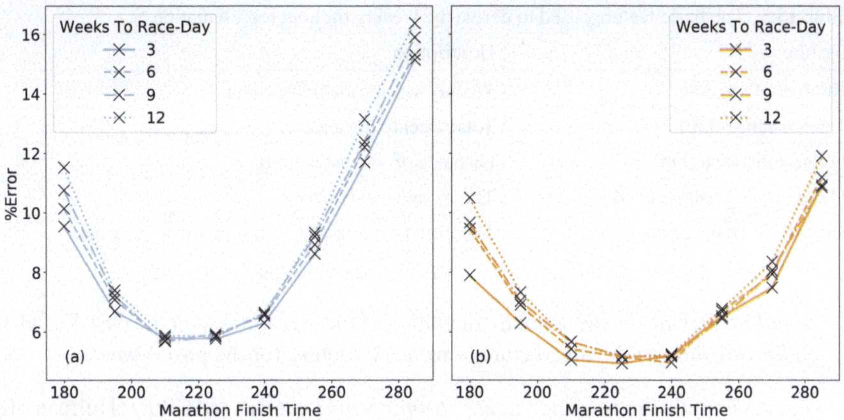

Fig. 13.3 Percentage error of the combined-features model by marathon finish times (mins) for males (**a**) and females (**b**) at 3, 6, 9 and 12 weeks from race day

finish time, to help ensure they execute a well-paced race and avoid hitting the wall (Smyth, 2021) late in the race.

13.5 Case Study 2: Forecasting Injury Risk

Injuries are an ever present risk for marathon runners (Kluitenberg et al., 2015). Identifying their cause is challenging and predicting the risk of injury is important (Bache-Mathiesen et al., 2023; Toresdahl et al., 2022; Lövdal et al., 2021). Here, we describe an attempt to forecast injury risk based on a runner's training history, using the Strava dataset. Since this dataset has no explicit information about injuries, we will use *training disruptions*—consecutive days without training—as a proxy for injuries, based on the work of (Feely et al., 2021).

13.5.1 Representing Disruption/Injury Cases

Once again, we adopt a CBR approach. Each case $C(r, w)$ consists of a set of training-related features $F(r, w)$ as well as an injury status indicator, which indicates whether the runner experienced a training disruption of at least 7 days [based on the consensus definition used by (Yamato et al., 2015)] in the weeks following. $F(r, w)$ are based on the features in Table 13.3, aggregated across the previous 4 weeks of training as follows:

1. *Average:* the mean total weekly distance, longest run distance, number of sessions etc. during the previous 4 weeks, $F(r, w-3), \ldots, F(r, w)$.

Table 13.3 The basic features used to derive the weekly training representation

Feature	Description
Number of sessions	Weekly sessions/activity count
Total distance (km)	Total weekly distance
Longest distance (km)	Distance of longest activity
Mean training pace (mins/km)	The mean weekly pace
Fastest 10 km pace (mins/km)	The pace of the fastest 10 km segment per week

2. *Standard Deviation*: the standard deviation of these features over the past 4 weeks.
3. *Relative Change:* the mean change for each feature for the past 4 weeks.

We also include the so-called *acute chronic workload ratio (ACWR)* (Hulin et al., 2016) as an additional case feature to measure the weekly training load of a runner. We calculate *ACWR* from the total training distance in the current week (the *acute load*) divided by the average weekly distance over the last 4 weeks (the *chronic load*); see Eq. 13.2. $ACWR > 1.1$ is usually not recommended and higher ACWR values are associated with a greater likelihood of injury (Toresdahl et al., 2022).

$$ACWR = \frac{dist_w}{(dist_w + \cdots + dist_{w-3})/4} \tag{13.2}$$

We use the Strava data to produce two types of cases. A *positive* disruption case $C^+(r, w)$ corresponds to a runner r who suffers a $\geq$7-day training disruption after week w, and is associated with two additional features: (i) $DW(r, w)$, the week in which the disruption occurred; and (ii) $DL(r, w)$ the length of the disruption in days; see Eq. 13.3 and note that we abbreviate $F(r, w)$ as F_w without loss of generality. A *negative* disruption case, $C^-(r, w)$, denotes a runner who does not experience a $\geq$7 day disruption after week w; see Eq. 13.4 Note that, for positive and negative cases, we use the training history features for the preceding 4 weeks (F_w, F_{w-1}, F_{w-2}, F_{w-3}).

$$C^+(r, w) = \{F_{w-3}, F_{w-2}, F_{w-1}, F_w\} \rightarrow disrupted, DW(r, w), DL(r, w) \tag{13.3}$$

$$C^-(r, w) = \{F_{w-3}, F_{w-2}, F_{w-1}, F_w\} \rightarrow undisrupted \tag{13.4}$$

During training, each runner can be associated with several different cases according to their future injury status. There are more negative (undisrupted) cases than positive ones, leading to an unbalanced case base. To address this, the case base was balanced by randomly *undersampling* the negative cases to produce the same number of negative cases as there are positive cases; see Hasanin and Khoshgoftaar (2018).

Table 13.4 Number of positive and negative cases for different weeks in training

Weeks to race	Positive	Negative
3	43,406	74,842
6	47,409	111,316
9	55,860	140,682
12	67,590	165,386

13.5.2 Predicting Training Disruptions

To predict the injury/disruption status for r_t at week w, we select the k most similar (week w) cases, using a standard Euclidean distance metric. The majority class (positive or negative) of these k cases is the predicted class, and the proportion of positive cases among these k cases is the disruption risk score.

13.5.3 Evaluation

We evaluate this approach using the Strava dataset to determine how reliably we can predict whether a runner will experience a training disruption given their training history.

13.5.3.1 Dataset

Table 13.4 summarises the dataset used in terms of the number of positive and negative cases at different key points in training (3, 6, 9, and 12 weeks from race day) prior to undersampling.

13.5.3.2 Method

We perform a standard tenfold cross-validation to evaluate the model's performance. For rt we identify the k nearest neighbours ($k = 15$) to use for classification and risk-score prediction. We compare the predicted class (positive or negative) with the actual class of the target case to calculate an accuracy score based on the fraction of correct classifications. Separately, to evaluate the accuracy of the risk score we calculate the correlation coefficient between the risk scores and the *actual* fraction of runners that experience a disruption for a given risk score range.

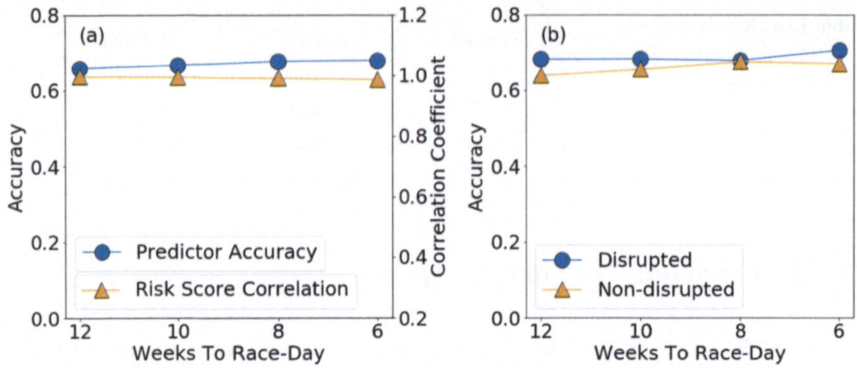

Fig. 13.4 **a** the prediction accuracy and the correlation coefficient for weeks leading up to race-day; **b** prediction accuracy for the undisrupted/negative and disrupted/positive classes

13.5.3.3 Results

Figure 13.4a shows how prediction accuracy and risk-score correlation vary with the number of weeks before race day. Prediction accuracy is modest ($\approx$68%), reflecting the challenging nature of the task but it improves slightly closer to race day. Figure 13.4b separates the prediction accuracy for the positive and negative classes (true positive and true negative rates). The model is slightly better at predicting disruptions than it is at predicting non-disruptions, but again the difference is modest.

13.5.4 Discussion

We have summarised recent work on predicting whether or not a runner is likely to experience a training disruption based on their training history as a proxy for predicting injuries. The lack of explicit injury data in the Strava dataset makes this task particularly challenging. However, the results show that it may be feasible to make reasonably accurate disruption predictions. In the future, we might expect more accurate predictions if more reliable labeled injury data becomes available.

13.6 Case Study 3: Recommending Pacing Adjustments

In our final case study, we turn our attention to race day and how runners pace their marathons. The prevailing wisdom is for runners to adopt an even pacing strategy, by running each segment of the race at a similar pace. The common mistake of starting too fast can lead to significant finish time costs and even cause runners to hit the dreaded wall (Smyth, 2018, 2021) later in the race, but saving energy for a fast finish is also problematic (Smyth, 2018). Even with an appropriate pacing plan, race day does not always go as expected, and runners often have to reevaluate if problems occur. In this final case study, which is based on work presented in Berndsen et al. (2019b), we attempt to help runners complete their marathons to the best of their ability even when problems occur. We use Machine Learning to predict whether a laterace slowdown is likely and then use ideas from recommender systems (Smyth, 2007) to suggest suitable pacing adaptations to avoid such slowdowns. We do this using Strava data from 7931 unique runners of New York, London and Dublin marathons, chosen because their marathon data includes cadence (steps per minute) and heart rate (HR) information, which allows us to track their effort during the race, in addition to the usual time, distance, and pacing data.

13.6.1 Predicting Late-Race Slowdowns

To predict late-race slowdowns, we extract several features from the pacing, cadence, and heart-rate time series. As an initial feature set, we use the average pace, cadence, and HR every 500 m of the race; we refer to these as the *original* features. We also produce an *extended* feature set by using the *TSFresh* time-series feature extraction method (Christ et al., 2018) to compute more detailed features from the pacing, HR and cadence data; because of the computational cost of this, we restrict it to the 10 km, half-way (21.1 km) and 30 km landmarks.

Then, for each point in the race (every 500 m for the original features and the landmarks for the extended features) we train an XGBoost (Chen & Guestrin, 2016) model to predict the second-half slowdown of a runner based on their race so far. The results of a tenfold cross-validation evaluation are shown in Fig. 13.5a as the mean absolute prediction error at different points in the race. The extended features offer improved performance, but at the expense of "granularity", because predictions can only be made every so often. In reality, it should be straightforward to make predictions at finer levels of granularity (e.g. every 5 km or even every 1 km) but it is unlikely that recreational runners will benefit from finer granularity than this in practice.

Predictions improve as the race unfolds. This is not surprising because the model has increasing information available. By the halfway mark the extended feature model can predict the slowdown magnitude with an error of about 6% which is sufficient in practice for alerting the runner to potential future pacing problems.

13.6.2 Recommending Pace Adaptions

Next, we suggest mitigating actions for runners who are predicted to slow. We do this by taking advantage of the fact that some past runners, whose early race data suggested they would slow, nevertheless made good decisions about their pacing,

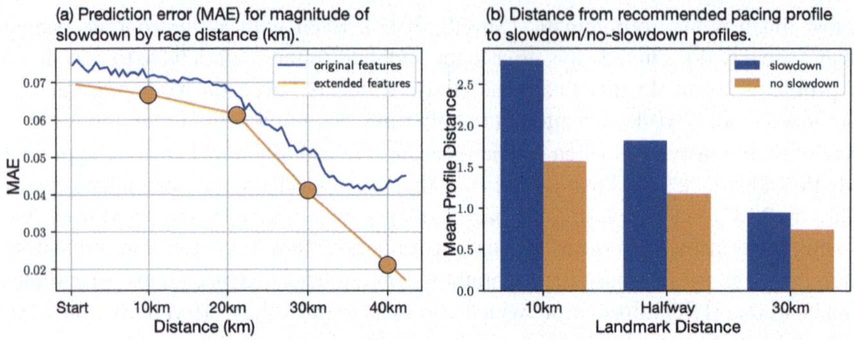

Fig. 13.5 **a** The prediction error (MAE) associated with late-race slowdowns when using the original and extended features; **b** The distance between recommended pacing profiles and those pacing profiles that mitigated slowdowns (no slowdown) and those that did not (slowdown). See (Berndsen et al., 2019b) for further details

and avoided this predicted slowing. We view their pacing decisions as examples of successful adaptions, which avoided late-race slowing, and we use these runners and their pacing decisions, as *mitigation* cases in a CBR system. If our model predicts a runner, r_t is at risk of slowing significantly, then we suggest a pacing adaptation based on the pacing of the most similar mitigation cases according to the following approach:

1. Find the k most similar runners, $\{r_1, \ldots, r_k\}$ to r_t;
2. Calculate the average pacing profile of these runners, $P\,(r_i)$;
3. Normalise the pacing profile of these similar runners with respect to r_t

$$P\prime(r_i) = \frac{P(r_i)}{P(r)}$$

4. Use the average finish time, for these similar runners as r_t's new target finish time;
5. Calculate the required pace, over the remaining race, for rt to finish in this target time.
6. Multiply this average pace by the normalised pacing profile to produce a personalized pacing profile for the remaining race for r.

To evaluate this approach, we begin with runners who were predicted to slow by our XGBoost model. They can be divided into (i) those who avoided slowing by adjusting their pace (*slowdown*) and (ii) those who did not (*no slowdown*). To evaluate our pacing recommendations for some rt we compare rt's remaining pacing to the corresponding pacing of these groups by computing the distance between the recommended pacing profile and the pacing profiles in (i) and (ii). We used a tenfold cross-validation procedure to produce the results in Fig. 13.5b. These results show that the recommended pacing profiles are closer to those found in the no-slowdown group than the slowdown group, at the 10 km, halfway, and 30 km landmarks and these differences were found to be statistically significant with $p < 0.0005$; see Berndsen et al. (2019b).

13.6.3 Discussion

This case study considered how to provide runners with guidance during a race to help them better optimise their finish times by predicting late-race slowdowns and suggesting useful mitigating pacing adjustments at several points in the marathon. A limitation of this study is that it is retrospective rather than prospective. It does not evaluate recommendations made to real runners in real-time as they race. However, the results are consistent with the hypothesis that, if runners adjust their pace as recommended, then they may avoid slowing later in the race. Nonetheless, additional work is required to establish whether this approach will deliver similar benefits in a real-world race setting.

13.7 Conclusions

This chapter highlights several ways Machine Learning and recommender systems can support recreational runners, as they train for, and participate in, marathon races. The case studies target different aspects of marathon preparation using a large-scale, real-world dataset. The findings show how marathon runners can benefit from performance prediction, injury risk assessment, and race planning techniques.

Although this work has focused on running marathons, the ideas presented also apply to several other endurance sports. For example, related challenges exist in skating (Smyth & Willemsen, 2020), cycling (Mattern et al., 2001), and multisport events such as triathlons (Wu et al., 2015) and adventure racing.

As the technology continues to improve—for example, new types of sensors are appearing frequently (e.g. blood oxygen, power meters, etc.)—it will be possible to measure and estimate many important physiological phenomena. And as the sports science community adapts to these ideas and results, we will likely benefit from important new insights into how we train, compete, and recover.

Acknowledgements The research underpinning this work is supported by funding provided by Science Foundation Ireland through the Insight Centre for Data Analytics (12/RC/2289 P2) and the SFI Centre for Research Training in Machine Learning (18/CRT/6183), and data provided by Strava Inc. as part of a data sharing agreement with the authors.

References

Abut, F., Akay, M. F., & George, J. (2016). Developing new vo2max prediction models from maximal, submaximal and questionnaire variables using support vector machines combined with feature selection. *Computers in Biology and Medicine, 79*, 182–192. https://doi.org/10.1016/j.compbiomed.2016.10.018

Akay, M. F., Aktürk, E., & Balıkcı, A. (2013). VO2max prediction from submaximal exercise test using artificial neural network. In *Proceedings of the 2013 21st signal processing and communications applications conference (SIU)* (pp. 1–3). https://doi.org/10.1109/SIU.2013.6531163

Akay, M. F., Zayid, E. I. M., Akturk, E., & George, J. D. (2011). Artificial neural network-based model for predicting VO2max from a submaximal exercise test. *Expert Systems with Applications, 38*(3), 2007–2010. https://doi.org/10.1016/j.eswa.2010.07.135

Álvarez, P., Guiu, A., Beltran, J. R., de Quiros, J. G., & Baldassarri, S. (2019). Dj-running: An emotion-based system for recommending spotify songs to runners. In *ICSPORTS* (pp. 55–63).

Álvarez, P., Zarazaga-Soria, F., & Baldassarri, S. (2020). Mobile music recommendations for runners based on location and emotions: The dj-running system. *Pervasive and Mobile Computing, 42*, 101242.

Bache-Mathiesen, L. K., Andersen, T. E., Dalen-Lorentsen, T., Tabben, M., Chamari, K., Clarsen, B., & Fagerland, M. W. (2023). A new statistical approach to training load and injury risk: Separating the acute from the chronic load. *Biology of Sport, 41*(1), 119–134.

Barros, E. S., Nascimento, D. C., Prestes, J., Nóbrega, O. T., Córdova, C., Sousa, F., & Boullosa, D. A. (2017). Acute and chronic effects of endurance running on inflammatory markers: A systematic review. *Frontiers in Physiology, 8*, 779. https://doi.org/10.3389/fphys.2017.00779

Bartolucci, F., & Murphy, T. B. (2015). A finite mixture latent trajectory model for modeling ultrarunners' behavior in a 24-hour race. *Journal of Quantitative Analysis in Sports, 11*(4), 193–203. https://doi.org/10.1515/jqas-2014-0060

Berndsen, J., Smyth, B., & Lawlor, A. (2019a). Pace my race: recommendations for marathon running. In T. Bogers, A. Said, P. Brusilovsky, & D. Tikk (Eds.), *Proceedings of the 13th ACM conference on recommender systems, recsys 2019, copenhagen, denmark, september 16–20, 2019* (pp. 246–250). ACM. https://doi.org/10.1145/3298689.3346991

Berndsen, J., Smyth, B., & Lawlor, A. (2019b). Pace my race: Recommendations for marathon running. In *Proceedings of the 13th ACM conference on recommender systems* (pp. 246–250).

Billat, V., Bernard, O., Pinoteau, J., Petit, B., & Koralsztein, J. (1994). Time to exhaustion at vo2max and lactate steady state velocity in sub elite long distance runners. *Archives Internationales De Physiologie, De Biochimie Et De Biophysique, 102*(3), 215–219.

Billat, V. L., Sirvent, P., Py, G., Koralsztein, J.-P., & Mercier, J. (2003). The concept of maximal lactate steady state. *Sports Medicine, 33*(6), 407–426.

Borràs, J., Moreno, A., & Valls, A. (2014). Intelligent tourism recommender systems: A survey. *Expert Systems with Applications, 41*(16), 7370–7389.

Bowen, L., Gross, A. S., Gimpel, M., Bruce-Low, S., & Li, F.-X. (2019). Spikes in acute: Chronic workload ratio (ACWR) associated with a 5–7 times greater injury rate in English Premier League football players: A comprehensive 3-year study. *British Journal of Sports Medicine, 321*, 099422. https://doi.org/10.1136/bjsports-2018-099422

Brady, S., Dunne, L. E., Tynan, R., Diamond, D., Smyth, B., & O'Hare, G. M. (2005). Garment-based monitoring of respiration rate using a foam pressure sensor. In *Ninth IEEE international symposium on wearable computers (iswc'05)* (pp. 214–215).

Bridge, D., Goker, M. H., McGinty, L., & Smyth, B. (2005). Case based recommender systems. *The Knowledge Engineering Review, 20*(3), 315–320. https://doi.org/10.1017/S0269888906000567

Buman, M. P., Brewer, B. W., Cornelius, A. E., Van Raalte, J. L., & Petitpas, A. J. (2008). Hitting the wall in the marathon: Phenomenological characteristics and associations with expectancy, gender, and running history. *Psychology of Sport and Exercise, 9*(2), 177–190.

Cantwell, J. D. (1985). Cardiovascular aspects of running. *Clinics in Sports Medicine, 4*(4), 627–640.

Carey, D. L., Ong, K.-L., Whiteley, R., Crossley, K. M., Crow, J., & Morris, M. E. (2017). Predictive modelling of training loads and injury in Australian football. arXiv preprint arXiv:1706.04336

Chakraborty, B. (2012). Integrating awareness in user-oriented route recommendation system. In *The 2012 international joint conference on neural networks (IJCNN)* (pp. 1–5).

Chen, T., & Guestrin, C. (2016). Xgboost: A scalable tree boosting system. In *Proceedings of the 22nd ACM sigkdd international conference on knowledge discovery and data mining* (pp. 785–794).

Chen, C.-W., Yang, L., Wen, H., Jones, R., Radosavljevic, V., & Bouchard, H. (2020). Podrecs: Workshop on podcast recommendations. In *Fourteenth ACM conference on recommender systems* (pp. 621–622).

Christ, M., Braun, N., Neuffer, J., & Kempa-Liehr, A. W. (2018). Time series feature extraction on basis of scalable hypothesis tests (tsfresh—a python package). *Neurocomputing, 307*, 72–77.

Claudino, J. G., Capanema, D. O., de Souza, T. V., Serrao, J. C., Machado-Pereira, A. C., & Nassis, G. P. (2019). Current approaches to the use of artificial intelligence for injury risk assessment and performance prediction in team sports: A systematic review. *Sports Medicine Open, 5*(1), 28. https://doi.org/10.1186/s40798-019-0202-3

Daniels, J. T. (2013). *Daniels' running formula*. Human Kinetics.

De Brabandere, A., De Beeck, T. O., Schütte, K. H., Meert, W., Vanwanseele, B., & Davis, J. (2018). Data fusion of body-worn accelerometers and heart rate to predict vo2max during submaximal running. *PLoS ONE, 13*(6), e0199509.

de Mántaras, R. L., McSherry, D., Bridge, D. G., Leake, D. B., Smyth, B., Craw, S., et al. (2005). Retrieval, reuse, revision and retention in case-based reasoning. *The Knowledge Engineering Review, 20*(3), 215–240. https://doi.org/10.1017/S0269888906000646

Doherty, C., Keogh, A., Davenport, J., Lawlor, A., Smyth, B., & Caulfield, B. (2019). An evaluation of the training determinants of marathon performance: A meta-analysis with meta-regression. *Journal of Science and Medicine in Sport, 421*, 11548.

Dunne, L. E., Ashdown, S. P., & Smyth, B. (2005). Expanding garment functionality through embedded electronic technology. *Journal of Textile and Apparel Technology and Management, 4*(3), 1–11.

Ely, M. R., Martin, D. E., Cheuvront, S. N., & Montain, S. J. (2008). Effect of ambient temperature on marathon pacing is dependent on runner ability. *Medicine and Science in Sports and Exercise, 40*(9), 1675–1680.

Faude, O., Kindermann, W., & Meyer, T. (2009). Lactate threshold concepts. *Sports Medicine, 39*(6), 469–490.

Feely, C., Caulfield, B., Lawlor, A., & Smyth, B. (2020a). Providing explainable racetime predictions and training plan recommendations to marathon runners. In *Fourteenth ACM conference on recommender systems* (pp. 539–544).

Feely, C., Caulfield, B., Lawlor, A., & Smyth, B. (2020b). Using case-based reasoning to predict marathon performance and recommend tailored training plans. In *International conference on case-based reasoning* (pp. 67–81).

Feely, C., Caulfield, B., Lawlor, A., & Smyth, B. (2021). A case-based reasoning approach to predicting and explaining running related injuries. In *Case based reasoning research and development: 29th international conference, ICCBR 2021, Salamanca, Spain, September 13–16, 2021, proceedings 29* (pp.79–93).

Feely, C., Caulfield, B., Lawlor, A., & Smyth, B. (2022). An extended case based approach to racetime prediction for recreational marathon runners. In *International conference on case-based reasoning* (pp. 335–349).

Feely, C., Caulfield, B., Lawlor, A., & Smyth, B. (2023). Modelling the training practices of recreational marathon runners to make personalised training recommendations. In *Proceedings of the 31st ACM conference on user modeling, adaptation and personalization* (pp. 183–193).

Fister, I., Rauter, S., Yang, X.-S., Ljubič, K., & Fister, I. (2015). Planning the sports training sessions with the bat algorithm. *Neurocomputing, 149*, 993–1002. https://doi.org/10.1016/j.neucom.2014.07.034

Frejlichowski, D., Czapiewski, P., & Hofman, R. (2016). Finding similar clothes based on semantic description for the purpose of fashion recommender system. In *Asian conference on intelligent information and database systems* (pp. 13–22).

Gabbett, T. J. (2016). The training—injury prevention paradox: Should athletes be training smarter and harder? *British Journal of Sports Medicines, 50*(5), 273–280.

Gavalas, D., Konstantopoulos, C., Mastakas, K., & Pantziou, G. (2014). Mobile recommender systems in tourism. *Journal of Network and Computer Applications, 39*, 319–333.

Glaros, C., Fotiadis, D. I., Likas, A., & Stafylopatis, A. (2003). A wearable intelligent system for monitoring health condition and rehabilitation of running athletes. In *Proceedings of the 4th international IEEE EMBS special topic conference on information technology applications in biomedicine, 2003.* (pp. 276–279). https://doi.org/10.1109/ITAB.2003.1222531

Goyal, P., Sapienza, A., & Ferrara, E. (2018). Recommending teammates with deep neural networks. In *Proceedings of the 29th on hypertext and social media* (pp. 57–61). ACM.

Grunseit, A., Richards, J., & Merom, D. (2018). Running on a high: Parkrun and personal well-being. *BMC Public Health, 18*(1), 1–11.

Han, Z., & Xu, J. (2016). *Recommending sports instructional content based on motion sensor data.* Google Patents. (US Patent 9,409,074)

Hasanin, T., & Khoshgoftaar, T. (2018). The effects of random undersampling with simulated class imbalance for big data. In *Proceedings of the 2018 IEEE international conference on information reuse and integration (IRI)* (pp. 70–79).

Hulin, B. T., Gabbett, T. J., Lawson, D. W., Caputi, P., & Sampson, J. A. (2016). The acute: chronic workload ratio predicts injury: High chronic workload may decrease injury risk in elite rugby league players. *British Journal of Sports Medicine, 50*(4), 231–236. https://doi.org/10.1136/bjsports-2015-094817

Hwangbo, H., Kim, Y. S., & Cha, K. J. (2018). Recommendation system development for fashion retail e-commerce. *Electronic Commerce Research and Applications, 28*, 94–101.

Kampakis, S. (2016). Predictive modelling of football injuries. arXiv preprint arXiv:1609.07480.

Keogh, A., Smyth, B., Caulfield, B., Lawlor, A., Berndsen, J., & Doherty, C. (2019). Prediction equations for marathon performance: A systematic review. *International Journal of Sports Physiology and Performance, 14*(9), 1159–1169.

Kiernan, D., Hawkins, D. A., Manoukian, M. A. C., McKallip, M., Oelsner, L., Caskey, C. F., & Coolbaugh, C. L. (2018). Accelerometer-based prediction of running injury in National Collegiate Athletic Association track athletes. *Journal of Biomechanics, 73*, 201–209. https://doi.org/10.1016/j.jbiomech.2018.04.001

Kluitenberg, B., van Middelkoop, M., Diercks, R., & van der Worp, H. (2015). What are the differences in injury proportions between different populations of runners? A systematic review and meta-analysis. *Sports Medicine, 45*, 1143–1161.

Kurade, N. P. (2014). An intelligent method for selecting and recommending best players to help build sports team. *International Journal of Computer Applications, 105*(7), 324.

Lazarus, B. H., Stewart, A. M., White, K. M., Rowell, A. E., Esmaeili, A., Hopkins, W. G., & Aughey, R. J. (2017). Proposal of a global training load measure predicting match performance in an elite team sport. *Frontiers in Physiology, 8*, 930.

Lieberman, D. E. (2015). Is exercise really medicine? An evolutionary perspective. *Current Sports Medicine Reports, 14*(4), 313–319.

Loepp, B., & Ziegler, J. (2018). Recommending running routes: framework and demonstrator. In *Workshop on recommendation in complex scenarios.*

López-Valenciano, A., Ayala, F., Puerta, J. M., De Ste-Croix, M. B. A., Vera-Garcia, F. J., Hernandez-Sanchez, S., et al. (2018). A preventive model for muscle injuries: A novel approach based on learning algorithms. *Medicine and Science in Sports and Exercise, 50*(5), 915–927. https://doi.org/10.1249/MSS.0000000000001535

Lövdal, S. S., Den Hartigh, R. J., & Azzopardi, G. (2021). Injury prediction in competitive runners with machine learning. *International Journal of Sports Physiology and Performance, 16*(10), 1522–1531.

Macedo, A. Q., Marinho, L. B., & Santos, R. L. (2015). Context-aware event recommendation in event-based social networks. In *Proceedings of the 9th ACM conference on recommender systems* (pp. 123–130).

Malisoux, L., Nielsen, R. O., Urhausen, A., & Theisen, D. (2015). A step towards understanding the mechanisms of running-related injuries. *Journal of Science and Medicine in Sport, 18*(5), 523–528. https://doi.org/10.1016/j.jsams.2014.07.014

Marks, W. H. (2017). *Footwear recommendations from foot scan data describing feet of a user.* Google Patents. (US Patent 9,648,926).

Mattern, C., Kenefick, R., Kertzer, R., & Quinn, T. (2001). Impact of starting strategy on cycling performance. *International Journal of Sports Medicine, 22*(05), 350–355.

Mc-Ginty, L., & Smyth, B. (2001). Collaborative case-based reasoning: Applications in personalised route planning. In *International conference on case-based reasoning* (pp. 362–376).

Minkov, E., Charrow, B., Ledlie, J., Teller, S., & Jaakkola, T. (2010). Collaborative future event recommendation. In *Proceedings of the 19th ACM international conference on information and knowledge management* (pp. 819–828).

Ni, J., Muhlstein, L., & McAuley, J. (2019). Modeling heart rate and activity data for personalized fitness recommendation. In *The world wide web conference* (pp. 1343–1353). Association for Computing Machinery. https://doi.org/10.1145/3308558.3313643

Noakes, T. (2003). *Lore of running*. Human Kinetics.

Noakes, T. (2000). Physiological models to understand exercise fatigue and the adaptations that predict or enhance athletic performance. *Scandinavian Journal of Medicine and Science in Sports: Review Article, 10*(3), 123–145.

O'Donovan, J., Smyth, B., Gretarsson, B., Bostandjiev, S., & Höllerer, T. (2008). Peerchooser: visual interactive recommendation. In *Proceedings of the Sigchi conference on human factors in computing systems* (pp. 1085–1088).

O'Donovan, J., Gretarsson, B., Bostandjiev, S., Höllerer, T., & Smyth, B. (2009). A visual interface for social information filtering. In *Proceedings of the 2009 international conference on computational science and engineering* (Vol. 4, pp. 74–81).

Pedisic, Z., Shrestha, N., Kovalchik, S., Stamatakis, E., Liangruenrom, N., Grgic, J., et al. (2020). Is running associated with a lower risk of all-cause, cardiovascular and cancer mortality, and is the more the better? A systematic review and meta-analysis. *British Journal of Sports Medicine, 54*(15), 898–905.

Pilloni, P., Piras, L., Boratto, L., Carta, S., Fenu, G., & Mulas, F. (2017). Recommendation in persuasive health systems: An effective strategy to spot users' losing motivation to exercise. In *Proceedings of the 2nd international workshop on health recommender systems, healthrecsys 2017* (Vol. 1953, pp. 6–9).

Poole, D. C., Wilkerson, D. P., & Jones, A. M. (2008). Validity of criteria for establishing maximal o2 uptake during ramp exercise tests. *European Journal of Applied Physiology, 102*(4), 403–410. https://doi.org/10.1007/s00421-007-0596-3

Pulkkinen, A., & Saarikoski, E. (2010). *System for monitoring and predicting physiological state under physical exercise.* Google Patents. (US Patent 7,805,186)

Qiao, Z., Zhang, P., Zhou, C., Cao, Y., Guo, L., & Zhang, Y. (2014). Event recommendation in event-based social networks. In *Twenty-eighth AAAI conference on artificial intelligence.*

Rauter, S. (2018). New approach for planning the mountain bike training with virtual coach. *TRENDS in Sport Sciences, 2* (25), 69–74. https://doi.org/10.23829/TSS.2018.25.2-2

Ricci, F. (2002). Travel recommender systems. *IEEE Intelligent Systems, 17*(6), 55–57.

Rossi, A., Pappalardo, L., Cintia, P., Iaia, F. M., Fernàndez, J., & Medina, D. (2018). Effective injury forecasting in soccer with GPS training data and machine learning. *PLoS ONE, 13*(7), e0201264.

Ryan, M. B., Valiant, G. A., McDonald, K., & Taunton, J. E. (2011). The effect of three different levels of footwear stability on pain outcomes in women runners: A randomised control trial. *British Journal of Sports Medicine, 45*(9), 715–721.

Schmid, W., Knechtle, B., Knechtle, P., Barandun, U., Rüst, C. A., Rosemann, T., & Lepers, R. (2012). Predictor variables for marathon race time in recreational female runners. *Asian Journal of Sports Medicine, 3*(2), 90.

Sharma, A., Madaan, V., & Petty, F. D. (2006). Exercise for mental health. *Primary Care Companion to the Journal of Clinical Psychiatry, 8*(2), 106.

Shipway, R., & Holloway, I. (2010). Running free: Embracing a healthy lifestyle through distance running. *Perspectives in Public Health, 130*(6), 270–276.

Smyth, B. (2007). Case-based recommendation. In *The adaptive web, methods and strategies of web personalization* (pp. 342–376).

Smyth, B., & Cunningham, P. (2017a). A novel recommender system for helping marathoners to achieve a new personal-best. In *Proceedings of the eleventh ACM conference on recommender systems, recsys 2017, Como, Italy, August 27–31, 2017* (pp. 116–120). https://doi.org/10.1145/3109859.3109874

Smyth, B., & Cunningham, P. (2017b). Running with cases: A CBR approach to running your best marathon. In *Case-based reasoning research and development—25th international conference, ICCBR 2017, Trondheim, Norway, June 26–28, 2017, proceedings* (pp. 360–374).

Smyth, B., & Cunningham, P. (2018a). An analysis of case representations for marathon race prediction and planning. In *Case-based reasoning research and development—26th international conference, ICCBR 2018, Stockholm, Sweden, July 9–12, 2018, proceedings* (pp. 369–384).

Smyth, B., & Cunningham, P. (2018b). Marathon race planning: A case-based reasoning approach. In *Proceedings of the twenty-seventh international joint conference on artificial intelligence, IJCAI 2018, July 13–19, 2018, Stockholm, Sweden* (pp. 5364–5368). https://doi.org/10.24963/ijcai.2018/754

Smyth, B., & Willemsen, M. (2020). Predicting the personal-best times of speed skaters using case-based reasoning. In *Case-based reasoning research and development—28th international conference, ICCBR 2020, Salamanca, Spain, June 8–12, 2020, proceedings.*

Smyth, B. (2018). Fast starters and slow finishers: A large-scale data analysis of pacing at the beginning and end of the marathon for recreational runners. *Journal of Sports Analytics, 4*(3), 229–242.

Smyth, B. (2021). How recreational marathon runners hit the wall: A large-scale data analysis of late-race pacing collapse in the marathon. *PLoS ONE, 16*(5), e0251513.

Smyth, B., Lawlor, A., Berndsen, J., & Feely, C. (2022). Recommendations for marathon runners: On the application of recommender systems and machine learning to support recreational marathon runners. *User Modeling and User-Adapted Interaction, 32*(5), 787–838.

Szabo, A., & Ábrahám, J. (2013). The psychological benefits of recreational running: A field study. *Psychology, Health and Medicine, 18*(3), 251–261.

Tang, J., Hu, X., & Liu, H. (2013). Social recommendation: A review. *Social Network Analysis and Mining, 3*(4), 1113–1133.

Thornton, H. R., Delaney, J. A., Duthie, G. M., & Dascombe, B. J. (2017). Importance of various training-load measures in injury incidence of professional rugby league athletes. *International Journal of Sports Physiology and Performance, 12*(6), 819–824. https://doi.org/10.1123/ijspp.2016-0326

Toresdahl, B. G., Metzl, J. D., Kinderknecht, J., McElheny, K., de Mille, P., Quijano, B., & Fontana, M. A. (2022). Training patterns associated with injury in New York city marathon runners. *British Journal of Sports Medicine.*

Tragos, E. Z., O'Reilly-Morgan, D., Geraci, J., Shi, B., Smyth, B., Doherty, C., et al. (2023). Keeping people active and healthy at home using a reinforcement learning-based fitness recommendation framework. In *Proceedings of the thirty-second international joint conference on artificial intelligence, IJCAI 2023, 19th–25th August 2023, Macao, SAR, China* (pp. 6237–6245).

Vall, A., Dorfer, M., Eghbal-Zadeh, H., Schedl, M., Burjorjee, K., & Widmer, G. (2019). Feature-combination hybrid recommender systems for automated music playlist continuation. *User Modeling and User-Adapted Interaction, 29*(2), 527–572.

Vina, J., Sanchis-Gomar, F., Martinez-Bello, V., & Gomez-Cabrera, M. (2012). Exercise acts as a drug; the pharmacological benefits of exercise. *British Journal of Pharmacology, 167*(1), 1–12.

Wakita, Y., Oku, K., Huang, H.-H., & Kawagoe, K. (2015). A fashion-brand recommender system using brand association rules and features. In *Proceedings of the 2015 IIAI 4th international congress on advanced applied informatics* (pp. 719–720).

Webb, C., Vehrs, P. R., George, J. D., & Hager, R. (2014). Estimating vo2max using a personalized step test. *Measurement in Physical Education and Exercise Science, 18*(3), 184–197. https://doi.org/10.1080/1091367X.2014.912985

Werthner, H., & Ricci, F. (2004). E-commerce and tourism. *Communications of the ACM, 47*(12), 101–105.

Willy, R. W. (2018). Innovations and pitfalls in the use of wearable devices in the prevention and rehabilitation of running related injuries. *Physical Therapy in Sport: Official Journal of the Association of Chartered Physiotherapists in Sports Medicine, 29*, 26–33. https://doi.org/10.1016/j.ptsp.2017.10.003

Wu, S. S. X., Peiffer, J. J., Brisswalter, J., Nosaka, K., Lau, W. Y., & Abbiss, C. R. (2015). Pacing strategies during the swim, cycle and run disciplines of sprint, Olympic and half-ironman triathlons. *European Journal of Applied Physiology, 115*(5), 1147–1154.

Yamato, T. P., Saragiotto, B. T., & Lopes, A. D. (2015). A consensus definition of running-related injury in recreational runners: A modified Delphi approach. *The Journal of Orthopaedic and Sports Physical Therapy, 45*(5), 375–380. https://doi.org/10.2519/jospt.2015.5741

Zrenner, M., Ullrich, M., Zobel, P., Jensen, U., Laser, F., Groh, B. H., et al. (2018). Kinematic parameter evaluation for the purpose of a wearable running shoe recommendation. In *Proceedings of the 2018 IEEE 15th international conference on wearable and implantable body sensor networks (BSN)* (pp. 106–109).

Chapter 14
Data-Driven Methods for Soccer Analysis

Sylvio Barbon Junior, Felipe Arruda Moura, and Ricardo da Silva Torres

Abstract This chapter delves into the potential of utilising data-driven methods for soccer analysis. Particularly soccer, with its intricate player interactions and abundant data sources, serves as an ideal canvas for applying these methodologies. The core concept of the chapter revolves around establishing a data-driven pipeline in soccer and sports science. This pipeline automates the collection, transformation, processing, and analysis of data, creating a systematic flow from raw data to insightful decision-making. We aim to provide a comprehensive overview of how data-driven techniques are revolutionising soccer performance analysis. This chapter covers the promises and possibilities that the confluence of Artificial Intelligence (AI) and sports science holds, offering a roadmap for optimising athlete and team performance.

Keywords Soccer Analysis · Data Science · Artificial Intelligence · Machine Learning · Deep Learning

14.1 Introduction to Data-Driven Methods

Data-driven methods in the scope of Artificial Intelligence (AI) refer to approaches that rely heavily on data to support decisions, draw insights, and improve systems performance. These methods utilise extensive datasets to train Machine Learning models, extract patterns, and generate predictions or decisions based on the collected data. Particularly, the field of sports science has undergone a profound transformation propelled by the integration of cutting-edge data-driven methods. This paradigm

S. Barbon Junior (✉)
Dipartimento di Ingegneria e Architettura, Università Degli Studi Di Trieste (UNITS), 34127 Trieste, Italy
e-mail: sylvio.barbonjunior@units.it

F. A. Moura
Sport Sciences Department, State University of Londrina (UEL), Londrina, Brazil

R. da Silva Torres
Department of ICT and Naural Sciences, Norwegian University of Science and Technology (NTNU), Alesund, Norway

C. Dindorf et al. (eds.), *Artificial Intelligence in Sports, Movement, and Health*,
https://doi.org/10.1007/978-3-031-67256-9_14

shift represents a departure from conventional approaches, as researchers and practitioners increasingly rely on data analytics, Machine Learning, and advanced sensing technologies (e.g., wearable) to unravel the complexities of athletic performance, injury prevention, and coaching strategies.

Data-driven solutions in soccer for engineers refer to the innovative integration of data analytics, sensor technologies, and computational methods to optimise player performance, injury prevention, and strategic decision-making (Gamble et al., 2020). Soccer, in particular, has become a focal point for data-driven methods owing to the intricate nature of the game, characterised by dynamic player interactions that traditional analysis struggles to capture comprehensively. The sport offers an abundance of rich data sources, including player tracking through GPS devices, video footage, and detailed match statistics, providing a robust foundation for sophisticated analysis (Goes et al., 2021a, b). Advancements in technology, such as wearable sensors and high-resolution cameras, have made data collection more accessible, allowing soccer teams to implement advanced methods for real-time and post-match analysis. In the fiercely competitive world of soccer, teams are incessantly searching for strategic advantage, and data-driven methods offer insights into opponents' strategies, optimise player performance, and enhance overall team dynamics.

Beyond the competitive realm, data-driven approaches play a pivotal role in injury prevention and player health by monitoring physical conditions, workload, and recovery patterns (Huang & Jiang, 2021). Coaches and analysts leverage data-driven insights to understand patterns of play, player positioning, and team formations, enabling them to devise effective game plans and make strategic decisions during matches (Shaw & Glickman, 2019). The global popularity of soccer contributes to the demand for an engaging fan experience, and data-driven methods provide advanced analytics, statistics, and visualisations that deepen fans' understanding of the game. Moreover, these methods are instrumental in talent identification and player recruitment, allowing clubs to assess player performance, potential, and suitability for their teams through informed decisions in the transfer market (Larkin & O'Connor, 2017).

In essence, soccer's embrace of data-driven methods based on data processing pipelines to support competitive advantage. A data-driven pipeline, also known as a data pipeline, refers to a series of processes and tools that are orchestrated to automate the collection, transformation, processing, and analysis of data. The goal of a data-driven pipeline is to efficiently and reliably move data from diverse sources to its destination, making it accessible and usable for analytics, decision-making, and other applications. This concept is particularly prevalent in the fields of data engineering, data science, and business intelligence.

Figure 14.1 shows the traditional data-driven pipeline in soccer and sports science involves a systematic flow of processes and tools to collect, process, analyse, and derive insights from data related to soccer performance and athlete well-being. The exemplified pipeline has the initial phase regarding the collection of raw data from diverse sources. This includes extracting information, for example, from player tracking devices, wearable sensors worn by athletes, recorded video footage of matches, health monitoring, and detailed match statistics. The gathered data encompasses a broad spectrum of information crucial for analysis. This includes tracking player movements on the field, capturing physiological parameters, such as heart rate and distance covered, logging various game events, and considering contextual factors like weather conditions and team dynamics. In the next step, following the collection phase, the raw data undergoes meticulous processing to ensure its cleanliness, proper formatting, and standardisation. This preparation is vital for maintaining consistency and creating a uniform dataset suitable for analysis. Subsequently, the processed data becomes the subject of in-depth analysis. Statistical methods and exploratory data analysis are applied to unveil patterns, identify trends, and extract key performance indicators. This stage provides a comprehensive understanding of the intricacies of players' performance and match dynamics, which could open the possibility for two different branches: Data Visualisation and Data (or Predictive) Modelling.

Data Visualisation provides insights gained from the analysis; results are often visualised using charts, graphs, dashboards, or other visual representations. Visualisation tools assist coaches, analysts, and stakeholders in interpreting complex data and making informed decisions. On the other hand, the predictive modelling phase involves the application of techniques by data scientists and sports analysts. Machine Learning models, statistical models, and domain-specific algorithms are employed to derive actionable insights from the processed data. These models serve various purposes, including predicting injuries, profiling player attributes, conducting tactical analyses, and addressing other aspects of sports science. Both phases compose Decision Support Tools, aiding coaches, analysts, and stakeholders in making informed decisions related to player development, game strategy, and overall team performance.

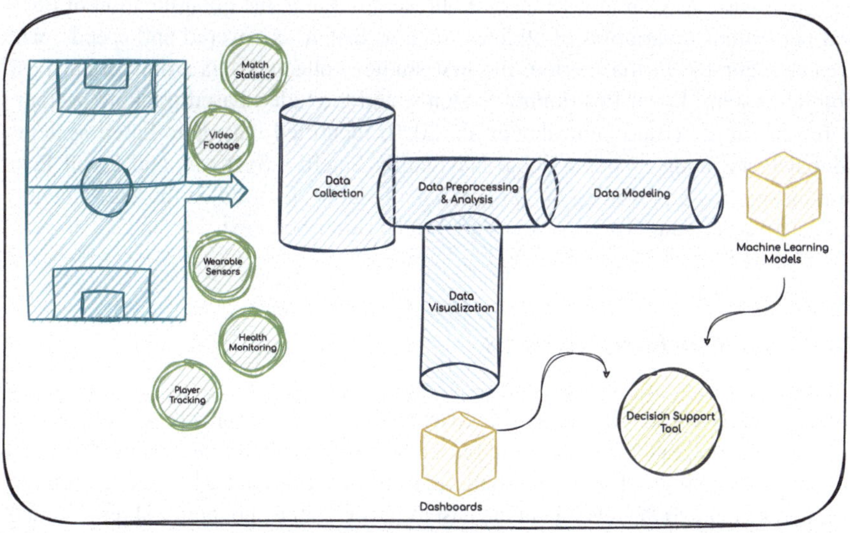

Fig. 14.1 General pipeline for a data-driven soccer analysis

This chapter endeavours to provide an in-depth exploration of the multifaceted applications of data-driven techniques within the realm of sports science, focusing on soccer to elucidate how these methodologies contribute to a holistic understanding of athlete dynamics and pave the way for optimised solutions. The confluence of AI and sports holds the promise of refining performance analysis and revolutionising athlete management, AI-based, and strategic decision-making in individual and soccer teams.

14.2 Data Collection

For a quantitative analysis of athletes' performance during competition and training situations, a series of manual and computational tools have been developed over the years since 1960s (Hughes & Franks, 1997; Reep & Benjamin, 1968). The first studies that sought to analyse the movements of players on the field used a methodology that consisted of, initially, quantifying the stride length of football athletes at different speeds. Then, the researchers filmed all the athlete's movements during the game and, using the images, estimated how many steps the player took at each speed. Despite the inherent errors associated with this type of data collection, such as the manual nature of the process, the authors were able to provide records of the distances covered by professional football players during an entire match at the time (Reilly, 1976; Withers, 1982).

In the late 1990s and early 2000s, several methods were developed with the main objective of identifying the player's position on the field as a function of time. Once players' positions were determined, it allowed, initially, the quantification of physical performance variables of athletes, such as distances covered and speeds, with greater accuracy. In that period, the first studies collected data from Global Positioning System, Local Positioning Systems, and the video-based tracking systems. A recent survey (Rico-González et al., 2020) identified that optic-based systems, Global Positioning System/Global Navigation Satellite Systems, and Local Positioning systems represented 60, 33, and 7% of studies focused on the assessment of collective behaviour. These systems are briefly described next.

14.2.1 *Video-Based Systems*

Since the early 2000s, advances in video technology and computer processing performance have motivated the interest of researchers in using computer vision and image processing techniques for the automatic analysis of sports games by videogrammetry (Figueroa et al., 2006b). While in the past the poor spatial and temporal resolution of the cameras represented a challenge to efficiently identify players for every frame, the current commercial and mobile phone cameras provide great spatial (4 K or more) and temporal (120 Hz or more) resolution. Thus, considering the cameras and the computational resources available at each moment of the timeline regarding data collection in sports, different methods have been developed in thc last two decades.

One of the first studies (Intille & Bobick, 1994) dealing with the automatic tracking of American Football players presented the concept of a closed-world tracking method, referred to as a space–time region in an image in which the taxonomy of all objects are known and all pixels of this region is associated with one of those objects. The key idea of the algorithm was (1) to compute the closed-world region around the players for the current frame, (2) to assign each pixel of the region to one of the objects within the closed-world region, (3) to determine context-specific features for the creation of a template of each player within the closed-world region, and (4) to track the player on the next frame based on the previous templates. A few years later, tracking soccer players was possible (Taki et al., 1996) based on the extraction of the static objects of the image by thresholding and line detection based on Hough transformation. Then, a body part of the player was manually identified as the initial template and players were tracked frame by frame by correlation-based template matching. Other studies (Matsui et al., 1998; Seo et al., 1997) proposed tracking players from TV broadcast images, however, considering that performance analysis is dependent on determining the positions of all players, these methods are limited. For most of the studies, the methods performed well for isolated players, but for regions with more than one player, tracking was challenging.

To improve the tracking methods, Figueroa et al. (2006b) proposed a method based on at least four static cameras which together cover the whole pitch.

Each camera had its own unique approach to image segmentation, diverging from the methods reported in the literature (Choi & Seo, 2011; Martín & Martínez, 2014; Xu et al., 2004), by background extraction based on a non-parametric morphological levelling operation (which deals with the specific problem of lighting changes in the scene during the match) (Figueroa et al., 2006a). By considering a model of the players and specific morphological operations, occlusion problems were treated by splitting segmented blobs. The splitting process was done using a graph representation in which the nodes were represented by the players' blobs and the edges were defined considering the information regarding the blobs, such as distance between blobs, colour, and movement direction. Although applied studies (Barros et al., 2007; Moura et al., n.d.) using this method reported the best automatic tracking rate as 94%, in general, manual operator intervention is excessively high and prone to errors. Additionally, image segmentation may compromise several hours considering image spatial and temporal resolutions, and the computational resources available. In this sense, recent advances in Deep Learning and Machine Vision Algorithms allowed the capture of relevant data (e.g., positional data) based on automatic segmentation and/or detection for both fixed cameras and TV broadcasts. Developments in such areas fostered scaling-up analysis based on large volumes of data. Soccer analysis using machine vision has been associated with SOTA results in several applications (Manafifard et al., 2017), ranging from dribbling detection (Barbon et al., 2022) to the prediction of successful actions (Stival et al., 2023) based on spatiotemporal patterns. More recently, studies proposed the concept of pose detection, motivated by biomechanical research questions related to limb kinematics and estimated kinetics, with relevant applications in soccer (Monteiro et al., 2022).

14.2.2 Time Series

Time series data comprises a sequence of data points recorded at regular time intervals, showcasing the evolution of variables over time. Each data point is associated with a specific timestamp or time period, creating a temporal order. The granularity of the data is determined by the time interval between consecutive observations, exemplified by instances like player tracking data recorded every second during a soccer match. Individual observations, such as scores, player positions, ball trajectories, or physiological metrics, are captured at specific time instances, contributing to the dynamic nature of the dataset.

Temporal patterns, both seasonal and long-term trends, are evident in time series data (Borrie et al., 2002). Seasonal patterns reveal recurring trends within specific time periods, exemplified by teams performing differently in certain seasons due to factors like weather conditions or player form. Long-term trends, on the other hand, depict gradual improvements or changes in team performance over extended periods, influenced by strategic alterations or player development.

Event sequences, capturing the order of occurrences could encompass player movements, such as dribbling (Barbon et al., 2022), providing insights into the dynamic buildup during a match. Each data observation is accompanied by a timestamp, indicating when player performance metrics or other variables were recorded. Periodic events, like matches scheduled weekly during a league season, contribute to the structured nature of time series data.

Anomalies in time series data denote unusual or unexpected patterns, serving as indicators of noteworthy occurrences. For instance, sudden spikes in player heart rate or unexpected changes in team performance can be identified through anomaly detection techniques.

A diverse array of sensors is employed to capture a comprehensive range of data. General Positioning Systems (GPS) trackers, worn by players, furnish real-time data on their positioning, distance covered, speed, and acceleration during both training sessions and matches (Buchheit et al., 2014). Wearable accelerometers complement this by measuring accelerations, decelerations, and changes in direction, offering valuable insights into physical exertion and workload. Heart rate monitors, another integral component, track players' heart rates, delivering critical information on cardiovascular load, fatigue, and overall fitness levels. Smart jerseys, equipped with sensors, capture data on players' movements, posture, and biomechanics, thereby aiding in injury prevention and performance optimization (McDevitt et al., 2022).

Ball tracking systems employ cameras and sensors to monitor the movement of the ball, providing insights into ball possession, trajectory, and pivotal events such as shots on goal. Furthermore, pressure sensors embedded in cleats measure foot pressure and offer insights into players' stride patterns, balance, and ground contact forces. Environmental sensors are important to capture data on factors like temperature, humidity, and altitude, influencing player performance and contributing to injury prevention strategies. Also, biomechanical sensors attached to players' bodies capture data on joint movements and muscle activation, providing insights into biomechanics and potential injury risks. Inertial Measurement Units (IMUs) worn by players capture data on movement, orientation, and changes in velocity, contributing to a detailed analysis of player kinetics (Zhang, 2014).

14.2.3 Tabular Data

Tabular data refers to information organised in a table-like structure, where data is presented in rows and columns. This format is highly structured, making it suitable for various analytical and computational purposes. Each row typically represents an individual record or observation, while columns correspond to different attributes or variables associated with those records. Tabular data is prevalent in numerous domains, including databases, spreadsheets, and datasets used in machine learning and data analysis.

Tabular data is amenable to various data analysis techniques, including statistical analysis, the creation of Machine Learning models, and exploratory data analysis. The structured nature of tabular data simplifies tasks like filtering, sorting, and aggregating information. Additionally, it serves as a foundational format for creating datasets that can be utilised to train machine learning models for predicting outcomes, uncovering patterns, and making informed decisions in the realm of soccer analytics and sports science.

Consider player statistics, where each row is dedicated to a specific player, and columns encapsulate essential attributes such as player ID, name, position, goals scored, and assists. This tabular arrangement offers a comprehensive overview of individual player performance metrics, creating datasets (Brooks et al., 2016).

Similarly, when examining match data, the tabular format aligns each row with a distinct match, while columns detail pertinent information including match ID, date, participating teams, and the final score. This structured presentation enables a systematic evaluation of match-related variables, aiding in comprehensive match analysis.

Team performance metrics, another crucial facet, are encapsulated within rows representing individual teams. Within this tabular construct, columns house attributes such as team ID, name, points earned, and goals conceded, providing a systematic and detailed portrayal of team-level performance. Delving into injury records, for example, the tabular structure organises data by allocating each row to a specific instance of a player's injury. Associated columns document pertinent information such as player ID, injury type, date of occurrence, and recovery time. This systematic arrangement facilitates a detailed examination of player injuries, contributing to injury prevention strategies and player well-being assessments.

The utilisation of tabular data in these contexts adheres to structured principles, allowing for systematic organisation and analysis of pertinent information critical for sports analytics and decision-making processes within the realm of soccer and sports science.

14.2.4 Graph Representations

Another recent trend relies on using graphs to model players in their interactions. In existing formulations, players are modelled as vertices, and edges are used to represent their relationships. Examples of applications include pass exchange analysis based on passing graphs (Zhou et al., 2023) or tactical analysis based on player location on the field (an edge exists if two players are close to each other) (Stival et al., 2023; Rodrigues et al., 2019).

14.3 Process and Analysis Techniques

Data processing and analysis is a step of the data-driven pipeline, which plays a pivotal role in transforming raw data into meaningful insights, providing models to automatise complex tasks and even discover patterns. Finally, this phase transforms all collected data into actionable insights, ranging from heatmaps to Machine Learning models. Preprocessing, in which data is cleaned and formatted; feature engineering, enhancing data representation for visualisation and Machine Learning modelling; data modelling for model selection and optimisation, choosing and fine-tuning the right model.

14.3.1 Data Preprocessing

The goal of data preprocessing is to improve data quality, revolving around the idea of preparing and cleaning raw data to make it suitable for analysis or modelling. Common issues found in raw data include missing values, the presence of noise, and lack of normalization. To address those challenges, several data transformation methods are employed, and their choice depends on the kind of data (e.g., image, time series, structure data) and the sensors' quality (e.g., noise, missing values, and resolution). The main tasks that need to be handled, include the following:

- Handling Missing Values: Identification and treatment of missing data points to avoid biases and inaccuracies in subsequent analyses (Emmanuel et al., 2021). Handling missing values can be addressed through deletion methods, like listwise or pairwise deletion, where rows or pairs with missing values are removed. Imputation methods include mean, median, or mode imputation, forward and backwards fill, Linear Regression, K-Nearest Neighbours, and multiple imputations, each replacing missing values based on specific criteria.

- Data Cleaning: Removal of irrelevant or redundant information, correction of errors, and addressing inconsistencies in the dataset to improve overall data quality (Chu et al., 2016). Principal Component Analysis (PCA) for feature reduction, spell-checking algorithms for textual data correction, statistical outlier detection for numerical inconsistencies, cross-validation with external sources for verification, and rule-based validation checks based on domain knowledge can be employed.
- Normalisation and Standardisation: Conversion of categorical variables into numerical representations for compatibility with Machine Learning methods. Normalisation is the process of scaling numerical features to a standard range, typically between 0 and 1. The goal is to ensure that all features contribute equally to the model training process, preventing certain features with larger scales from dominating the learning process. Standardisation involves transforming numerical features to have a mean of 0 and a standard deviation of 1. Machine Learning models often require numerical input, making the conversion of categorical variables necessary.
- Feature Engineering: Creation of new features or transformation of existing ones to enhance the representation of information, improving the learning capabilities of Machine Learning models (Nargesian et al., 2017). Techniques include creating polynomial features to capture non-linear relationships, introducing interaction terms to represent synergies between features, discretising numerical features into bins for non-linear relationship capture, log-transforming numerical features for symmetry, scaling features to ensure uniformity, generating time-based features like lag features for time-series data, encoding categorical variables into numerical forms using techniques like One-Hot Encoding, and extracting features from text data using methods like TF-IDF or word embeddings. These techniques collectively improve the learning capabilities of Machine Learning models by providing more informative and relevant features. The choice of methods depends on the nature of the data and the specific modelling goals.
- Handling Imbalanced Data: Addressing class imbalances in the dataset to prevent models from being skewed towards the majority class (Rout, Mishra, & Mallick, 2018). Various methods for handling imbalanced data include resampling techniques such as over-sampling (e.g., SMOTE) and under-sampling, ensemble methods like Balanced Random Forest and Easy Ensemble, and anomaly detection with techniques like Isolation Forest. The goal is to handle imbalanced data, allowing for improved recognition of patterns in minority classes.
- Noise Reduction: Identification and removal of noisy data or outliers that may distort the analysis or training of Machine Learning models (Garcia et al., 2016). Common methods for the identification and removal of noisy data or outliers in a dataset include visual inspection through plots such as box plots, statistical approaches based on measures like z-scores or IQR, and Machine Learning models

such as Isolation Forests and Local Outlier Factor (LOF). The choice of method often involves a balance between statistical rigour and practical considerations based on the data at hand.

- Frequent Pattern Analysis Preprocessing: In the context of frequent pattern analysis (e.g., association rule mining), preprocessing may involve the discretisation of continuous variables and the conversion of data into a transactional format suitable for pattern discovery (Aggarwal, 2014).

The aforementioned methods are crucial to tackling different challenges in preparing soccer and sports data for analysis, visualisation, and modelling. Diverse sensor data and acquisition systems may necessitate distinct preprocessing approaches, yet they simultaneously face common challenges. Presently, the primary challenges in preprocessing revolve around ensuring the quality and consistency of data, particularly when confronted with diverse sources and formats. Inaccurate or inconsistent data has the potential to introduce biases in analyses and generate unreliable insights. Furthermore, delayed or outdated information can significantly constrain the effectiveness of in-game decision making processes. Addressing these challenges through robust preprocessing methodologies is paramount to fostering accurate, reliable, and timely analyses in the realm of sports data analytics.

Additionally, it is crucial to employ methods aimed at mitigating temporal misalignment. For instance, utilising techniques like Dynamic Time Warping (DTW) (Barbon et al., 2009) for aligning temporal data, including events and player movements, ensures synchronisation and diminishes the likelihood of misaligned temporal data. Addressing misalignment is imperative, as it can otherwise lead to erroneous conclusions and impede the accurate analysis of sequential events. By incorporating robust methods to reduce temporal misalignment, sports data analysts can enhance the reliability and precision of their analyses, contributing to a more accurate understanding of the dynamics unfolding during matches.

14.3.2 Data Visualisation

Data visualisation can be performed along several stages of the data-driven pipeline. Employing Exploratory Data Analysis (EDA) methods, such as histograms and scatter plots, allows for an initial understanding of the distribution of player statistics and match events. For instance, employing dimensionality reduction techniques like t-Distributed Stochastic Neighbour Embedding (t-SNE) (Soni et al., 2020) aids in visualising high-dimensional player data, providing an intuitive representation of player similarities and differences.

Performance metrics illustration, encompassing bar graphs or radar charts, facilitates the representation of crucial statistics, such as player ratings or team rankings. The comparative analysis benefits from visualisation techniques like radar charts, enabling side-by-side assessments of player or team attributes. This visual approach empowers coaches and analysts to discern strengths and weaknesses across various performance dimensions. Player trajectory mapping, exemplified in (Mehrasa et al., 2018), leverages spatial visualisation techniques such as heatmaps and trajectory plots. The utilisation of algorithms like kernel density estimation enhances the portrayal of player movement patterns, aiding in the identification of strategic hotspots on the field. Moreover, the application of clustering algorithms like K-Means facilitates the grouping of player trajectories based on movement similarities.

In-game decision support necessitates real-time visualisations, incorporating methods like dynamic shot maps or live player performance updates. Machine Learning models, including those for predictive analytics like player performance forecasting, can be seamlessly integrated into these visualisations to assist coaches in making informed decisions during matches. On the other hand, post-match analysis benefits from animated replays, utilising methods like data-driven animations to recreate key moments. Tactical diagrams, generated through algorithms like graph visual rhythms (Rodrigues et al., 2019), Voronoi diagrams, or models based on players' kinematics (Caetano et al., 2021) (as illustrated in Fig. 14.2), contribute to visualising team formations and player positioning during specific game phases.

The integration of data visualisation methods and algorithms throughout the pipeline enhances the interpretation, communication, and utilisation of soccer-related data. The combination of EDA, dimensionality reduction, clustering, and interactive visualisation techniques contributes to a comprehensive and impactful data-driven analysis in the domain of soccer.

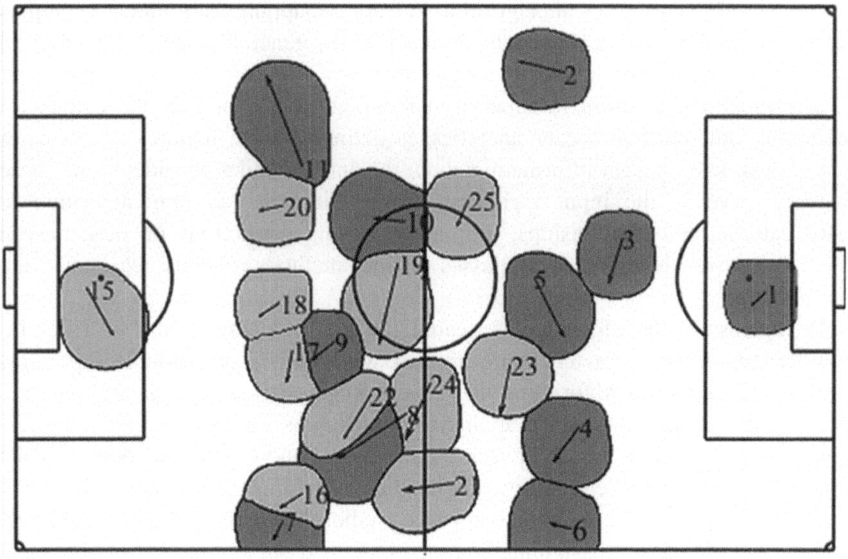

Fig. 14.2 Dominant regions for all players of the two teams based on kinetmatic data (Caetano et al., 2021)

14.3.3 Data Modelling

Data modelling is a process of creating representations that mirror real-world context, their patterns, and the governing constraints. It involves generating an abstract representation, such as decision tables, mathematical functions, or data structures, to comprehend the interrelationships among data elements. The primary objective is to support various applications and business requirements by providing a structured and organised view of the data. This section covers three primary approaches: supervised learning, semi-supervised learning, and unsupervised learning. Within these overarching topics, the methodologies and algorithms tailored to soccer analytics will be explored, providing an understanding of the diverse techniques employed for predictive modelling and pattern discovery in soccer-related data.

14.3.3.1 Supervised Learning

Machine Learning algorithms allow the creation of models able to predict outcomes, such as player performance, match results, or injury likelihood (Fister et al., 2015). Particularly, supervised learning aids in making informed decisions regarding player selection, game strategy, and overall team performance. Supervised learning stands as a fundamental paradigm predicting or estimating an output variable based on input features in a labelled dataset. This dataset comprises pairs of input–output examples, providing a foundation for the algorithm to learn a mapping from inputs to outputs during the training phase, ultimately allowing for the generalisation of this acquired knowledge to make predictions on unseen data.

The input composition in supervised learning, particularly in the context of predicting outcomes in soccer analytics, is defined by the features or attributes that encapsulate relevant information about the entities under consideration. These features serve as the input variables for the Machine Learning algorithm to learn patterns and relationships, ultimately making predictions on new, unseen data. Supervised learning encompasses distinct methods, namely regression and classification.

In regression, the algorithm is geared towards mapping inputs to a continuous range of values, a technique applied when the target variable represents a numerical quantity. Algorithms like Linear Regression, Ridge Regression, and Gradient Boosting are frequently applied to create regression models. Linear Regression models the relationship between input features and continuous output, while Ridge Regression adds regularisation to handle multicollinearity. Gradient Boosting combines multiple weak learners to improve predictive accuracy. On the other hand, classification focuses on assigning inputs to predefined categorical classes, making it suitable for scenarios where the target variable represents labels or classes. For classification tasks, where the goal is to categorise inputs into predefined classes, algorithms like Support Vector Machines (SVM), Decision Trees, and Random Forests

(RF) are commonly utilised. SVM finds a hyperplane that best separates classes, while Decision Trees and Random Forests create tree-like structures to classify data.

Algorithms are often referred to as versatile or hybrid models, and they can be applied to different types of predictive tasks. One such example is the RF algorithm. RF is an ensemble learning method that builds a collection of decision trees during training. In the context of regression, it can predict a numerical outcome, while in classification, it can categorise inputs into different classes. The versatility of RF makes it applicable to a wide range of tasks, making it a popular choice in various domains, including soccer analytics. Another example is Gradient Boosting, which is primarily used for regression but can be adapted for classification tasks as well. Gradient Boosting builds a series of weak learners to improve overall predictive performance. When used for regression, it predicts a continuous output, and when used for classification, it assigns inputs to predefined classes.

Another important class of algorithms is Artificial Neural Networks (Perl & Dauscher, 2006), especially to create deep learning models. They can learn complex patterns and relationships in the data, making them adaptable to diverse tasks within the domain, whether it involves predicting match outcomes, player performance, or other relevant metrics. The flexibility and expressive power of neural networks contribute to their effectiveness in handling both regression and classification challenges. Deep Learning approaches, such as Convolutional Neural Networks (CNNs) (Russo et al., 2019), play an important role in supervised learning when dealing with image data. The importance of CNNs in this context lies in their ability to effectively extract hierarchical and spatial features from images, providing valuable insights for various tasks in soccer analytics, such as player tracking, movement analysis, and spatial pattern recognition. In simpler terms, CNNs can directly take images as input and generate the desired output without the need for an extensive preprocessing pipeline.

The choice of the most suitable algorithm is contingent upon the specific characteristics of the task, the nature of the data, and the overarching objectives of the analysis. Different algorithms exhibit varying strengths and considerations in different scenarios. The determination of the best algorithm involves experimentation and comparison of their performance in the specific context of the data-driven soccer application. Factors such as hyperparameter tuning, cross-validation, and the interpretability of the model also play pivotal roles in the decision-making process.

14.3.3.2 Unsupervised Learning

Unsupervised learning, another category of machine learning methods used in the sports and soccer context, focuses on extracting patterns and relationships from unlabelled data. Various strategies and algorithms are employed in unsupervised learning for tasks such as clustering and association rule mining (Celebi & Aydin, 2016).

One prevalent strategy in unsupervised learning is clustering, an approach that involves grouping similar data points based on underlying patterns in the data. K-Means clustering is a widely employed algorithm in this context. It partitions the data into clusters, each represented by a centroid. The K-Means algorithm iteratively assigns data points to the nearest cluster centroid and updates the centroids to minimise the within-cluster variance. This process continues until convergence, resulting in distinct clusters. In addition to K-Means, Density-Based Spatial Clustering of Applications with Noise (DBSCAN) is another notable clustering algorithm. DBSCAN identifies clusters based on the density of data points, allowing for the detection of clusters of arbitrary shapes. Unlike K-Means, DBSCAN does not require the specification of the number of clusters beforehand. Instead, it categorises points as core, border, or noise points, adapting to variations in cluster density.

Finally, association rule mining serves as another valuable unsupervised learning strategy for uncovering intriguing relationships between variables in large datasets. Apriori, a widely adopted algorithm in association rule mining, plays a pivotal role in this process. It excels in identifying frequent itemsets within the data, thereby establishing patterns of co-occurrence among different variables.

In addition to Apriori, FP-growth (Frequent Pattern growth) stands out as another influential algorithm in association rule mining. FP-growth employs a different approach compared to Apriori, utilizing a frequent pattern tree structure to efficiently mine frequent itemsets. By avoiding the generation of candidate itemsets, FP-growth enhances computational efficiency, particularly in scenarios involving large datasets with extensive itemset combinations.

14.3.3.3 Semi-supervised Learning

Semi-supervised learning is a paradigm that leverages both labelled and unlabelled data for training Machine Learning models. In the context of data-driven soccer applications, semi-supervised learning can be valuable when labelled data is limited, but a larger pool of unlabelled data is available (Vandeghen et al., 2022). The goal is to exploit the unlabelled data to enhance the model's performance and generalisation. The utilisation of a combination of labelled and unlabelled data presents the opportunity for a potential reduction in the costs associated with the manual annotation of data. This reduction is particularly significant in scenarios where the annotation process is resource intensive.

Semi-supervised learning encompasses some strategies and algorithms designed to leverage the availability of data labels for model training. One prominent strategy is self-training (Rosenberg et al., 2005), which involves iterative model training on labelled data, followed by the assignment of pseudo-labels to unlabelled instances with high confidence. Another approach, co-training, simultaneously trains multiple models on different feature subsets or representations, with the agreement between models used for labelling unlabelled instances. Multi-view learning is a strategy that utilises different data representations or views to enhance model performance by capturing complementary information.

14.4 Applications

Several works in soccer analytics apply a great part of the methods and concepts presented in the previous sections. Over the past 70 years, performance analysis in soccer changed from simple registering of match-related statistics (such as absolute and relative frequencies of passes, shots, fouls, goals scored, etc.) to complex data treatment generated from raw tracking data and events registering associated. Notation systems developed to register information on players' actions during matches are traditional for both soccer professionals and specialised sports media. The outcome is tabular data generally used for descriptive purposes. More recently, multivariate techniques have been applied to discriminate winning from drawing and losing teams or to classify playing styles (Moura et al., 2014; Ruan et al., 2022).

For instance, Principal Component Analysis and K-Means clustering applied to tabular data of game-related individual and team performance of 2006 World Cup allowed to identify $\approx$70% of the winning teams into the same group. Another way to better interpret the game-related statistics is to associate the players' actions with the pitch local where every event was performed. This application was proposed previously for the full development of the tracking systems. From the coordinates of the event location associated with the pitch coordinate system, PCA was applied to represent the regions where the players visited most with ball possession, the variability of these locations, and to make inferences about team system of play (Barros et al., 2006). With the development of the tracking systems, the identification of the system of play was possible for each timestamp via K-Means clustering from players' coordinates, allowing a more in-depth tactical analysis during attacking and defending sequences (Machado et al., 2017). Since the 2010s, world-class championships like UEFA European Championship, FIFA World Cup, and UEFA Champions League have provided in their official website information about team and player performances. One of these performance indicators is the 'heat map' of each player, a coloured representation of the pitch of the frequency of the player position at a given location. From the coordinates of the region where a given player visited most, PCA was also applied to represent not only the player position variability during the match, but also throughout the championship (Moura et al., n.d.).

From players' position as a function of the time, teams' tactical behaviour started to be explored in the early 2010s as time series. Players' distribution on the pitch has been represented by the surface area (represented by the area of the convex hull), spread (as a general measure of the distances between team-mates), stretch index (a measure of distance among players and team centroid), and coupling distances, among others (Caetano et al., 2020; Moura et al., n.d.; Rico-González et al., n.d). From the identification of discrete values of the time series, previous studies showed the relation between tactical variables and the success during attacking and defending actions in soccer (Moura et al., n.d.). Frequency-domain analysis using Fast Fourier Transformation also showed that soccer professional teams increase the lower frequencies of the teams spread time series during the second half of the matches, suggesting that teams decrease the tactical performance in terms of organising the players while defending and attacking (Moura et al., n.d.). The same analysis was sensitive to show the variability of the tactical features time series, and how different categories of futsal matches (indoor soccer) present different behavioural demands (Bueno et al., n.d).

The relationship between time series was also the focus of previous studies on tactical analysis in soccer. In terms of a systematic approach, during the match teams are conflicting and interacting, and attempts are made to perturb the stability of the opponent's defensive system. Considering that tactical features describe how teammates and opponents behave, previous works presented different methods to measure the synchronisation between tactical time series, and its relation with performance. For instance, during the early stages, attacking sequences ending in shots on goal present greater anti-phase between teams' spread time series, compared to sequences ending in tackles, suggesting that success is associated with a break in the opponent stability (Moura et al., n.d.). For the movements performed by subgroups (defenders, midfielders, and attackers), a recent study reported a decreased inter- and intra-team synchrony of interactions involving the defenders of the attacking team during successful attacks in the longitudinal direction (Goes et al., 2021a, b). Using similar methods, (Duarte et al., 2013) showed large synergistic relations within teams from the English Premier League, considering the longitudinal movements that the players perform during the matches. The synchronisation of the movement between pairs of opponents, labelled as dyads, was also extensively explored in literature. For instance, a recent investigation showed that the offensive players of the dyads tend to'surprise' the opponent causing greater disruptions on the dyad relation during sequences ending in shot to goal compared to the ones ending in defensive tackle (Caetano et al., 2023). Together, all these studies present a clear application of the time, frequency, and phase domain analysis to understand individual and collective behaviour in soccer.

Since the development of tracking systems, millions of data have been generated with each match. Thus, providing objective feedback to players and coaches became challenging, especially in selecting the relevant moments of the match. Data visualisation tools help describe players' behaviour and relations using simple representations. For instance, the concept of visual rhythm (Rodrigues et al., 2019) was used for a visual representation of temporal graphs. In soccer, graph is usually modelled having players as nodes and the edges represent a given relation among the players. Considering that players move and interact in every frame, temporal graphs are generated from which complex network measurements are extracted to represent the features of individual and team behaviour. These features were then used as a column of a new image, named visual rhythm image, a compact representation that allows efficient processing and analysis of huge volumes of sequential data (Rodrigues et al., 2019). Similar representations were reported also for the association of the players' coordinates time series and teams' tactical formation during the entire match (Machado et al., 2017), and for the shape description of the tactical organisation during the match (Bueno et al., n.d), using unique images. Some examples are available in Fig. 14.3.

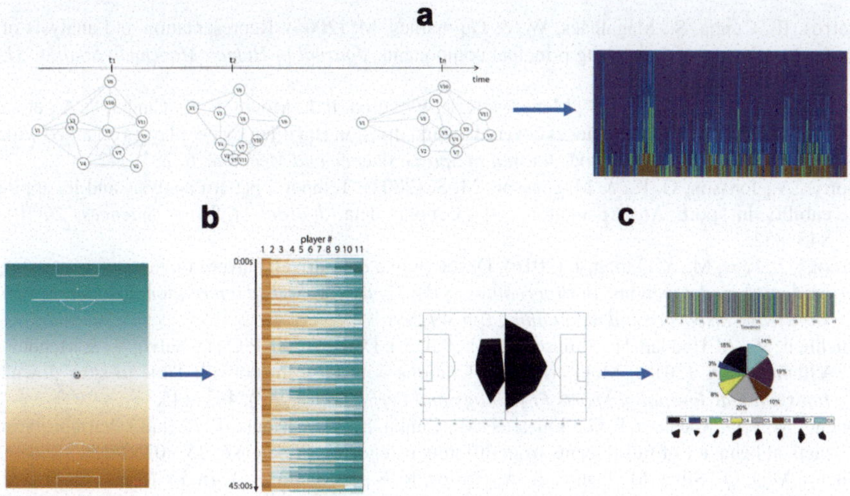

Fig. 14.3 Representation of visual rhythm applied to temporal graphs **a** Uchoa Maia Rodrigues et al. (2019), to players' coordinates time series **b** Machado et al. (2017) and to shape description of the tactical organisation **c** Bueno et al. (n.d.)

14.5 Conclusion

The integration of data-driven methods within the scope of AI has not only revolutionised sports science but has become the driving force behind transformative changes in the intricate realm of soccer. This chapter has unravelled the profound impact of data-driven solutions, emphasising their crucial role in optimising player performance, preventing injuries, and informing strategic decisions. Soccer, with its dynamic player interactions and diverse data sources, stands as a forefront area for benefiting from this data-driven revolution. As the soccer community continues to navigate the dynamic landscape of sports science, the integration of data-driven methodologies is poised to be an enduring catalyst for innovation, excellence, and success in the world's most beloved sport.

References

Aggarwal, C. C. (2014). Applications of frequent pattern mining. *Frequent Pattern Mining, 32*, 443–467.

Barbon, S., Guido, R. C., Vieira, L. S., Fonseca, E. S., Sanchez, F. L., Scalassara, P. R., et al. (2009). Wavelet-based dynamic time warping. *Journal of Computational and Applied Mathematics, 227*(2), 271–287.

Barbon, S., Pinto, A., Barroso, J. V., Caetano, F. G., Moura, F. A., Cunha, S. A., & Torres, R. S. (2022). Sport action mining: Dribbling recognition in soccer. *Multimedia Tools and Applications, 81*(3), 4341–4364.

Barros, R., Cunha, S., Magalhães, W., & Guimarães, M. (2006). Representation and analysis of soccer players' actions using principal components. *Journal of Human Movement Studies, 51*, 103–116.

Barros, R. M. L., Misuta, M. S., Menezes, R. P., Figueroa, P. J., Moura, F. A., Cunha, S. A., et al. (2007). Analysis of the distances covered by first division Brazilian soccer players obtained with an automatic tracking method. *Journal of Sports Science and Medicine, 6*, 233–242.

Borrie, A., Jonsson, G. K., & Magnusson, M. S. (2002). Temporal pattern analysis and its applicability in sport: An explanation and exemplar data. *Journal of Sports Sciences, 20*(10), 845–852.

Brooks, J., Kerr, M., & Guttag, J. (2016). Developing a data-driven player ranking in soccer using predictive model weights. In *Proceedings of the 22nd ACM Sigkdd international conference on knowledge discovery and data mining* (pp. 49–55).

Buchheit, M., Al-Haddad, H., Simpson, B. M., Palazzi, D., Bourdon, P. C., Di Salvo, V., & Mendez-Villanueva, A. (2014). Monitoring accelerations with GPS in football: Time to slow down? *International Journal of Sports Physiology and Performance, 9*(3), 442–445.

Bueno, M. J. O., Caetano, F. G., Souza, N. M., Cunha, S. A., & Moura, F. A. (n.d.). Variability in tactical behavior of futsal teams from different categories. *PLoS ONE, 15*, e0230513.

Bueno, M. J. O., Silva, M., Cunha, S. A., Torres, R. S., & Moura, F. A. (n.d.). Multiscale fractal dimension applied to tactical analysis in football: A novel approach to evaluate the shapes of team organization on the pitch. *PLoS ONE, 16*(9), 1–14. https://doi.org/10.1371/journal.pone.0256771

Caetano, F. G., Barbon, S., Torres, R. S., Cunha, S. A., Ruffino, P. R. C., Martins, L. E. B., & Moura, F. A. (2021). Football player dominant region determined by a novel model based on instantaneous kinematics variables. *Scientific Reports, 11*(1), 18209.

Caetano, F. G., de Souza, N. M., de Oliveira-Bueno, M. J., Cunha, S. A., & Moura, F. A. (2020). Interpersonal interaction during official soccer matches considering the coupling of different playing positions. *International Journal of Performance Analysis in Sport, 20*(4), 646–658. https://doi.org/10.1080/24748668.2020.1775412

Caetano, F. G., Santiago, P. R. P., da Silva-Torres, R., Cunha, S. A., & Moura, F. A. (2023). Interpersonal coordination of opposing player dyads during attacks performed in official football matches. *Sports Biomechanics, 2*(35), 1–16. https://doi.org/10.1080/14763141.2023

Celebi, M. E., & Aydin, K. (2016). *Unsupervised learning algorithms* (Vol. 9). Springer.

Choi, K., & Seo, Y. (2011). Automatic initialization for 3D soccer player tracking. *Pattern Recognition Letters, 32*(9), 1274–1282. https://doi.org/10.1016/j.patrec.2011.03.009

Chu, X., Ilyas, I. F., Krishnan, S., & Wang, J. (2016). Data cleaning: Overview and emerging challenges. In *Proceedings of the 2016 international conference on management of data* (pp. 2201–2206).

Duarte, R., Araújo, D., Correia, V., Davids, K., Marques, P., & Richardson, M. J. (2013). Competing together: Assessing the dynamics of team–team and player–team synchrony in professional association football. *Human Movement Science, 32*(4), 555–566. https://doi.org/10.1016/j.humov.2013.01.011

Emmanuel, T., Maupong, T., Mpoeleng, D., Semong, T., Mphago, B., & Tabona, O. (2021). A survey on missing data in machine learning. *Journal of Big Data, 8*(1), 1–37.

Figueroa, P. J., Leite, N. J., & Barros, R. M. (2006a). Background recovering in outdoor image sequences: An example of soccer players segmentation. *Image and Vision Computing, 24*(4), 363–374. https://doi.org/10.1016/j.imavis.2005.12.012

Figueroa, P. J., Leite, N. J., & Barros, R. M. (2006b). Tracking soccer players aiming their kinematical motion analysis. *Computer Vision and Image Understanding, 101*(2), 122–135. https://doi.org/10.1016/j.cviu.2005.07.006

Fister, I., Ljubič, K., Suganthan, P. N., Perc, M., & Fister, I. (2015). Computational intelligence in sports: Challenges and opportunities within a new research domain. *Applied Mathematics and Computation, 262*, 178–186.

Gamble, P., Chia, L., & Allen, S. (2020). The illogic of being data-driven: Reasserting control and restoring balance in our relationship with data and technology in football. *Science and Medicine in Football, 4*(4), 338–341.

Garcia, L. P., de Carvalho, A. C., & Lorena, A. C. (2016). Noise detection in the meta-learning level. *Neurocomputing, 176*, 14–25.

Goes, F. R., Brink, M. S., Elferink-Gemser, M. T., Kempe, M., & Lemmink, K. A. P. M. (2021a). The tactics of successful attacks in professional association football: Large-scale spatiotemporal analysis of dynamic subgroups using position tracking data. *Journal of Sports Sciences, 39*(5), 523–532. https://doi.org/10.1080/02640414.2020.1834689

Goes, F. R., Meerhoff, L., de Oliveira-Bueno, M. J., Rodrigues, D. M., Moura, F. A., Brink, M. S., et al. (2021b). Unlocking the potential of big data to support tactical performance analysis in professional soccer: A systematic review. *European Journal of Sport Science, 21*(4), 481–496. https://doi.org/10.1080/17461391.2020.1747552

Huang, C., & Jiang, L. (2021). Data monitoring and sports injury prediction model based on embedded system and machine learning algorithm. *Microprocessors and Microsystems, 81*, 103654.

Hughes, M., & Franks, I. M. (1997). *Notational analysis of sport*. E & FN Spon.

Intille, S., & Bobick, A. (1994). *Visual tracking using closed-worlds* (Technical Report No. 294). M.I.T Media Laboratory Perceptual Computing Section.

Larkin, P., & O'Connor, D. (2017). Talent identification and recruitment in youth soccer: Recruiter's perceptions of the key attributes for player recruitment. *PLoS ONE, 12*(4), e0175716.

Machado, V., Leite, R., Moura, F., Cunha, S., Sadlo, F., & Comba, J. L. (2017). Visual soccer match analysis using spatiotemporal positions of players. *Computers and Graphics, 68*, 84–95. https://doi.org/10.1016/j.cag.2017.08.006

Manafifard, M., Ebadi, H., & Abrishami-Moghaddam, H. (2017). A survey on player tracking in soccer videos. *Computer Vision and Image Understanding, 159*, 19–46. https://doi.org/10.1016/j.cviu.2017.02.002

Martín, R., & Martínez, J. M. (2014). A semi-supervised system for players detection and tracking in multi-camera soccer videos. *Multimedia Tools and Applications, 73*(3), 1617–1642. https://doi.org/10.1007/s11042-013-1659-6

Matsui, K., Iwase, M., Agata, M., Tanaka, T., & Ohnishi, N. (1998). Soccer image sequence computed by a virtual camera. In *Proceedings 1998 IEEE computer society conference on computer vision and pattern recognition (cat. no. 98cb36231)* (pp. 860–865). https://doi.org/10.1109/CVPR.1998.698705

McDevitt, S., Hernandez, H., Hicks, J., Lowell, R., Bentahaikt, H., Burch, R., et al. (2022). Wearables for biomechanical performance optimization and risk assessment in industrial and sports applications. *Bioengineering, 9*(1), 33.

Mehrasa, N., Zhong, Y., Tung, F., Bornn, L., & Mori, G. (2018). Deep learning of player trajectory representations for team activity analysis. In *Proceedings of the 11th MIT Sloan sports analytics conference* (Vol. 2, p. 3).

Monteiro, R. L. M., Bedo, B. L. S., Monteiro, P. H. M., de Andrade, F. S. P., Moura, F. A., Cunha, S. A., et al. (2022). Penalty feet positioning rule modification and laterality effect on soccer goalkeepers' diving kinematics. *Scientific Reports, 12*, 18493. https://doi.org/10.1038/s41598-022-21508-6

Moura, F. A., Martins, L. E. B., Anido, R. O., de Barros, R. M. L., & Cunha, S. A. (n.d.). Quantitative analysis of Brazilian football players' organisation on the pitch. *PLoS ONE, 11*, 85–96.

Moura, F. A., Martins, L. E. B., Anido, R. O., Ruffino, P. R. C., Barros, R. M. L., & Cunha, S. A. (n.d.). A spectral analysis of team dynamics and tactics in Brazilian football, *31*, 1568–77.

Moura, F. A., Santana, J. E., Vieira, N. A., Santiago, P. R. P., & Cunha, S. A. (n.d.). Analysis of soccer players' positional variability during the 2012 UEFA European championship: A case study, *47*(1), 225–236. https://doi.org/10.1515/hukin-2015-0078

Moura, F. A., van Emmerik, R. E. A., Santana, J. E., Martins, L. E. B., Barros, R. M. L., & Cunha, S. A. (n.d.). Coordination analysis of players' distribution in football using cross-correlation and vector coding techniques, *34*, 2224–2232.

Moura, F. A., Martins, L. E. B., & Cunha, S. A. (2014). Analysis of football game-related statistics using multivariate techniques. *Journal of Sports Sciences, 32*, 1881–1887. https://doi.org/10.1080/02640414.2013.853130

Nargesian, F., Samulowitz, H., Khurana, U., Khalil, E. B., & Turaga, D. S. (2017). Learning feature engineering for classification. In *IJCAI* (Vol. 17, pp. 2529–2535).

Perl, J., & Dauscher, P. (2006). Dynamic pattern recognition in sport by means of artificial neural networks. In *Computational intelligence for movement sciences: Neural networks and other emerging techniques* (pp. 299–319). IGI Global.

Reep, C., & Benjamin, B. (1968). Skill and chance in association football. *Journal of the Royal Statistical Society Series A, 131*(4), 581–585.

Reilly, T. (1976). *A motion analysis of work-rate in different positional roles in professional football match-play*. https://api.semanticscholar.org/CorpusID:210568281

Rico-González, M., Ortega, J. P., Nakamura, F. Y., Moura, F. A., & Arcos, A. L. (n.d.). Identification, computational examination, critical assessment and future considerations of spatial tactical variables to assess the use of space in team sports by positional data: A systematic review. *Journal of Human Kinetic, 77*(1), 205–221

Rico-González, M., Pino-Ortega, J., Nakamura, F. Y., Moura, F. A., Rojas-Valverde, D., & Arcos, A. L. (2020). Past, present, and future of the technological tracking methods to assess tactical variables in team sports: A systematic review. *Proceedings of the Institution of Mechanical Engineers, Part p: Journal of Sports Engineering and Technology, 234*(4), 281–290. https://doi.org/10.1177/1754337120932023

Rodrigues, D. C. U. M., Moura, F. A., Cunha, S. A., & Torres, R. S. (2019). Graph visual rhythms in temporal network analyses. *Graphical Models, 103*, 101021. https://doi.org/10.1016/j.gmod.2019.101021

Rosenberg, C., Hebert, M., & Schneiderman, H. (2005). Semi-supervised self-training of object detection models.

Rout, N., Mishra, D., & Mallick, M. K. (2018). Handling imbalanced data: a survey. In *International proceedings on advances in soft computing, intelligent systems and applications: Asisa 2016* (pp. 431–443).

Ruan, L., Ge, H., Shen, Y., Pu, Z., Zong, S., & Cui, Y. (2022). Quantifying the effectiveness of defensive playing styles in the Chinese football super league. *Frontiers in Psychology, 13*, 199. https://doi.org/10.3389/fpsyg.2022.899199

Russo, M. A., Kurnianggoro, L., & Jo, K.-H. (2019). Classification of sports videos with combination of deep learning models and transfer learning. In *Proceedings of the 2019 international conference on electrical, computer and communication engineering (ECCE)* (pp. 1–5).

Seo, Y., Choi, S., Kim, H., & Hong, K.-S. (1997). Where are the ball and players? Soccer game analysis with color-based tracking and image mosaick. In A. Del Bimbo (Ed.), *Image analysis and processing* (pp. 196–203). Springer.

Shaw, L., & Glickman, M. (2019). Dynamic analysis of team strategy in professional football. *Barca Sports Analytics Summit, 13*, 1154.

Soni, J., Prabakar, N., & Upadhyay, H. (2020). Visualizing high-dimensional data using t-distributed stochastic neighbor embedding algorithm. *Principles of Data Science*, 189–206.

Stival, L., Pinto, A., Andrade, F. S. P., Santiago, P. R. P., Biermann, H., Torres, R. S., & Dias, U. (2023). Using machine learning pipeline to predict entry into the attack zone in football. *PLoS ONE, 18*(1), 1–24. https://doi.org/10.1371/journal.pone.0265372

Taki, T., Hasegawa, J., & Fukumura, T. (1996). Development of motion analysis system for quantitative evaluation of teamwork in soccer games. In *Proceedings of 3rd IEEE international conference on image processing* (Vol. 3, pp. 815–818). https://doi.org/10.1109/ICIP.1996.560865

Uchoa Maia Rodrigues, D. C., Moura, F. A., Cunha, S. A., & Torres, R. S. (2019). Graph visual rhythms in temporal network analyses. *Graphical Models,* 103, 101021. https://doi.org/10.1016/j.gmod.2019.101021

Vandeghen, R., Cioppa, A., & Van Droogenbroeck, M. (2022). Semi-supervised training to improve player and ball detection in soccer. In *Proceedings of the IEEE/cvf conference on computer vision and pattern recognition* (pp. 3481–3490).

Withers, R. (1982). Match analyses of Australian professional soccer players. *Journal of Human Movement Studies, 8*(4), 159–176.

Xu, M., Orwell, J., & Jones, G. (2004). Tracking football players with multiple cameras. In *Proceedings of the 2004 international conference on image processing, 2004.* ICIP'04 (Vol. 5, pp. 2909–2912). https://doi.org/10.1109/ICIP.2004.1421721

Zhang, M. (2014). Multi-sensor inertial measurement system for analysis of sports motion (Unpublished doctoral dissertation). University of Pittsburgh.

Zhou, W., Yu, G., You, S., & Wang, Z. (2023). An improved passing network for evaluating football team performance. *Applied Sciences, 13*(2), 84. https://doi.org/10.3390/app1302084

Chapter 15
Artificial Intelligence in Talent Identification and Development in Sport

Alexander B. T. McAuley, Joe Baker, Kathryn Johnston, and Adam L. Kelly

Abstract Talent identification and development in sport are complex processes that often produce large, multidimensional datasets. Technological approaches powered by Artificial Intelligence (AI) potentially offer an effective and efficient method to help interpret such information. Research conducted on talent identification and development processes in youth sport contexts using AI have not been well synthesised. As such, the primary purpose of the present chapter is to provide an overview of contemporary investigations in this particular field of research. The chapter begins by outlining talent identification and development systems in sport before briefly describing the concept of AI. Subsequently, studies using AI to investigate research questions related to any of the inter-connected phases within talent identification and development processes are summarised. This is followed by an example of how AI is currently being employed in youth sport settings to support recruitment strategies. Finally, some strengths, weaknesses, opportunities, and threats of AI in this field of research are highlighted.

Keywords Artificial Intelligence · Machine Learning · Athlete Development · Expertise · Talent Selection

15.1 Talent Identification and Development Systems

Contemporary high-performance sports settings are extremely competitive, with substantial commercial and financial rewards accompanying success. This has resulted in large resource investments within professional sports organisations as

A. B. T. McAuley (✉) · A. L. Kelly (✉)
Birmingham City University, Birmingham, England
e-mail: alex.mcauley@mail.bcu.ac.uk

A. L. Kelly
e-mail: adam.kelly@bcu.ac.uk

J. Baker · K. Johnston
University of Toronto, Toronto, ON, Canada

C. Dindorf et al. (eds.), *Artificial Intelligence in Sports, Movement, and Health*,
https://doi.org/10.1007/978-3-031-67256-9_15

well as [inter]national governing bodies to improve prospects on the global and national stage (Till & Baker, 2020). A principal area of focus has been recognising and nurturing young athletes with the potential to achieve expertise in the future through the design and implementation of Talent Identification and Development Systems (TIDS) (McAuley et al., 2023a). In the United Kingdom, for instance, approximately £300 million was invested in sports throughout the last Olympic and Paralympic cycles for both summer and winter games, as well as £70 million in direct athlete funding to develop potential high performers (UK Sport, 2023). From a sport-specific perspective, several English soccer academies have reportedly spent up to approximately £5 million per annum on the development of their players (Larkin & Reeves, 2018).

The processes within TIDS typically comprise the following series of progressive and inter-connected phases: (a) *detection*, discovering individuals with the potential to progress in the development environment of a respective sport but are not currently participating; (b) *identification*, recognising which current participants have the potential to become high performers in the future; (c) *development*, providing an optimal learning environment for performers to facilitate development and express their full potential; (d) *selection*, a cyclical procedure of choosing which participants within development programmes have displayed a requisite measure of performance to progress further and receive greater support; and (e) *transfer*, an opportunity for participants to switch to another sport where their unique characteristics and skills may be better suited to potentially achieve expertise (Collins et al., 2014; van Harten et al., 2021; Williams & Reilly, 2000; Williams et al., 2020).

A central pillar underpinning the framework of TIDS is the concept of 'talent'. However, despite being the cornerstone of integrating these recruitment and promotion related processes, talent remains poorly understood and operationalised both in science and practice (Baker et al., 2024; Johnston et al., 2023; McAuley et al., 2022a). Researchers have positioned talent at each end of the development continuum (i.e., the starting point and end product), and practitioner descriptions have often been grounded in the nature (i.e., absence or presence of specific biological material) or nurture (i.e., opportunity and engagement with environmental affordances) dichotomy (Baker et al., 2023; Baker & Wattie, 2018; Johnston & Baker, 2022; Jones et al., 2020a, b). These inconsistencies in the application and interpretation of key terminology creates confusion, limits measurement precision, and makes performance forecasting more difficult (Johnston et al., 2023; McAuley et al., 2022a).

To capture the nuances of the sporting domain, Baker et al. (2019) suggested conceptualising talent as: (a) *innate*, originating in biological elements present at birth; (b) *multi-dimensional*, consisting of capacities from a range of broad cognitive, physical, and psychological categories; (c) *emergenic*, involving interactions among factors that combine multiplicatively; (d) *dynamic*, evolving across developmental time due to interactions with environments and random gene expression; and (e) *symbiotic*, emphasising that cultural and social factors determine the ultimate value of an individual's talent. Indeed, research has shown that athletic development is multifactorial, influenced by a number of performer constraints (e.g., anthropometric, genetic, physiological, and psychological factors), task constraints (e.g., engagement in deliberate practice and play as well as specialisation and sampling pathways), and environmental constraints (e.g., birthdate, birthplace, cultural, and socioeconomic effects) (Dimundo et al., 2021a; Kelly et al., 2020, 2022a, 2022b; McAuley et al., 2023c; Murata et al., 2023; Wattie et al., 2015).

An impressive number of studies have been conducted on these constraints and their associations with an individual's developmental journey in sport. A scoping review of talent research in sport found nearly 2000 peer-reviewed articles written in English had been published between the years 1990 and 2018 (Baker et al., 2020). Other research syntheses highlighting the quality of evidence within and across different contextual settings have also been performed, with a marked increase over recent years (e.g., Barraclough et al., 2022; Bergkamp et al., 2019; Brown et al., 2023; Dimundo et al., 2021b; McAuley et al., 2022b; Johnston et al., 2018; Sarmento et al., 2018; Verbeek et al., 2023; Williams et al., 2020). Despite numerous empirical investigations and having the results well-amalgamated, *how* and *to what extent* these elements of performance interact during development to facilitate expertise remains unclear (McAuley et al., 2021, 2023a).

This ambiguity in the extant literature makes it challenging for decision makers within TIDS to make precise measurements and correct judgements regarding the prospective ability of young athletes. For instance, the efficacy of North American major professional sport draft systems has been questioned from an economic and performance perspective, as a recent review reported the majority of rounds are not very accurate in relation to measures of future success (e.g., career length, number of games played, and performance statistics) (Johnston et al., 2022). Furthermore, across soccer academies in England, only ~3% of players who progress through these TIDS play a match in the highest senior league, whereas only 30% attain a professional contract (Cunningham, 2022). Conventional prediction methods of athletic 'potential' are therefore considered unreliable, with poor validity (Baker et al., 2018; Till & Baker, 2020).

The poor accuracy and low junior-to-senior transition rates reported are, in part, due to the combination of static measurements at one-off timepoints and the weak relationship that exists between early and future success (McAuley et al., 2023a). More specifically, to become a high performer at a senior level, it is not a prerequisite for an athlete to be a high performer at a junior level. For instance, a recent meta-analysis found the performance of over 13,000 Olympic athletes at junior ages accounted for just 2% of the performance variance observed at senior level (Barth et al., 2023). Another review of approximately 60,000 multi-sport athletes also reported that only 18% of senior international performers had achieved international status at U17/18 level (Güllich et al., 2023). Currently implemented approaches appear to assume talent is a fixed capacity that remains stable over time instead of dynamic, emergent, and non-linear (Baker et al., 2023).

Trying to predict an individual's potential to achieve expertise, alongside how the demands of specific sports will evolve in the future, is clearly a difficult undertaking. This task is further confounded by the activities employed at present, as they create biased contexts where being relatively older (i.e., relative age effects) and/or maturing earlier are advantageous (Brown et al., 2023; Dimundo et al., 2021a, b; Hill et al.,

2020; Johnston et al., 2018; Kelly et al., 2022a, b; McAuley et al., 2022b; Radnor et al., 2021). These environments also allow a wide range of cognitive biases (e.g., conformation bias, endowment effect, primacy effect, sunk-cost fallacy) to unconsciously affect the efficiency of decisions (Johnston & Baker, 2020). Despite these issues, however, having individuals enter into TIDS at early ages is often viewed as a necessary evil due to resource constraints (i.e., limited number of personnel and facilities as well as available finances) (Till & Baker, 2020).

Since this approach is unlikely to change in the short-term across many sport settings, it is imperative researchers strive to establish clear variables associated with the long-term development of expertise to increase the effectiveness and efficiency of TIDS. Research conducted in this area, however, has several methodological limitations. For instance, a number of reviews on talent identification and development in sport reported most studies used cross-sectional and mono-disciplinary designs (Baker et al., 2020; Barraclough et al., 2022; Johnston et al., 2018; Verbeek et al., 2023). Similar observations have been made in sports genomics, as limited research exists on epistatic and epigenetic mechanisms, with most studies investigating genetic variants independently using case–control designs (McAuley et al., 2022b, 2023b, 2024). This means there is a lack of longitudinal, multidisciplinary, and gene-environmental research, despite the previous emphasis on talent being dynamic and multidimensional (Baker et al., 2019).

Previously cited explanations for the underrepresentation of these methodologies include the difficulty associated with their administration and analysis requirements in terms of user knowledge, statistical power, and computational capacity (Barraclough et al., 2022; Johnston et al., 2018). However, irrespective of the complexities involved, and as a way to improve accuracy in determining (and eventually applying) causality to specific developmental variables, methodological approaches such as these will be necessary (McAuley et al., 2021). One potential avenue being explored by researchers in sport over recent years is the adoption and application of technological approaches powered by Artificial Intelligence (AI) (Chmait and Westerbeek, 2021; Hammes et al., 2022; Rico-González et al., 2022; Sperlich et al., 2023). The purpose of the present chapter, therefore, is to provide an overview of contemporary investigations in this field of research.

We begin by outlining the concept of AI, including the way it is defined, a brief history of its evolution to date, and how it has been implemented in the sports domain. Next, we explore and summarise studies that have used AI to specifically investigate research questions related to any of the inter-connected phases within a TIDS. Following this overview, we present some practical examples of how companies providing AI-powered technological solutions are being employed by sports organisations to support their athlete recruitment and promotion strategies. Finally, we provide an analysis on the strengths, weaknesses, opportunities, and threats of AI in TIDS before concluding.

15.2 Definition and History of Artificial Intelligence

AI has been defined as the theory and development of computer systems able to perform tasks that normally require human intelligence (Sperlich et al., 2023). For instance, comprehending natural language, decision-making, learning from experiences, recognizing patterns, solving problems, and video analysis (Cossich et al., 2023). From a sports perspective, Hammes et al. (2022) proposed the 'Sense-Model-Plan-Act' concept, whereby AI is viewed as a loop beginning with observation, creating a model based on these observations, developing a plan from this model, then exerting an action on the world. AI encompasses all forms of classical Machine Learning (ML), Deep Learning (DL), and modern Artificial Neural Networks (ANN), with the combination of amplified computational power and overall digitisation enabling the processing of large amounts of information (i.e., Big Data) (Chmait and Westerbeek, 2021).

The field of AI emerged in the 1950s, and despite the significantly reduced interest and funding in the 1970s and 1980s (i.e., a period referred to as the "AI winters"), by the end of the 1990s, AI research was at the forefront of technological innovation (Hammes et al., 2022). Since the early 2000s, AI began to infiltrate various sectors to different degrees, with a notable area being its performance in board (e.g., Checkers, Chess, GO, Shogi) and virtual (e.g., Dota2 and StarCraft) games. For instance, AI developed computer programmes have evolved to the point that they almost always defeat human world champions, with some updated algorithms (e.g., AlphaZero) believed to be unbeatable by humans (Chmait and Westerbeek, 2021). In aspects more central to everyday life, however, AI-powered technology has now been made more accessible and usable by the general population through virtual assistants (e.g., Amazon Alexa, Siri, Cortana) and many aspects of autonomous driving, as well as the unprecedented proliferation of large language models such as ChatGPT (Cossich et al., 2023).

There are also many cases of AI being integrated into the present sporting landscape. In Formula 1, for instance, AI algorithms can enhance the efficiency of tactical decisions during races, such as automating an optimal tyre strategy by modelling the frequency and timing of pit-stops as a sequential decision-making problem (Piccinotti, 2021). In tennis, an AI algorithm has been used to develop a recommended-racket procedure, whereby an individual's movements and swing patterns as well as their general playing style are analysed to advise on an ideal racket type (Krause, 2019). In gymnastics, a judging system has been created to score a routine by having AI analyse 3D laser sensors that capture the joint angles of a gymnast (Atikovic et al., 2020). More common processes in sport are also influenced by aspects of AI, such as Hawk-eye and goal-line technologies to model the precise positioning of the ball at a specific time-point in tennis and soccer, respectively (Hammes et al., 2022).

Perhaps one of the more well-known examples of AI in sports, however, was its use by the Oakland Athletics Major League Baseball (MLB) team in the early 2000s. Using a novel ML approach to analyse in-game playing statistics to inform their recruitment and selection decisions, Oakland Athletics assembled a team that made the playoffs in 2002 despite possessing a relatively small budget. Commonly referred to as "Moneyball" (Lewis, 2004), this approach to analysis identified and exploited an information gap that has led to its implementation throughout MLB and across other sports (Chmait and Westerbeek, 2021). The use of AI for athlete recruitment and performance at senior levels as well as its general application across sports has since been well reviewed (e.g., Beal et al., 2019; Claudino et al., 2019; Rico-González et al., 2022). However, the feasibility and value of AI research with young athletes and within TIDS have not been well synthesised. Given the benefits of AI in professional sport and their potential relevance across TIDS, this will be an important area to consider moving forward.

15.3 Overview of Artificial Intelligence Research on TIDS Processes: Talent Identification

Talent identification and development are inherently complex and multifactorial (Kelly, 2023). Based on the complexities of TIDS coupled with the large, multi-dimensional datasets that are often collected within these settings, AI has the potential to offer effective and efficient approaches to help researchers and practitioners interpret such information. From an analysis perspective, since traditional regression approaches lack the capability to estimate model coefficients when the number of independent variables is similar to the number of observations, the emerging family of feature selection algorithms from AI offer alternative techniques (Tibshirani, 1996). Indeed, as explorative studies within the field of TIDS must employ statistical approaches that can handle multiple competing, possibly correlated, features, AI techniques may be more suited (Oquendo et al., 2012). Whilst identifying talented athletes at a young age is an interesting, but difficult, problem to be successfully solved by AI, more accurate identification using such techniques may enable better career development and performance (Jauhiainen et al., 2019). Despite the surge in AI research due to recent technological advancements in sport, such studies in TIDS remain limited—although we predict this will significantly increase over the forthcoming years. Amongst the research that exists, ML seems to be the most common statistical analyses method used.

Corresponding with conventional talent research in sport (see Baker et al., 2020), soccer appears to be a popular choice for the use of AI techniques. For example, Jauhiainen et al. (2019) trained a nonlinear One Class Support Vector Machine on a dataset from 14-year-old Finland male youth soccer players ($n = 951$) to detect possible future 'elite' players (i.e., those who subsequently signed for an academy at 16-years-old). Findings revealed the most accurate model was obtained when physical tests measuring technical skills, speed, and agility were used. In a two-fold study, our research group (Kelly et al., 2022a, b) used a cross-validated Lasso regression using the glmnet package in R to examine factors that contributed to: (a) player review ratings in U9–U16 England male academy soccer players (n = 98), and (b) the characteristics of selected (i.e., offered a professional contract) and deselected (i.e., not offered a professional contract) U18 England male academy soccer players. First, improvement in subjective performance was found in 15 out of the 53 analysed features, with key findings showing advanced maturation, greater lob pass score via skill testing, higher average dribble completion percentage during competitive match-play, more competitive match-play hours, and being relatively older (i.e., born earlier in the selection year) were the most important features that contributed towards player review ratings. Second, greater 'perceived ability to cope with performance and developmental pressures' as well as perceived 'ability to organise and engage in quality practice' were important contributing factors towards gaining a professional contract. Most recently, Duncan et al. (2023) determined the contributors towards technical skills in English male grassroots soccer players (n = 162) aged 8–14 years. They used a stepwise recursive feature elimination with a fivefold cross-validation method followed by five models (Linear Regression, Ridge Regression, Lasso Regression, Random Forest, and Boosted Trees) in a heuristic approach with a small subset of suitable algorithms. Their results indicated that the total functional movement screening (FMS) score was the most important feature in predicting technical soccer skills, followed by coach rating of player skills for their age, years of playing experience, and age at peak height velocity.

Research on TIDS in cricket has also been at the fore of ML techniques. Jones et al. (2019), for instance, used non-linear pattern recognition to analyse 93 features from senior international (n = 15) and professional (i.e., first-class county; n = 13) male cricket spin bowlers in England. They revealed that a subset of twelve developmental features discriminated between the international and professional groups, reflecting the international players' earlier engagement in cricket, greater quantity of domain-specific practice and competition, and superior adaptability to new levels of competition. Thereafter, Jones et al. (2020a, b) used a similar approach to analyse 658 features from 'super-elite' (i.e., predetermined high-profile senior international; n = 10) and 'elite' (i.e., predetermined high-profile domestic senior professional; n = 10) England male cricket batters. They showed how a subset of 18 features differentiated the two groups, whereby 'super-elite' batters undertook a larger volume of skills-based practice that was both more random and varied in nature at age 16 years. Currently under peer review, our research group (Brown et al., in press) performed a Bayesian Binomial Regression using rSTAN following a clustering approach to observe what differentiated selected (n = 33) and non-selected (n = 49) England male academy players aged 14–17 years based on 104 features. Results highlighted that superior athleticism, greater wellbeing and cohesion, higher number of older brothers, and being born in birth quarters two and three were positively correlated with player selection.

Researchers have also used ML techniques to investigate a handful of other team sports in TIDS, including handball (Oytun et al., 2020), rowing (Liu et al., 2023), rugby league (Till et al., 2016), rugby union (Owen et al., 2022), and volleyball (Musa et al., 2023). As an example, Owen et al. (2022) assessed Welsh U16–U18 age-grade club rugby union players (n = 104) for physiological and psychosocial features during regional talent selection days. They developed predictive models to compare selected and non-selected players using a Bayesian ML approach. The generated physiological models correctly classified 67.6% of all players, with greater hand-grip strength, faster 10 and 40 m sprint, and power as common features for selection. Moreover, the generated psychosocial models correctly classified 62.3% of all players, with reduced burnout, reduced emotional exhaustion, and lower reduced sense of accomplishment as common features for selection. Like more traditional 'team' sports, a small number of primary investigations of more traditional 'individual' sports in TIDS have utilised ML approaches, including archery (Musa et al., 2019), skateboarding (Ab Rasid et al., 2024), and tennis (Siener et al., 2021). As an example, Musa et al. (2019) used a variation of k-NN algorithms and Logistic Regression in Malaysian 'talented' archers aged 13–20 years ($n = 50$; male $n = 37$, female $n = 13$) to predict high and low 'potential' (i.e., based on their archery shooting scores). The weighted k-NN outperformed all the tested models with reasonably good accuracy (83%) for the prediction of 'high potential' (i.e., top of group) and 'low-potential' (i.e., bottom of group), whilst showing how physical fitness features (i.e., vertical jump and the core muscle strength) influenced the determination of the archers' performance quality.

Due to the rarity of high-performing athletes, datasets are inherently imbalanced, making classical statistical inference difficult. Therefore, research in TIDS could be considered as an anomaly detection problem (Jauhiainen et al., 2019). The ML studies in TIDS showcase the modelling and comprehension of such approaches to help better understand both between group differences and possible research methodologies (Auletta et al., 2023). What is apparent within existing TIDS research is that ML approaches do not aim to answer the questions of what leads to optimal performance, but instead seek to outline a method to leverage some of the quantities of available data to generate new hypotheses and insights (Kelly et al., 2022a, b). Therefore, the methodological techniques used in these studies might best serve as an impetus for researchers to adopt a ML approach to TIDS, whilst they could be useful to support decision-makers in the process of TIDS when identifying and developing future athletes. More research in TIDS using AI approaches is required to better understand its reliability and validity in the long-term, whilst there should also be an emphasis on utilising these techniques in female TIDS due to the imbalance in the current samples.

15.4 Overview of Artificial Intelligence Research on TIDS Processes: Talent Development

In the context of athlete development, AI/MI has been used to better understand developmental participation patterns. For example, in the work by Barth et al. (2019), a methodical approach combining Decision Trees and Gradient Boosting to data from a previously published study was used to identify differences between international and national-level athletes across various sports, in the volume of the athlete's main-sport and other-sports practiced. The authors argued that this was superior to more traditional statistical approaches, and offers value to researchers looking to re-investigate previously published studies. Building on this work, Barth et al. (2020), applied a supervised machine learning approach to investigate the effects of supervised and coach-guided practice in athletes' main sport (and other sports), on a sample of athletes with podium performances (i.e., international medals). This approach helped to identify that 'coach-led other-sports practice' until age 14 years was the most important feature relating to podium performance. Through both these research investigations, the research teams promote the approach of combining traditional statistics with advanced supervised ML as a way to improve both testing and discovering patterns among variables.

Similarly, Güllich et al. (2019) used AI/ML to examine the developmental biographies of 16 Great British Olympic and World Champions, and 16 international athletes (who had not won major medals). The data were analysed using pattern recognition analysis—a ML approach developed in bioinformatics to solve the problem of classifying objects by the features that they possess (for more details please see Duda et al., 2001). By using this approach, the authors were able to identify multiple intriguing differences between the two groups. More specifically, compared to athletes who had not won a major medal, those who did had characteristics such as: (a) having experienced an early negative life experience at a time point that was neighbouring a significant positive sport-related event, (b) having a higher relative importance of 'sport over other aspects of life', stronger obsessiveness/ perfectionism, and sport-related ruthlessness/selfishness, and (c) having coaches who better met their physical and psychosocial needs (amongst other key findings, see full paper for details). The authors acknowledge that one of the strengths of the study is the advanced data analysis using pattern recognition procedures, which illuminates fruitful areas of future exploration for AI and developmental modelling.

AI/ML has also been used to provide a set of 'rules' for determining group membership between high performers and lower performing athletes. For instance, the work by Anderson et al. (2022) employed a multi-level methodology using parameter optimization, calculation of odds ratios, feature selection, and feature classification to help understand the development of 'talent' in Olympic Weightlifting. The variables under consideration included: (a) demographics and family sport participation, (b) anthropometrics and physiological factors, (c) psychosocial characteristics, (d) sport participation history, and (e) weightlifting specific practice activities (Anderson et al., 2022). ML helped to analyse a wide number of features (i.e., 648 variables in their study), over a relatively long period of time (athlete tracked for nearly two years), and suggests this could be a valuable tool for such research questions.

Another recent ML investigation explored the extent to which different generic characteristics vary between sports to generate unique profiles by classifying coaches' perceptions of the individual, task, and environmental requirements (Teunissen et al., 2023). The researchers asked 1247 coaches from 34 sports to rank the importance (i.e., 0 = not important – 10 = very important) of 18 characteristics in their sports using a validated survey. To distinguish between each response per sport, a Discriminant Analysis (DA) and Uniform Manifold Approximation and Projection (UMAP) with CatBoost classifier was performed, as well as the generation of a confusion-matrix. The cross-validated DA revealed 70.2% of the coaches were correctly classified to their sport and the UMAP/CatBoost technique showed 75.1% accuracy, with correctly predicted responses per sport ranging from 18.2 (sailing) to 98.2% (soccer). Such approaches provide an insight into the distinctions and parallels between sports that may facilitate greater detection, development, and transfer affinity by optimising the alignment of athlete and sport profiles.

15.5 Applications in Youth Sport Contexts

Unsurprisingly, explorations of AI and advanced technologies have proliferated in youth sport contexts as well as in professional settings. In January 2024, for example, news reports described a new software—aiScout—being used by Premier League football club Chelsea. The app allows players to upload video clips of themselves doing specific drills and skills that clubs can assess far away from the playing field. Not wanting to be left behind, other clubs are following suit (see Smith, 2024).

While many sport scientists, especially those in the fields of athlete development, talent identification, and sport expertise were quick to criticize this and similar approaches, the reality is the technologies are becoming part of many TIDS around the world. However, are there any positives associated with their use? For instance, technologies like aiScout have the advantage of easy access to athlete data, a key limitation for many researchers using traditional research designs. Currently, thousands of players can upload their data to the platform for further assessment by coaches, analysts, and other stakeholders. Although the technology may lack the measurement precision and sensitivity of established approaches, the power of large samples may offset this limitation. Obviously, the reliability and long-term validity of these approaches remains to be seen and can only come from appropriate evaluations using robust scientific methods, but there may be some upside to the changing landscape of high-performance athlete development.

Acknowledging that any emerging technology comes with a range of potential costs and benefits, it may be useful to consider an assessment of AI approaches in youth sport contexts. Fortunately, Sperlich et al. (2023) conducted just such an assessment using a SWOT (Strengths, Weaknesses, Opportunities, Threats) framework. In Fig. 15.1 below, we summarize and extend the assessment conducted by Sperlich et al. (2023). In a related paper, Hammes et al. (2022) examined the success and challenges associated with AI in sports. Amongst a broad discussion of the potential of this technology for improving how sport scientists conduct their work, the authors highlighted five broad challenges: (a) assessing the right types and amounts of data for AI to be useful, (b) linking communities of stakeholders in the AI and sport communities to allow creation of, and access to, the data required, (c) allowing

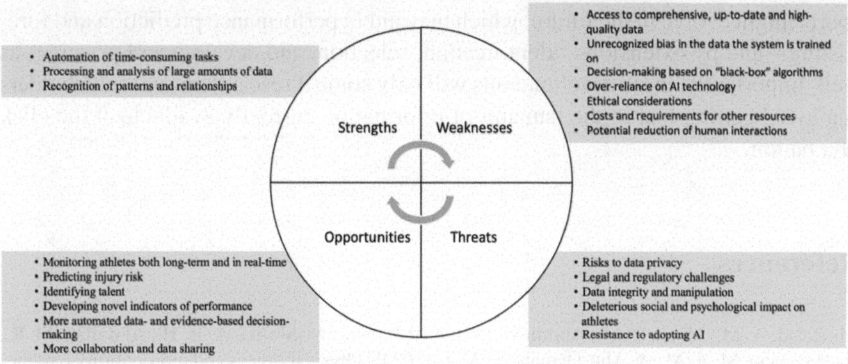

Fig. 15.1 SWOT Analysis of Use of AI in Sport (adapted from Sperlich et al., 2023)

practitioners to maintain a sense of control, (d) ensuring AI outputs are explainable without the need for specialized knowledge, and (e) creating predictive rather than explanatory models, which remains a problem for much work in sport contexts.

15.6 Conclusion

The purpose of the present chapter was to provide an overview of contemporary research that has used technological approaches powered by AI to specifically investigate any of the inter-connected phases within a TIDS. Although it seems to be quickly and widely used in applied settings, this field of research is currently in its infancy. This current evidence-base, however, has been conducted on a wide range of individual (e.g., archery, skateboarding, tennis, weightlifting) and team sports (e.g., cricket, rugby league, rugby union, soccer), as well as used a variety of methodological approaches (e.g., mono-disciplinary, multi-disciplinary, cross-sectional, longitudinal, quantitative, qualitative) and AI procedures (e.g., ML, DL, ANN, Decision Trees, Markov Process, Support Vector Machine) that have produced varying statistical associations. In the future, it is important that studies in this field continue to address the shortcomings of conventional analyses by performing investigations with research designs that advance our understanding of the dynamic, emergent, multi-dimensional, and non-linear process of athlete development.

The current moment in time is characterized by a seemingly ever-increasing torrent of performance- and development-related data for sport researchers and analysts to make sense of. However, in an environment where such value is available and highly sought after, the challenge becomes increasing the capacity for stakeholders to be able to filter through these sources to find information of value. AI and ML have considerable potential to improve the methods used by sport researchers and practitioners. They can assist with the small sample limitations that have plagued this area of research for decades, and they may be useful for developing models of how sports might evolve in the future, which may aid in performance prediction and forecasting—and by extension—identification, selection, and development practices as well. Importantly, these developments will only come if researchers and stakeholders can avoid getting lost in the tsunami of information currently available at the click of a button.

References

Ab-Rasid, A. M., Musa, R. M., Abdul-Majeed, A. P. P., Musawi-Maliki, A. B. H., Abdullah, M. R., Razmaan, M. A. M., & Abu-Osman, N. A. A. (2024). Physical fitness and motor ability parameters as predictors for skateboarding performance: A logistic regression modelling analysis. *PLoS ONE, 19*(2), e0296467. https://doi.org/10.1371/journal.pone.0296467

Anderson, D. N. J., Gottwald, V. M., & Lawrence, G. P. (2022). Capturing the holistic profile of high performance Olympic weightlifting development. *Frontiers in Sports and Active Living, 4*, 6134. https://doi.org/10.3389/fspor.2022.986134

Atiković, A., Kamenjašević, E., Mujanović, A. N., Užičanin, E., Tabaković, M., & Ćurić, M. (2020). Differences between all-around results in women's artistic gymnastics and ways of minimizing them. *Baltic Journal of Health and Physical Activity, 12*(3), 80–91.

Auletta, F., Kallen, R. W., di Bernardo, M., & Richardson, M. J. (2023). Predicting and understanding human action decisions during skillful joint-action using supervised machine learning and explainable-AI. *Scientific Reports, 13*, 4992. https://doi.org/10.1038/s41598-023-31807-1

Baker, J., Johnston, K., & Till, K. (2023). Is it time to retire 'talent' from discussions of athlete development? *High Ability Studies*. https://doi.org/10.1080/13598139.2023.2295320

Baker, J., Kelly, A. L., McAuley, A. B. T., & Wattie, N. (2024). Language games: Improving the words we use in soccer research and practice. In A. L. Kelly (Ed.), *Talent identification and development in youth soccer* (pp. 316–326). Routledge.

Baker, J., Schorer, J., & Wattie, N. (2018). Compromising talent: Issues in identifying and selecting talent in sport. *Quest, 70*(1), 48–63. https://doi.org/10.1080/00336297.2017.1333438

Baker, J., & Wattie, N. (2018). Innate talent in sport: Separating myth from reality. *Current Issues in Sport Science, 3*, 006.

Baker, J., Wattie, N., & Schorer, J. (2019). A proposed conceptualization of talent in sport: The first step in a long and winding road. *Psychology of Sport and Exercise, 43*, 27–33. https://doi.org/10.1016/j.psychsport.2018.12.016

Baker, J., Wilson, S., Johnston, K., Dehghansai, N., Koenigsberg, A., de Vegt, S., & Wattie, N. (2020). Talent research in sport 1990–2018: A scoping review. *Frontiers in Psychology, 11*, 607710. https://doi.org/10.3389/fpsyg.2020.607710

Barraclough, S., Till, K., Kerr, A., & Emmonds, S. (2022). Methodological approaches to talent identification in team sports: A narrative review. *Sports, 10*(6), 81. https://doi.org/10.3390/sports10060081

Barth, M., Emrich, E., & Güllich, A. (2019). A machine learning approach to "revisit" specialization and sampling in institutionalized practice. *SAGE Open, 9*(2), 2158244019840554. https://doi.org/10.1177/2158244019840554

Barth, M., Güllich, A., Macnamara, B. N., & Hambrick, D. Z. (2023). Quantifying the extent to which junior performance predicts senior performance in olympic sports: A systematic review and meta-analysis. *Sports Medicine*. https://doi.org/10.1007/s40279-023-01906-0

Barth, M., Güllich, A., Raschner, C., & Emrich, E. (2020). The path to international medals: A supervised machine learning approach to explore the impact of coach-led sport-specific and non-specific practice. *PLoS ONE, 15*(9), e0239378. https://doi.org/10.1371/journal.pone.0239378

Beal, R., Norman, T. J., & Ramchurn, S. D. (2019). Artificial intelligence for team sports: A survey. *The Knowledge Engineering Review, 34*, e28. https://doi.org/10.1017/S0269888919000225

Bergkamp, T. L. G., Niessen, A. S. M., den Hartigh, R. J. R., Frencken, W. G. P., & Meijer, R. R. (2019). Methodological issues in soccer talent identification research. *Sports Medicine, 49*(9), 1317–1335. https://doi.org/10.1007/s40279-019-01113-w

Brown, T., Cook, R., Gough, L. A., Khawaja, I., McAuley, A. B. T., & Kelly, A. L. (in press) Exploring the multidimensional characteristics of selected and non-selected White British and British South Asian youth cricketers: An exploratory machine learning approach.

Brown, T., McAuley, A. B. T., Khawaja, I., Gough, L. A., & Kelly, A. L. (2023). Talent identification and development in male cricket: A systematic review. *Journal of Expertise, 6*(2), 176–206.

Chmait, N., & Westerbeek, H. (2021). Artificial intelligence and machine learning in sport research: An introduction for non-data scientists. *Frontiers in Sports and Active Living, 3*, 82287. https://doi.org/10.3389/fspor.2021.682287

Claudino, J. G., Capanema, D. O., de Souza, T. V., Serrão, J. C., Machado Pereira, A. C., & Nassis, G. P. (2019). Current approaches to the use of artificial intelligence for injury risk assessment and performance prediction in team sports: A systematic review. *Sports Medicine Open, 5*(1), 28. https://doi.org/10.1186/s40798-019-0202-3

Collins, R., Collins, D., MacNamara, Á., & Jones, M. I. (2014). Change of plans: An evaluation of the effectiveness and underlying mechanisms of successful talent transfer. *Journal of Sports Sciences, 32*(17), 1621–1630. https://doi.org/10.1080/02640414.2014.908324

Cossich, V. R. A., Carlgren, D., Holash, R. J., & Katz, L. (2023). Technological breakthroughs in sport: Current practice and future potential of artificial intelligence, virtual reality, augmented reality, and modern data visualization in performance analysis. *Applied Sciences, 13*(23), 2965. https://doi.org/10.3390/app132312965

Cunningham, S. (2022). *97% of Premier League academy players never play a minute in top flight, new analysis reveals*. Inews.Co.Uk. https://inews.co.uk/sport/football/premier-league-academy-players-figures-appearances-numbers-1387302

Dimundo, F., Cole, M., Blagrove, R. C., McAuley, A. B. T., Till, K., & Kelly, A. L. (2021a). Talent identification in an English premiership rugby union academy: Multidisciplinary characteristics of selected and non-selected male Under-15 players. *Frontiers in Sports and Active Living, 3*, 162.

Dimundo, F., Cole, M., Blagrove, R., Till, K., McAuley, A. B. T., Hall, M., Gale, C., & Kelly, A. (2021b). Talent identification and development in male rugby union: A systematic review. *Journal of Expertise, 4*(1), 33–55.

Duda, R. O., Hart, P. E., & Stork, D. G. (2001). *Pattern classification* (2nd ed.). Wiley.

Duncan, M. J., Eyre, E. L. J., Clarke, N., Hamid, A., & Jing, Y. (2023). Importance of fundamental movement skills to predict technical skills in youth grassroots soccer: A machine learning approach. *International Journal of Sports Science and Coaching*. https://doi.org/10.1177/17479541231202015

Güllich, A., Barth, M., Macnamara, B. N., & Hambrick, D. Z. (2023). Quantifying the extent to which successful juniors and successful seniors are two disparate populations: A systematic review and synthesis of findings. *Sports Medicine, 53*(6), 1201–1217. https://doi.org/10.1007/s40279-023-01840-1

Güllich, A., Hardy, L., Kuncheva, L., Laing, S., Evans, L., Rees, T., Abernethy, B., Côté, J., Warr, C., & Wraith, L. (2019). Developmental biographies of Olympic super-elite and elite athletes: A multidisciplinary pattern recognition analysis. *Journal of Expertise, 2*(1), 23–46.

Hammes, F., Hagg, A., Asteroth, A., & Link, D. (2022). Artificial intelligence in elite sports: A narrative review of success stories and challenges. *Frontiers in Sports and Active Living, 4*, 1466. https://doi.org/10.3389/fspor.2022.861466

Harten, K., Bool, K., Vlijmen, J., & Elferink-Gemser, M. (2021). Talent transfer: A systematic review. *Current Issues in Sport Science (CISS), 6*, 006.

Hill, M., Scott, S., Malina, R. M., McGee, D., & Cumming, S. P. (2020). Relative age and maturation selection biases in academy football. *Journal of Sports Sciences, 38*(11–12), 1359–1367. https://doi.org/10.1080/02640414.2019.1649524

Jauhiainen, S., Äyrämö, S., Forsman, H., & Kauppi, J.-P. (2019). Talent identification in soccer using a one-class support vector machine. *International Journal of Computer Science in Sport, 18*(3), 125–136. https://doi.org/10.2478/ijcss-2019-0021

Johnston, K., & Baker, J. (2020). Waste reduction strategies: Factors affecting talent wastage and the efficacy of talent selection in sport. *Frontiers in Psychology, 10*, 2925. https://doi.org/10.3389/fpsyg.2019.02925

Johnston, K., & Baker, J. (2022). The complex and (sometimes) conflicting beliefs about talent: A case study of elite distance running coaches. *Journal of Expertise, 5*(1), 38–57.

Johnston, K., Farah, L., Ghuman, H., & Baker, J. (2022). To draft or not to draft? A systematic review of North American sports' entry draft. *Scandinavian Journal of Medicine and Science in Sports, 32*(1), 4–17. https://doi.org/10.1111/sms.14076

Johnston, K., McAuley, A. B. T., Kelly, A. L., & Baker, J. (2023). Language games and blurry terminology: Can clarity enhance athlete development? *Frontiers in Sports and Active Living, 5*, 1150047. https://doi.org/10.3389/fspor.2023.1150047

Johnston, K., Wattie, N., Schorer, J., & Baker, J. (2018). Talent identification in sport: A systematic review. *Sports Medicine, 48*(1), 97–109. https://doi.org/10.1007/s40279-017-0803-2

Jones, B. D., Hardy, L., Lawrence, G., Kuncheva, L. I., Du Preez, T., Brandon, R., Such, P., & Bobat, M. (2019). The identification of "game changers" in England cricket's developmental pathway for elite spin bowling: A machine learning approach. *Journal of Expertise, 2*(2), 92–120.

Jones, B. D., Hardy, L., Lawrence, G., Kuncheva, L. I., Brandon, R., Bobat, M., & Thorpe, G. (2020a). It ain't what you do—It's the way that you do it: Is optimizing challenge key in the development of super-elite batsmen? *Journal of Expertise, 3*(2), 144–168.

Jones, J., Johnston, K., & Baker, J. (2020b). "I can't teach you to be taller": How Canadian, collegiate-level coaches construct talent in sport. *Case Studies in Sport and Exercise Psychology, 4*(1), 84–94. https://doi.org/10.1123/cssep.2020-0003

Kelly, A. L. (2023). *Talent identification and development in youth soccer: A guide for researchers and practitioners.* Routledge.

Kelly, A. L., McAuley, A. B. T., Dimundo, F., & Till, K. (2022a). Talent identification in male youth rugby: An ecological perspective. In K. Till, J. Weakley, S. Whitehead, & B. Jones (Eds.), *Youth Rugby* (pp. 40–55). Routledge.

Kelly, A. L., Williams, C. A., Cook, R., Jiménez, S. L., & Wilson, M. R. (2022b). A multidisciplinary investigation into the talent development processes at an English football academy: A machine learning approach. *Sports, 10*(10), 159. https://doi.org/10.3390/sports10100159

Kelly, A. L., Wilson, M. R., Gough, L. A., Knapman, H., Morgan, P., Cole, M., Jackson, D. T., & Williams, C. A. (2020). A longitudinal investigation into the relative age effect in an English professional football club: Exploring the 'underdog hypothesis.' *Science and Medicine in Football, 4*(2), 111–118. https://doi.org/10.1080/24733938.2019.1694169

Krause, L. (2019). *Exploring the influence of practice design on the development of tennis players.* Victoria University.

Larkin, P., & Reeves, M. J. (2018). Junior-elite football: Time to re-position talent identification? *Soccer and Society, 19*(8), 1183–1192. https://doi.org/10.1080/14660970.2018.1432389

Lewis, M. (2004). *Moneyball: The art of winning an unfair game.* W. W. Norton & Company.

Liu, J. W., Chen, S. H., Chen, C. H., & Huang, T.-H. (2023). Constructing an artificial intelligence strategy algorithm for the identification of talented rowing athletes. *Soft Computing, 27*, 1743–1750. https://doi.org/10.1007/s00500-021-06050-3

McAuley, A. B. T., Baker, J., & Kelly, A. L. (2021). How nature and nurture conspire to influence athletic success. In A. L. Kelly, J. Côté, M. Jeffreys, & J. Turnnidge (Eds.), *Birth advantages and relative age effects in sport: Exploring organizational structures and creating appropriate settings* (pp. 159–183). Routledge.

McAuley, A. B. T., Baker, J., & Kelly, A. L. (2022a). Defining "elite" status in sport: From chaos to clarity. *German Journal of Exercise and Sport Research, 52*(1), 193–197. https://doi.org/10.1007/s12662-021-00737-3

McAuley, A. B. T., Hughes, D. C., Tsaprouni, L. G., Varley, I., Suraci, B., Baker, J., Herbert, A. J., & Kelly, A. L. (2022b). Genetic associations with technical capabilities in English academy football players: A preliminary study. *The Journal of Sports Medicine and Physical Fitness.* https://doi.org/10.23736/S0022-4707.22.13945-9

McAuley, A. B. T., Baker, J., Johnston, K., Varley, I., Herbert, A. J., Suraci, B., Hughes, D. C., Tsaprouni, L. G., & Kelly, A. L. (2023a). Talent inclusion and genetic testing in sport: A practitioner's guide. *Current Issues in Sport Science (CISS), 8*(1), 008.

McAuley, A. B. T., Hughes, D. C., Tsaprouni, L. G., Varley, I., Suraci, B., Roos, T. R., Herbert, A. J., Jackson, D. T., & Kelly, A. L. (2023b). A systematic review of the genetic predisposition to injury in football. *Journal of Science in Sport and Exercise, 5*(2), 97–115. https://doi.org/10.1007/s42978-022-00187-9

McAuley, A. B. T., Varley, I., Herbert, A. J., Suraci, B., Baker, J., Johnston, K., & Kelly, A. L. (2023c). Maturity-associated polygenic profiles of under 12–16-compared to under 17–23-year-old male English academy football players. *Genes, 14*(7), 431. https://doi.org/10.3390/genes14071431

McAuley, A. B. T., Hughes, D. C., Tsaprouni, L. G., Varley, I., Suraci, B., Bradley, B., Baker, J., Herbert, A. J., & Kelly, A. L. (2024). Genetic associations with acceleration, change of direction, jump height, and speed in English academy football players. *The Journal of Strength and Conditioning Research, 38*(2), 350–359. https://doi.org/10.1519/JSC.0000000000004634

Murata, A., McAuley, A. B. T., Ferguson, M., Toms, M., & Kelly, A. L. (2023). Activities and trajectories: Exploring pathways of athlete development in youth soccer. In A. L. Kelly (Ed.), *Talent identification and development in youth soccer* (pp. 109–120). Routledge.

Musa, R. M., Abdul Majeed, A. P. P., Suhaimi, M. Z., Abdullah, M. R., Razman, M. A. M., Abdelhakim, D., & Abu Osman, N. A. (2023). Identification of high-performance volleyball players from anthropometric variables and psychological readiness: A machine-learning approach. *Journal of Sports Engineering and Technology, 237*(4), 317–324. https://doi.org/10.1177/17543371211045451

Musa, R. M., Abdul Majeed, A. P. P., Taha, Z., Chang, S. W., Nasir, A. F. A., & Abdullah, M. R. (2019). A machine learning approach of predicting high potential archers by means of physical fitness indicators. *PLoS ONE, 14*(1), e0209638. https://doi.org/10.1371/journal.pone.0209638

Oquendo, M. A., Baca-Garcia, E., Artes-Rodriguez, A., Perez-Cruz, F., Galfalvy, H. C., Blasco-Fontecilla, H., Madigan, D., & Duan, N. (2012). Machine learning and data mining: Strategies for hypothesis generation. *Molecular Psychiatry, 17*(10), 956–959. https://doi.org/10.1038/mp.2011.173

Owen, J., Owen, R., Hughes, J., Leach, J., Anderson, D., & Jones, E. (2022). Psychosocial and physiological factors affecting selection to regional age-grade rugby union squads: A machine learning approach. *Sports, 10*(3), 35. https://doi.org/10.3390/sports10030035

Oytun, M., Tinazci, C., Sekeroglu, B., Acikada, C., & Yavuz, H. U. (2020). Performance prediction and evaluation in female handball players using machine learning models. *IEEE Access, 8*, 116321–116335. https://doi.org/10.1109/ACCESS.2020.3004182

Piccinotti, D. (2021). *Open loop planning for formula 1 race strategy identification.* Association for the Advancement of Artificial Intelligence.

Radnor, J. M., Staines, J., Bevan, J., Cumming, S. P., Kelly, A. L., Lloyd, R. S., & Oliver, J. L. (2021). Maturity has a greater association than relative age with physical performance in English male academy soccer players. *Sports, 9*(12), 171. https://doi.org/10.3390/sports9120171

Rico-González, M., Pino-Ortega, J., Méndez, A., Clemente, F. M., & Baca, A. (2022). Machine learning application in soccer: A systematic review. *Biology of Sport, 40*(1), 249–263. https://doi.org/10.5114/biolsport.2023.112970

Sarmento, H., Anguera, M. T., Pereira, A., & Araújo, D. (2018). Talent identification and development in male football: A systematic review. *Sports Medicine, 48*(4), 907–931. https://doi.org/10.1007/s40279-017-0851-7

Siener, M., Faber, I., & Hohmann, A. (2021). Prognostic validity of statistical prediction methods used for talent identification in youth tennis players based on motor abilities. *Applied Sciences, 11*(15), 7051. https://doi.org/10.3390/app11157051

Smith, A. (2024). *Chelsea leave Man Utd in their wake with 'revolutionary' new recruitment tool.* The Mirror. https://www.mirror.co.uk/sport/football/news/chelsea-take-lead-revolutionary-new-31918442

Sperlich, B., Düking, P., Leppich, R., & Holmberg, H.-C. (2023). Strengths, weaknesses, opportunities, and threats associated with the application of artificial intelligence in connection with sport research, coaching, and optimization of athletic performance: A brief SWOT analysis. *Frontiers in Sports and Active Living, 5*, 8562. https://doi.org/10.3389/fspor.2023.1258562

Teunissen, J. W., Faber, I. R., De Bock, J., Slembrouck, M., Verstockt, S., Lenoir, M., & Pion, J. (2023). A machine learning approach for the classification of sports based on a coaches' perspective of environmental, individual and task requirements: A sports profile analysis. *Journal of Sports Sciences*. https://doi.org/10.1080/02640414.2023.2271706

Tibshirani, R. (1996). Regression shrinkage and selection via the Lasso. *Journal of the Royal Statistical Society: Series B (methodological), 58*, 267–288. https://doi.org/10.1111/j.2517-6161.1996.tb02080.x

Till, K., & Baker, J. (2020). Challenges and [possible] solutions to optimizing talent identification and development in sport. *Frontiers in Psychology, 11*, 664. https://doi.org/10.3389/fpsyg.2020.00664

Till, K., Jones, B. L., Cobley, S., Morley, D., O'Hara, J., Chapman, C., Cooke, C., & Beggs, C. B. (2016). Identifying talent in youth sport: A novel methodology using higher-dimensional analysis. *PLoS ONE, 11*(5), e0155047. https://doi.org/10.1371/journal.pone.0155047

UK Sport. (2023). *Historical funding figures.* https://www.uksport.gov.uk/our-work/investing-in-sport/historical-funding-figures

Verbeek, J., Van Der Steen, S., Van Yperen, N. W., & Den Hartigh, R. J. R. (2023). What do we currently know about the development of talent? A systematic review in the soccer context. *International Review of Sport and Exercise Psychology*. https://doi.org/10.1080/1750984X.2023.2283874

Wattie, N., Schorer, J., & Baker, J. (2015). The relative age effect in sport: A developmental systems model. *Sports Medicine, 45*(1), 83–94. https://doi.org/10.1007/s40279-014-0248-9

Williams, A. M., Ford, P. R., & Drust, B. (2020). Talent identification and development in soccer since the millennium. *Journal of Sports Sciences, 38*(11–12), 1199–1210. https://doi.org/10.1080/02640414.2020.1766647

Williams, A. M., & Reilly, T. (2000). Talent identification and development in soccer. *Journal of Sports Sciences, 18*(9), 657–667. https://doi.org/10.1080/02640410050120041

SPRINGER NATURE

GPSR Compliance

The European Union's (EU) General Product Safety Regulation (GPSR) is a set of rules that requires consumer products to be safe and our obligations to ensure this.

If you have any concerns about our products, you can contact us on ProductSafety@springernature.com

In case Publisher is established outside the EU, the EU authorized representative is:

Springer Nature Customer Service Center GmbH
Europaplatz 3
69115 Heidelberg, Germany

The manufacturer's authorised representative in the EU is Springer Nature Customer Service Centre GmbH, Europaplatz 3, 69115 Heidelberg, Germany. If you have any concerns regarding our products, please contact ProductSafety@springernature.com

Printed and bound by CPI Group (UK) Ltd, Croydon, CR0 4YY
30/09/2026
02225564-0010